Exam Preparatory Manual for Undergraduates

Fixed Partial Dentures

Exam Preparatory Manual for Undergraduates
Fixed Partial Dentures

Lovely M
MDS Dip NB (Prosth) PhD
Professor
Department of Prosthodontics
Sree Mookambika Institute of Dental Sciences
Kanyakumari, Tamil Nadu, India

Foreword
NS Azhagarasan

JAYPEE *The Health Sciences Publisher*
New Delhi | London | Philadelphia | Panama

Jaypee Brothers Medical Publishers (P) Ltd

Headquarters

Jaypee Brothers Medical Publishers (P) Ltd
4838/24, Ansari Road, Daryaganj
New Delhi 110 002, India
Phone: +91-11-43574357
Fax: +91-11-43574314
Email: jaypee@jaypeebrothers.com

Overseas Offices

J.P. Medical Ltd
83 Victoria Street, London
SW1H 0HW (UK)
Phone: +44-20 3170 8910
Fax: +44 (0) 20 3008 6180
Email: info@jpmedpub.com

Jaypee-Highlights Medical Publishers Inc
City of Knowledge, Bld. 235, 2nd Floor, Clayton
Panama City, Panama
Phone: +1 507-301-0496
Fax: +1 507-301-0499
Email: cservice@jphmedical.com

Jaypee Medical Inc
325 Chestnut Street
Suite 412, Philadelphia, PA 19106, USA
Phone: +1 267-519-9789
Email: support@jpmedus.com

Jaypee Brothers Medical Publishers (P) Ltd
17/1-B Babar Road, Block-B, Shaymali
Mohammadpur, Dhaka-1207
Bangladesh
Mobile: +08801912003485
Email: jaypeedhaka@gmail.com

Jaypee Brothers Medical Publishers (P) Ltd
Bhotahity, Kathmandu, Nepal
Phone: +977-9741283608
Email: kathmandu@jaypeebrothers.com

Website: www.jaypeebrothers.com
Website: www.jaypeedigital.com

Inquiries for bulk sales may be solicited at: jaypee@jaypeebrothers.com

Exam Preparatory Manual for Undergraduates: Fixed Partial Dentures

First Edition: 2017

ISBN: 978-93-86107-99-2

Printed at Sanat Printers

Dedicated to

My Almighty God
and
My dear Husband Dr Biji Thomas George

Contributors

Added Essays and Short Notes in this Edition

V Vidyashree Nandini MDS DNB
Professor and Head
Department of Prosthodontics and Implantology
SRM Kattankulathur Dental College and Hospital
SRM University
Chennai, Tamil Nadu, India

Implantology Section

N Gopi Chander MDS
Department of Prosthodontics
SRM Dental College
Chennai, Tamil Nadu, India

MCQ Section

CS Rajmohan MDS
Fixed Partial Denture Coordinator
Oman Dental College
Muscat, Oman

Chapter on Laminate Veneers

Eldo Koshy MDS
Formerly, Professor and Head
Department of Prosthodontics and Implantology
Royal Dental College
Chaliserry, Palakkad, Kerala, India
Associate Fellow
American Academy of Implant Dentistry (AAID)

Fixed Partial Denture—An Insight

Manish Lahori MDS
Professor and Head
Department of Prosthodontics
KD Dental College
Mathura, Uttar Pradesh, India

Foreword

It gives me immense pleasure to see one of my brightest and earliest students—the author of this book Dr Lovely M, taking fixed prosthodontics subject to its next level. Today's students are flooded with information about the subject from several sources—Internet, journals and international books. Such available information is raw and has not been prepared for a young student. Dr Lovely M has handled with ease the responsibility of processing and moderating the concept, facts and the subject of the prosthodontics. *Exam Preparatory Manual for Undergraduates: Fixed Partial Dentures* is the revised version of its mother edition—Review of Fixed Partial Dentures.

The success of initial book, which was extremely well received by an increasing readership, speaks for the realization for their dreams and adapting to the perceived needs of those facing entrance and postgraduate examinations. I am in receipt of positive reviews of the initial review book and many messages from grateful readers who found the book very useful for the preparation of the examinations, many of them being my own students.

The current dental educational system demands and assesses the ability of knowledge in students using short notes and essay format. Given the vast information available in text and reference books, an average student finds it difficult to prioritize the scheme for answering. Dr Lovely M's current effort would lend a helping hand to prioritize information from the examination point of view. The current authors in unison have made all attempts to retain the strengths of previous print of the review book while making all sincere attempts to include all advancement in the field of FPD and implantology. The basic format of the book, being examination oriented would help the students to face the examination confidently. The inclusion of multiple choice questions (MCQs) and recent advances along with references is an added bonanza for students to keep themselves updated.

Undoubtedly, this book will be a good stepping stone for the beginners to understand this subject and will evoke more interest in reading further reference books. The book has been designed to contemporary syllabus of various Indian Universities and Dental Council of India, which is an added advantage. I am glad to introduce the *Exam Preparatory Manual for Undergraduates: Fixed Partial Dentures*, 1st edition, to the prosthodontic fraternity and I am sure this book will prove to be useful not only for undergraduates and postgraduates but also for practicing dentists.

I wish Dr Lovely M and all her co-authors, all success in this current and all their future endeavors.

NS Azhagarasan MDS
Professor and Head
Department of Prosthodontics and Crown & Bridge
Ragas Dental College and Hospital
Chennai, Tamil Nadu, India

Preface

I am grateful for the support of my dear colleagues and students who gave me valuable input in terms of the shortcomings in the first volume. Hence, in this manual, great care was taken to cover the left out questions and also a section on implant dentistry, newer techniques in fixed partial dentures and recent advances with references is added. Responding to many requests from students, a section on MCQ is added. The manual includes answers to the oldest and latest questions that could be asked in the final university question paper.

As requested by the postgraduates, the present manual has included references wherever required, an implant section and recent advances in fixed prosthesis topics have been added.

I am extremely grateful to the contributors for their academic contribution to the implant section, added essays and short notes, MCQ, and recent advances. This book as stated earlier is meant to be a revision tool and not to be considered as a textbook. I am especially indebted to my dear husband Dr Biji Thomas George, for his encouragement and timely support.

I am highly indebted to my teacher Professor K Chandrasekharan Nair, Head, Department of Prosthodontics, Maruthi Dental College, Bengaluru, Karnataka, India, and Professor Fazil Ghani, Head, Department of Prosthodontics, Khyber College of Dentistry, Peshawar, Pakistan, for their insight and constructive comments regarding the contents. Professor Ghani was kind enough to review the entire series of the review books and gave me constructive ideas on how to make it more resourceful. I am indebted to Professor Dr NS Azhagarasan, Vice-Principal and Head, Department of Prosthodontics, Ragas Dental College and Hospital, Chennai, Tamil Nadu, India, for going through the contents and giving valuable suggestions.

Finally, I owe my sincere gratitude to Shri Jitendar P Vij (Group Chairman), Mr Ankit Vij (Group President), Mr Tarun Duneja (Director–Publishing) and other members of M/s Jaypee Brothers Medical Publishers (P) Ltd, New Delhi, India, for making the contents more reader friendly. I am hoping that the changes made in this print will be more beneficial for the student fraternity and the entire dental faculty in all aspects.

Lovely M

Contents

SECTION 1: ESSAYS

SECTION 3: MCQ, EXTENDED MATCHING QUESTIONS, SHORT ANSWER QUESTIONS, LAMINATE VENEERS AND RECENT ADVANCES IN FIXED PARTIAL DENTURE

SECTION 1

Essays

1. Discuss the importance of diagnosis and treatment planning in fixed partial denture.
2. List the ideal requirements of an abutment tooth and describe the steps taken to maintain biological integrity while preparing teeth for fixed partial denture.
3. Describe various methods used for gingival retraction and add a note on the advantages of fluid control and tissue displacement.
4. Describe the methods used to classify fixed bridges. Add a note on types of retainers used in fixed partial dentures.
5. Define and classify retainers. List the advantages and disadvantages of partial veneer crown over other types of retainers. What are the factors that come into play in the selection of retainers?
6. Define retention and resistance form in fixed partial denture. What are the factors affecting retention and resistance in posterior tooth preparation?
7. Classify finish lines. Enumerate the functions, indications, advantages and disadvantages of finish lines. Add a note on selection of type of finish line to be used.
8. Illustrate with diagrams, the tooth preparation on right upper central incisor for receiving porcelain jacket crown. Add a note on the advantages, indications and contraindications of all-porcelain jacket crown.
9. Define a crown and mention the advantages, disadvantages and indications of a full metal crown. Describe in detail, with diagrams, the step-by-step procedure in the preparation of a full metal crown on a mandibular first molar.
10. Describe in detail, with diagrams, the step-by-step preparation of a maxillary canine to receive a three quarter crown. Explain and justify different impression techniques for fixed partial denture.
11. Name the component parts of a bridge. Define and classify pontics. Add a note on selection of pontic design in anterior and posterior teeth. What are the requirements of a pontic?

12. What are the biological, mechanical and esthetic considerations in designing a pontic? Add a note on fabrication of pontics.
13. Describe different types of provisional restorations. Describe various techniques used for making provisional restoration for anterior and posterior tooth preparation.
14. Describe ideal requirements of luting agents and various luting agents used in crown and bridge cementing. Explain the procedure and care to be taken to lute porcelain jacket crowns.
15. Classify adhesive bridges/resin bonded bridges. Cite the advantages, disadvantages, indications, contraindications and preparation steps. Add a note on types of bonding to metal and tooth.
16. What are the requirements of dies? Describe materials used in preparation of dies and few techniques used for preparing dies?
17. Classify ceramics. Enumerate its advantages and disadvantages. Explain the mechanism of bonding and describe the laboratory steps involved in fabrication of different ceramics.
18. What are the types of veneering materials? Describe their advantages, disadvantages and indications. Add a note on the recent advances in veneering materials used in fixed partial denture.
19. Discuss in detail failures in fixed dental prosthesis.

IMPLANT DENTISTRY

20. Classify and discuss on various impression procedures involved in implant-supported prosthesis.
21. Discuss on implants for fixed prosthesis work.
22. Classify types of implants and discuss the role of surface topography of implants in osseointegration.
23. Explain procedural options for single tooth implant prosthesis
24. Discuss the immediate loading and progressive loading of endosseous implants.
25. Occlusal consideration for implant-supported prosthesis.
26. Recent advances in surgical techniques.
27. Discuss implant failures and precautions that need to be taken.

ESSAYS

1. Discuss the importance of diagnosis and treatment planning in fixed partial denture.

Diagnosis is the examination of the physical state, evaluation of the mental or psychological makeup and understanding the needs of each patient to ensure a predictable result.

Treatment planning means developing a course of action that encompasses the ramifications and sequelae of treatment to serve the patient's needs.

Diagnosis

Diagnosis in fixed partial denture includes:

1. Chief complaints.
2. History taking of the patient.
3. Examination.
   - General examination
   - Temporomandibular joint examination
   - Extraoral examination
   - Intraoral examination
   - Occlusal evaluation
   - Abutment tooth evaluation.
4. Making of diagnostic casts.
5. Full-mouth radiographs.

Chief complaints

Are mainly of four categories:

1. Comfort (pain, sensitivity, swelling).
2. Function (difficulty in mastication or speech).
3. Social (bad taste or odor).
4. Appearance (fractured or discolored tooth).

Comfort

Pain

Location, character, severity and frequency of the pain should be noted as well as the first time it occurred, the factors increasing pain (e.g. hot or cold things) and any changes in its character.

Swelling

The location, size, consistency and color change during inflammation and the duration, and frequency of the swelling needs to be noted.

Function

Difficulties in chewing can be due to a fractured cusp or generalized malocclusion. Speech difficulty may be due to local cause or systemic problems.

Social

A bad taste or smell may be due to poor oral hygiene or periodontal disease.

Appearance

- Missing or crowded teeth
- Fractured tooth or restoration
- Malpositioned or discolored teeth
- Congenital anomalies of dentition.

History

1. Personal details (name, age, sex, address).
2. Medical history.
3. Drug history.
4. Dental history.
   - Periodontal history
   - Restorative history
   - Endodontic history
   - Orthodontic history
   - Removable prosthodontic history
   - Oral surgical history
   - Radiographic history
   - TMJ dysfunction history.

Medical history

- Any cardiac ailments, requiring antibiotic premedication before treatment, CNS disorders or other systemic diseases affecting treatment method. Hypertensive patients and coronary disease patients should not be given epinephrine
- Any previous radiation therapy, blood disorders, terminal illness affecting treatment plan
- Systemic conditions with oral manifestations
- Infective diseases as aids, hepatitis and syphilis needs to be evaluated.

Drug history

Previous medication history, drug allergies and if patient is taking any medicines routinely should be noted.

Dental history

Periodontal history

Oral hygiene status, any previous oral hygiene prophylaxis or any previous periodontal surgery is noted.

Restorative history

All restorations of amalgam and tooth-colored restorations along with time of these restorations are noted.

Endodontic history

If the endodontically restored tooth is a prospective abutment tooth then a radiographic evaluation of the periapical health is noted.

Orthodontic history

If radiographic evaluation shows root resorption, it can be due to previous orthodontic treatment. Occlusal adjustment with minor tooth movement can promote long-term positional stability of the teeth and reduce, or eliminate, parafunctional activity.

Removable prosthodontic history

Previous removable prostheses must be carefully evaluated and the duration of wear needs to be noted.

Oral surgical history

Missing teeth and period of edentulousness should be noted.

Radiographic history

Previous radiographs and current diagnostic radiographic series aids to assess the progress of the disease. It also aids in locating impacted tooth, root tips and cyst and tumours.

TMJ dysfunction history

1. Pain or clicking in the temporomandibular joints.
2. Tenderness to palpation.
3. Difficulty in opening the mouth.
4. Deviation while opening.
5. The above symptoms with any treatment done earlier for the dysfunction as occlusal appliances, medications, or exercises should be noted.

Examination

General examination

General appearance, gait, weight skin color (anemia or jaundice). Vital signs, such as respiration, pulse, temperature, and blood pressure, are measured and recorded.

Temporomandibular joint examination

- Bilateral palpation anterior to the auricular tragi while the patient opens and closes the mouth, can locate disorder in the posterior attachment of the disk
- Tenderness clicking, or pain is noted
- Jaw opening of less than 40 mm indicates restriction
- Deviation from midline is also recorded
- Maximum lateral movement can then be measured (normal is about 12 mm)
- Masseter and temporal muscles are palpated for signs of tenderness and classified as mild, moderate, or severe.

Extraoral examination

Includes noting of:

- Facial asymmetry
- Cervical lymph node palpation
- TMJs and the muscles of mastication
- Lips: Smile line, negative space between the maxillary and mandibular teeth when the patient laughs, missing teeth, diastemae and fractured or poorly restored teeth are noted.

Intraoral examination

Soft tissues, teeth and supporting structures as the tongue, floor of the mouth, vestibule, cheeks and hard and soft palates are examined and findings noted.

Periodontal examination

- Oral hygiene status assessment
- Examination of gingiva, periodontium and the response to the host tissues (BPE)
  - Healthy gingiva is pink, stippled and bound to the underlying connective tissue
  - The texture, size, contour, consistency, position and color are noted. Any exudate or pus is examined for
  - The width of the keratinized attached gingiva around each tooth is assessed.

Examination of teeth

- Absence of teeth, dental caries, any restorations, wear faceting, fractures, abrasions, malformations and erosions are noted
- Pocket depths (usually six per tooth) are recorded on a periodontal chart.

Occlusal examination

- General alignment
- Lateral and protrusive contacts
- Centric relation
- Jaw maneuverability.

General alignment

The teeth can be evaluated for crowding, rotation, over eruption, spacing, malocclusion and vertical and horizontal overlap.

Lateral and protrusive contacts

The presence or absence of tooth contact in eccentric movements is verified with a thin Mylar strip. Tooth movement (fremitus) should be identified by palpation.

Centric relation

The relationship of teeth in both centric and intercuspal position is assessed. If a slide from CR to IP is present, its horizontal and vertical components can be estimated and a note made of any lateral deviation.

Jaw manoeuvrability

The ability and ease with which the patient moves the jaw and the guiding movements should be assessed.

Check for habitual occlusion.

Abutment tooth evaluation

- Abutment teeth need to be strong enough to withstand the forces directed to the missing teeth in addition to those usually applied to the abutments
- Abutment teeth should not exhibit mobility
- An asymptomatic endodontically treated tooth can be considered for an abutment provided it can withstand the forces transmitted to it

- The supporting tissues surrounding the abutment teeth should be healthy and free from inflammation.

Evaluation of abutment teeth includes:
- Crown–root ratio
- Tooth configuration
- Periodontal surface area
- Vitality testing.

Crown–root ratio
An abutment teeth should have a combined pericemental area equal to or greater in pericemental area than the tooth or teeth to be replaced (Antes law).
Favorable crown-root ratio is 1:1.

Tooth configuration
- Root shape: Short conical roots give less support. Divergent multiple roots give good support.

Periodontal surface area
Root surface area: Larger teeth will have greater surface area and will handle stress better.

Vitality testing
Prior to any restorative treatment, pulpal health must be assessed by measuring the response to percussion as well as thermal and electrical stimulation.

Diagnostic casts
- Articulated diagnostic casts aid in planning treatment procedures, provide information about static and dynamic relationships of the teeth and help to view several aspects of the occlusion not detectable within the confines of the mouth.

Advantages of diagnostic cast
- Changing the arch relationship before orthognathic procedures
- Changing the tooth position prior to orthodontic procedures
- Modifying the occlusal scheme before attempting any selective occlusal adjustment
- Trial tooth preparation and waxing can be done before fixed restorative procedures
- Selection of an optimum path of withdrawal of a fixed partial denture can be assessed.

Radiographic examination
1. Periapical radiographs.
2. Bitewing radiographs.
3. Panoramic films.
4. Transcranial exposure, serial tomography, arthrography, CT scanning, or magnetic resonance imaging in case of TMJ disorders.

Periapical radiographs
(14 periapical radiographs help in complete examination)

Uses
- To assess the extent of bone support, quality of supporting bone

- Detailed root morphology of each abutment tooth
- Width of periodontal ligament space
- Bone resorption (vertical, horizontal)
- Inclination of teeth
- Continuity of lamina dura
- Pulpal morphology and previous endodontic treatment
- Any periapical pathology can be evaluated
- Evaluation of crown–root ratio
- Evaluation of the shape, length and direction of root
- Helps in checking for periodontal situation of the abutment tooth, as widening or thickening of lamina dura, occlusal prematurities or trauma can cause thickening.

Bitewings

Use

Evaluation of caries on proximal surfaces and secondary caries on previous restorations.

Panoramic films

Uses

- Evaluation of bone resorption, pattern of bone resorption and quality of bone support
- To check for presence of retained root tips, impacted tooth
- To determine the thickness of soft tissue on the ridge in area of pontic placement
- They do not provide a detailed view for assessing bone support, root morphology, or caries.

Treatment Planning

Treatment planning helps to design and select the material of choice for a particular situation.

The design and material choice depends on:

- Amount of tooth structure present
- Esthetics
- Plaque control.

Choice of restoration

In following situations, fixed partial denture is contraindicated and the restoration of choice is removable partial denture.

- Large edentulous space
- Edentulous space with no distal abutment
- Bilaterally edentulous with no distal abutment
- Grossly tipped teeth
- Periodontally weak teeth
- Teeth with short clinical crowns
- Severe bone resorption
- Young age
- Large tongue
- Extensive caries with poor oral hygiene.

2. List the ideal requirements of an abutment tooth and describe the steps taken to maintain biological integrity while preparing teeth for fixed partial denture.

Alternate form of the question

What are the biomechanical principles used in tooth preparation for a fixed partial denture?

Requirements of an Abutment Tooth

- Abutment teeth need to be strong enough to withstand the forces directed to the missing teeth in addition to those usually applied to the abutments
- Abutment teeth should not exhibit mobility
- An endodontically treated tooth can be considered if it is asymptomatic and if it can withstand the forces transmitted to it. The supporting tissues surrounding the abutment teeth should be healthy and free from inflammation.

Factors to be considered in abutment selection

- Crown–root ratio
- Tooth configuration
- Periodontal surface area
- The length of the pontic span
- Forces
- Oral hygiene measures.

Crown–root ratio

- An abutment teeth should have a combined pericemental area equal to or greater in pericemental area than the tooth or teeth to be replaced (Antes' law)
- The optimum crown–root ratio is 2:3. A root ratio of 1:1 at least needs to be present for a prospective abutment
- If coronal structure is less, core build up or crown lengthening needs to be done to fulfil the crown–root ratio.

Tooth configuration

Root shape and angulation

A molar with divergent roots, single-rooted tooth with an elliptic cross section (broader labiolingually than mesiodistally), a long root or multiple roots provide better support than a root surface area with circular cross section.

Periodontal surface area

Root surface area

Larger teeth will have greater surface area and will handle stress better.

Bone support

Teeth with vertical and horizontal resorption give less support.

The length of the pontic span

- Two abutment teeth can support two pontics
- Failures due to abnormal stress have been attributed to increased length of the span.

Forces

Varying the occlusal scheme by altering the occlusal table or plane can decrease the load on abutment teeth.

Oral hygiene

Teeth with slight mobility can be used as abutments if stabilised and if oral hygiene is maintained.

Principles of Tooth Preparation

1. Biologic considerations.
2. Mechanical considerations.
3. Esthetic considerations.

Biologic considerations

(Are factors that affect the health of the oral tissues)

1. Prevention of damage during tooth preparation to:
   - Adjacent teeth
   - Soft tissues
   - Pulp of the tooth being prepared.
2. Conservation of tooth structure.
3. Margin placement.
4. Finish lines.
5. Occlusal consideration.

1. Prevention of damage during tooth preparation to:

Adjacent teeth

If the proximal contact area is damaged during preparation it needs to be reshaped and polished otherwise it is susceptible to dental caries.

To prevent damage:

- A metal matrix band needs to be used around the adjacent tooth
- A thin tapered diamond is used to break the inter-proximal contact.

Soft tissues

Damage to the tongue and cheeks can be prevented by careful retraction with an aspirator tip, mouth mirror or flanged saliva ejector.

Pulp

Extreme temperatures, chemical irritation can cause pulpal damage.

Prevention

- Assess morphology of the dental pulp chamber before preparation with the help of a radiograph
- Use new and perfect abrasives while reducing the tooth. This reduces the heat that is generated

- Apply gentle pressure while preparation of tooth
- Use copious amount of water spray directed at the area of contact between tooth and bur. This removes clogging and prevents desiccation of the dentin
- All retention grooves and polishing need to be done with a slow-speed handpiece with adequate amount of water spray
- Avoid use of chemical agents for cleaning.

Conservation of tooth structure:
- Use of partial veneer crowns instead of full veneer crowns
- Minimum taper between axial walls
- Occlusal surface reduction following anatomic planes
- Tilted tooth to be repositioned, so that less tooth structure is removed during preparation
- A conservative margin finish
- Supra gingival or crest of the gingival margin finish line.

Failures due to improper preparation of tooth:
- Insufficient axial reduction with an over contoured restoration can cause periodontal disease or dental caries
- Inadequate occlusal reduction can cause occlusal dysfunction and poor margin placement
- Excessive axial contours can cause gingival inflammation.

Margin placement

Requirements
- Ease of preparation without overextension
- Easy to identify in the impression and on the die
- Easy to finish on wax pattern
- Sufficient bulk of material
- Preserve tooth structure.

Types
1. Supragingival.
2. Subgingival.
3. At the crest of the gingiva.

Supragingival margins
- They can be easily finished
- They are more easily kept clean
- Impressions are more easily made with less potential for soft tissue damage
- Restorations can be easily evaluated at recall appointments.

Subgingival margins
- Subgingival margins are often on dentin or cementum
- They are done when cervical erosion or restorations extend subgingivally and when a crown-lengthening procedure cannot be carried out

- A well-designed preparation has a margin that is smooth and will provide the patient with a longer-lasting restoration.

Finish lines

Types

1. Featheredge or shoulderless crown preparations: Conservative but not to be used.
2. Chisel edge: Only on tilted tooth.
3. Chamfer: All metal restorations.
4. Shoulder: All ceramic restorations and not conservative.
5. Sloped shoulder: Reduces possibility of leaving unsupported enamel and leaves sufficient bulk to allow thinning of the metal framework to a knife-edge for good esthetics.
6. Shoulder with bevel: In subgingivally extended finish lines due to cervical erosion. A bevelled shoulder margin is used for the facial surface of a metal–ceramic restoration where a metal collar is to be used.

Advantages of a bevel

- Easy burnishing of the cast metal margin
- Decreases marginal discrepancy
- Protects unprepared tooth structure from chipping.

Occlusal considerations

If occlusion is disrupted by supra-erupted or tilted teeth either uprighting of tooth or a modified restoration should be considered after endodontic treatment.

Adequate occlusal clearance is required for an optimal occlusion.

Mechanical Considerations

1. Providing retention form.
2. Providing resistance form.
3. Preventing deformation of the restoration.

Providing Retention form:

This is the quality of a preparation that prevents the restoration from becoming dislodged by such forces parallel to the path of withdrawal.

Factors affecting retention:

- Magnitude of the dislodging forces
- Geometry of the tooth preparation
- Roughness of the fitting surface of the restoration
- Materials being cemented
- Type of luting agent
- Film thickness of the luting agent.

Magnitude of the dislodging forces

Great removal forces occur with sticky food. The magnitude of the dislodging forces depends on the stickiness of the food and the surface area and texture of the restoration being pulled.

Geometry of the tooth preparation

Fixed prostheses depend on the geometric form rather than on adhesion for retention as majority of the luting agents are non-adhesive like zinc phosphate.

Factors
- Taper
- Surface area
- Stress concentration
- Type of preparation.

Taper
- Maximum retention is obtained if a tooth preparation has parallel walls
- Smaller degrees of taper have more retention
- As the taper increases, however, so does the free movement of the restoration and retention will be reduced
- The recommended convergence between opposing walls is 6 degrees.

Surface area
Provided the restoration has a limited path of withdrawal, its retention is dependent on the length of this path in sliding contact. Therefore, crowns with long axial walls are more retentive than those with short axial walls.

Stress concentration
Round margins may reduce stress concentrations and hence, increase the retention of the restoration.

Type of preparation
Retention is increased by adding grooves and boxes to a preparation with a limited path of withdrawal.

Roughness of the surfaces
Retention is increased if the restoration is roughened or grooved by air-abrading the fitting surface with alumina.

Materials being cemented
- More reactive the alloy, more adhesion with certain luting agents
- Base-metal alloys are better retained than less reactive high-gold content metals
- Cement adheres better to amalgam than to composite resin or cast gold
- Crowns adhere better with composite resin than with amalgam cores.

Type of luting agent
Adhesive resin cements are the most retentive, with less bond during long-term.

Providing Resistance form
Lateral forces tend to displace the restoration by causing rotation around the gingival margin which is prevented by any areas of the tooth preparation that are placed in compression called resistance area.

Resistance depends on:

- Magnitude and direction of the dislodging forces
- Geometry of the tooth preparation: Increased taper and rounding of axial angles, short tooth preparations with large diameters reduce resistance
- Physical properties of the luting agent: Zinc phosphate cements have a higher modulus of elasticity than polycarboxylate cements, hence polycarboxylate cement depends more on the taper of the preparation than zinc phosphate cement.

Preventing deformation of the restoration

Restoration must have sufficient strength to prevent it from being permanently deformed during function.

Factors

- Alloy selection
- Adequate tooth reduction
- Margin design.

Alloys

Type III or Type IV gold alloys. High-noble metal content metal–ceramic alloys have a hardness equivalent to Type IV golds and nickel–chromium alloys are more hard and can be used in long-span fixed partial dentures (FPD).

Adequate tooth reduction

A minimum alloy thickness of about 1.5 mm over centric cusps (buccal in the mandible and lingual in the maxillae) and 1 mm in non-functional cusps. Occlusal reduction should follow the morphology of tooth.

Margin design

Depending on the type of restoration the ideal margin design needs to be followed.

Esthetic considerations

1. Complete examination and assessment of teeth during smiling, talking, and laughing.
2. Find the patient's esthetic requirements.
3. Type of restoration selected.

Partial-coverage restorations

Proximal margin

Place proximal margin just buccal to the maximal contact area where metal will be hidden by the distal line angle of the neighbouring tooth.

Facial margin

The facial margin of a maxillary partial-coverage restoration should be extended just beyond the occlusofacial line angle. A short bevel is needed to prevent enamel chipping. A chamfer can be placed where appearance is less important (e. g., on molars) because this will provide greater bulk of metal for strength.

Metal–ceramic restorations

Facial tooth reduction

A minimum reduction of 1.5 mm is required for sufficient bulk of porcelain and metal for strength.

Labial margin placement

Supragingival margin placements are easier to prepare properly and easier to keep clean.
After observing the patient's smile, margins should be placed.
Margins should not be placed subgingivally encroaching on the attachment. If it extends within 1.5 mm of the alveolar crest bone resorption tends to occur.

3. Describe various methods used for gingival retraction and add a note on the advantages of fluid control and tissue displacement.

Definition

Gingival retraction is a process of exposing margins when making impressions of prepared teeth.

Other names

Tissue dilation, tissue retraction and tissue displacement.

Advantages of gingival retraction

- Duplicating subgingival margins in impressions
- Copying the unprepared tooth surface to aid in evaluating the marginal finish line accurately
- Helps in accuracy of wax pattern fabrication and location of finish line
- Final restoration tends to have better marginal adaptation
- To alter the contour of the gingival tissue around the teeth or edentulous ridge.

Classification of Gingival Displacement

Generally classified as non surgical and surgical

Nonsurgical

- Mechanical: Retracted by mechanical methods
- Chemical: Dilation with help of certain dilatants
- Mechanical–chemical: Retracted with a cord impregnated with a chemical for hemostasis.

Surgical

- Rotary
- Conventional (gingivoplasty, gingivectomy and periodontal flap procedures)
- Electrosurgery
- Lasers (CO_2, argon, diode and Nd:YAG).

Mechanical methods

1. Retraction by modified temporay crown or impression caps.
2. Modified impression techniques
   - Oversized copper bands with elastomeric impression materials
   - Temporary acrylic coping
   - Modified custom tray technique
   - Matrix impression system.

3. Mechanical retraction
   - Gingival protectors
   - Matrices and wedges/rubber dam
   - Strips (hydroxylate polyvinyl acetate)/paste
   - Syringed PVS/aluminium chloride.
4. Mechanochemical methods
   - Retracting with hemostatic agents
   - Retracting with paste and hemostatic agent.

Mechanical methods

Impression techniques

Oversized copper bands

- Are placed on the prepared tooth and either impression compound or elastomeric impression material supported by acrylic with adhesive is used to make an impression of the prepared tooth which retracts the gingiva under pressure
- Time consuming and can cause trauma to tissue.

Temporary acrylic coping

Acrylic coping is relieved by 1 mm and an adhesive is used followed by an elastomeric impression material.

Matrix Impression system (MIS)[1]

- Three impression procedures using three viscosities of impression materials
- Technique—A matrix fitting the tooth preparation is made using a semi-rigid elastomeric material before gingival retraction
- After gingival retraction a definitive impression is made with the matrix using a high-viscosity elastomeric impression material
- Pick up with the matrix impression seated a stock tray filled with a medium-viscosity elastomeric impression material is used to make the entire arch impression
- Advantage—The design of matrix gently forces the high-viscosity impression material into the sulcus, which does not allow it to collapse as the medium-viscosity material in the stock tray is seated for the pick-up impression
- Disadvantage—Increased chair side time.

Modified custom tray Technique[2]

- Custom tray is modified by intra oral relining with autopolymerising acrylic resin
- The relined custom tray is trimmed by 2 mm to obtain clearance for elastomeric impression material
- In case of subgingival finish lines that area is only trimmed by 0.5 mm so that the elastomeric impression material is directed into sulcus
- Advantages—Time saving, accurate and retraction cord can be avoided.

Chemical methods

1. Anti-sialogogues.
2. Local anesthetics.
3. Anticholinergics: Methantheline bromide (50 mg), propantheline bromide (15 mg), atropin, etc.
4. Antihypertensives as clonidine hydrochloride (0.2 mg).

Chemical methods are done when mechanical methods cannot be achieved. Each of the drugs has side effects, which need to be critically evaluated.

Mechanical–Chemical Methods

This technique consists of using impregnated cords with chemicals.

Chemicals that are used are:

- Racemic epinephrine: Contraindicated in cardiac, hypertensive and diabetic patients
- Aluminium potassium sulphate (least inflammation and little sulcus collapse after cord removal)
- Aluminium chloride and ferric sulphate (inhibits set of polyvinyl siloxane and polyether impressions)
- Phenylephrine hydrochloride
- Others as inert matrix polyvinyl-siloxane (generates hydrogen that causes expansion of material against sulcus walls)
- Injection of 15% aluminum chloride in Kaolin matrix (easy, no pain, no trauma but inhibits polyether and polyvinyl siloxane).

Armamentarium

1. Saliva ejector.
2. Mouth mirror.
3. Explorer.
4. Scissors.
5. Cord packing instrument.
6. Retraction cord.
7. Hemodent liquid.
8. Cotton pliers.
9. Cotton rolls.
10. Dappen dish.
11. Cotton pellets.
12. 2×2 gauze sponges.

Method of Gingival Retraction

1. The prepared tooth area is dried and isolated with cotton rolls.
2. A retraction cord of two-inch length is drawn out from the dispenser bottle held with sterile pliers and cut with scissors.
3. The retraction cord is dipped in 25% aluminium chloride solution or 8% epinephrine.
4. The excess amount of aluminium chloride is squeezed out with a gauze piece.

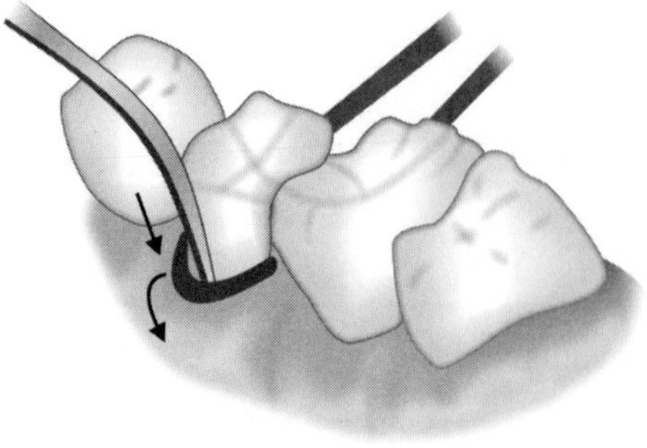

Fig. 1: The cord is first secured in the mesial interproximal area and the distal interproximal area with a cord-packing instrument

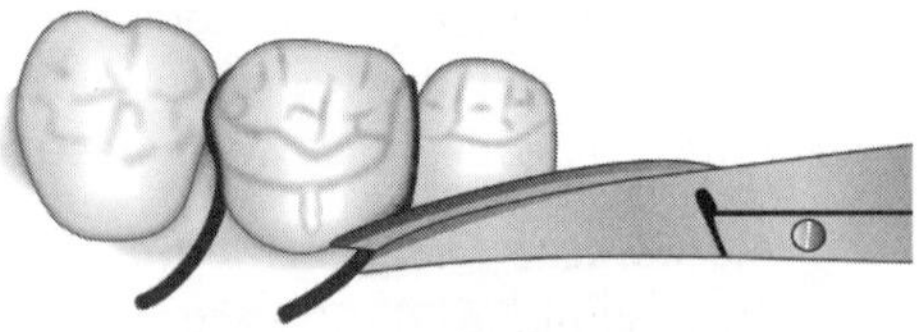

Fig. 2: Cut the excess amount of cord in the mesial interproximal area

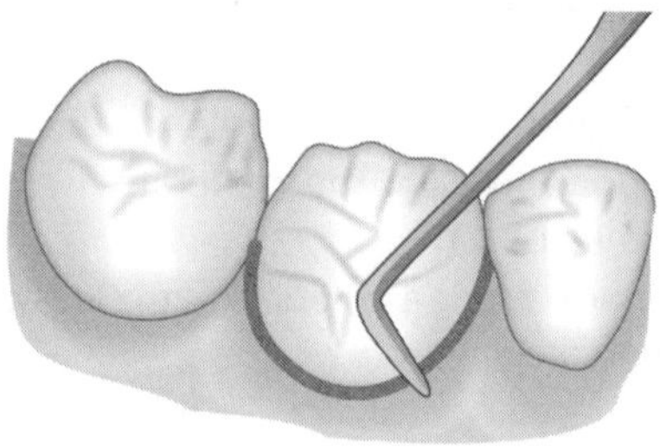

Fig. 3: Complete the placement of cord on the buccal side from the distal end to the mesial side until it overlaps the mesial portion

5. The cord is made into a "u", and looped around the prepared tooth. Only the end of the cord is to be touched (Fig. 1).
6. The cord is first secured in the mesial interproximal area and the distal interproximal area with a cord-packing instrument.
7. After the cord is secured in the distal interproximal area, the cord is inserted from the mesiolingual to distolingual corner. While tucking in the cord the tip of the packing instrument should be angled towards the area where the cord has been placed.
8. Cut the excess amount of cord in the mesial interproximal area (Fig. 2) and complete the placement of cord on the buccal side from the distal end to the mesial side until it overlaps the mesial. A minimum bulk of 0.2 mm sulcular width is essential to make an undistorted impression (Fig. 3).
9. After 5–10 minutes, the cord is gently removed with the sulcus around the prepared tooth exposed and hemostasis maintained.
10. This is followed by the impression of the arch.

Double cord technique

Advantage—Declines the tendency of gingival cuff to recoil and partially displace the impression material as it sets.

This is a technique in which a thin cord is placed initially and over which a large cord is placed. Thin cord remains during impression making. Hansen et al. observed that 98% of prosthodontists use cords of which 48% use a dual cord technique.[3]

Surgical Tissue Dilation

Electrosurgery/Surgical diathermy

(Introduced by D'Arsenal).

An electrosurgery unit is a high-frequency oscillator or radio transmitter which uses either a vacuum tube or a transmitter for delivering a high-frequency electric current of at least 1 Mega Hertz.

An electrosurgical unit consist of oscillator, active electrode and a ground electrode for the safety of the patient.

Types of electrode

- Coagulating electrode: Controls hemorrhage
- Small wire-loop electrode: Used for sulcular enlargement
- Round electrode: Removes gingival tissue
- Large loop electrode: Is used to remove large amount of tissue
- Straight electrode: By angling the working electrode at approximately 15–20 degrees and carrying the tip through the tissue, a small wedge of tissue can be removed. In anterior quadrants, the angle of the working electrode is positioned parallel to the long axis of the tooth.

Posner Electrode

With the AP 1 ½ electrode, the insulated portion of the electrode is directed around the tooth, removing the gingival sulcular epithelium. If less trough depth is desired, part of the tip is removed to create the desired depth at 0.5 mm, 0.75 mm, or 1.0 mm.

Types of current

- Monoterminal: Used for fulguration, removal of papillomas and fistulous tract
- Biterminal: For coagulation, removal of granulation tissue
- Unrectified damped current: Not used in dental treatments
- Fully-rectified full-wave modulated current: Good for gingival enlargement
- Fully-rectified filtered current: Is the best current source.

Method

1. Profound local anesthesia is given and a pleasant smelling aromatic oil is applied on the vermilion border of upper lip.
2. Plastic suction tips and plastic-mounted mouth mirrors are used. Odor is controlled by an outside ventilated oral evacuator system.
3. An adequate power is set on the unit. Electrode is passed quickly over the tissue to be removed. Adequate time interval between each stroke needs to be followed.
4. Fragments of tissue are removed with an alcohol-soaked sponge.

Indications

- Minor tissue removal before impression procedures

- Removal of granulation or inflamed tissue around a given tooth
- For enlargement of gingival sulcus in some cases
- Crown lengthening.

Contraindications

- In cardiac pacemaker patients
- Not to use on thin attached gingiva.

Rules

1. Profound anesthesia.
2. No metal instruments should be used.
3. Proper grounding should be done.
4. A fully-rectified filtered current should be used.
5. Electrode should not make contact with any metal restorations in the patients mouth.
6. A light stroke with a 5 second time interval between applications of the electrode.
7. If the tip drags, the instrument is at too low a setting and the current should be increased.
8. If sparking is visible the current level is set high and need to be decreased.
9. A cutting stroke should not be repeated within 5 seconds.
10. The electrode must remain clean of tissue fragments.
11. The sulcus should be swabbed with hydrogen peroxide before the displacement cord is placed.
12. Maintaining the biologic width after tissue healing.
13. After the impression is made tincture of myrrh and benzoin is placed till healing completes in 5–10 days.

Rotary curettage/Gingettage

(Introduced by Amsterdam in 1954)

- This is a troughing technique to remove limited amount of epithelial tissue in the sulcus while chamfer finish line is prepared.
- This technique needs to be done on healthy, non-inflamed gingiva to avoid tissue shrinkage after healing of the diseased tissue.

Lasers[4]

Diode lasers, such as neodymium: yttrium-aluminum-garnet (Nd-YAG), Erbium: yttrium-aluminum-garnet (Er:YAG) and CO_2 laser are commonly used for gingival retraction around natural teeth.

Advantage

Less bleeding (CO_2 laser), gingival recession, painless and sterilizes sulcus.

Disadvantages

- Er:YAG laser is not as good at hemostasis as CO_2 laser
- CO_2 laser provides no tactile feedback hence, can damage junctional epithelium.

Advantages of Fluid Control and Tissue Management

- Patient comfort

- Safety for patient
- Good visibility while doing clinical procedures
- Clear the area of saliva and water, for better visibility.

Fluid control attained by:

- Rubber dam
- Cotton rolls
- High-volume vacuum
- Saliva ejector
- Svedopter
- Vac-ejector
- Moisture absorbing cords.

Rubber dam

Punch holes are made in the area of preparation site of the rubber dam and clamped in position.

Uses

- While removing old restorations
- While preparing onlay or inlay
- For endodontic procedures as a safety measure
- While using pin-retained restoration.

Disadvantages

- Difficult to use while preparing crowns and FPD
- Reacts with polyvinyl siloxane impression materials.

Cotton rolls

Absorbent cotton rolls are placed in the area where saliva pools (in maxillary arch, a single cotton roll is used in buccal vestibule and in mandibular arch in lingual sulcus).

Placement of cotton roll

One or two cotton rolls are placed vertically against the horizontally placed cotton rolls or one single horse-shaped roll can be used.

Limitation

The entire saliva and water soaked roll needs to be removed each time.

High-volume vacuum

Can be used as a retractor as well as for clearing saliva and water during preparation.

Saliva ejector

- Useful for maxillary arch along with cotton rolls
- Placed in the corner of mouth opposite the quadrant being operated with the patient's head towards that side.

Svedopter/Speejector

Svedopter consist of a metal saliva ejector with a tongue deflector. Effectively used in mandibular arch. Effective fluid control along with cotton rolls. The patient is seated in an upright position.

Positioning

Placed in the incisor region with the tubing under the patient's arm.

Disadvantages

- Access to lingual aspect is limited
- Metal surface can cause tissue irritation
- Can cause gagging in some patients
- Cannot use in mandibular tori patients.

Vac-ejector

Tongue control and high-volume evacuation along with a bite block. It aids in removing large volumes of fluid. Tongue deflectors and bite blocks are available in several sizes. The tongue deflectors are made of plastic.

Moisture absorbing cords

Consist of pressed paper wafers covered on one side with a reflective foil. The wafer side is placed facing the tissues. Used along with cotton rolls to control saliva and retract cheek laterally.

References

1. Livaditis GJ. The matrix impression system for fixed prosthodontics. J Prosthet Dent. 1998;79:208-16.
2. Ortensi L, Stocchi ML. Modified custom tray. J Prosthet Dent. 2000;84(2):237-40.
3. Hansen PA, Tira DE, Barlow J. Current methods of finish-line exposure by practicing prosthodontists. J Prosthodont. 1999;8:163-70.
4. Martin E, Parker S. The use of lasers in fixed prosthodontics. Dent Clin North Am. 2004;48:971-98.

4. Describe the methods used to classify fixed bridges. Add a note on types of retainers used in fixed partial dentures.

Classifications of Fixed Bridges

- Classification depending on edentulous spaces/site
- Classification based on type of connector
- Classification based on type of abutments
- Classification based on retention
- Classification based on materials used
- Classification based on temporary and permanent nature of bridges
- Classification based on span length.

Classification depending on edentulous spaces

Class 1: Posterior edentulous space.

Class 2: Anterior edentulous space.

Class 3: Anterior and posterior edentulous spaces.
Each of these classifications has divisions and subdivisions.

Divisions

To get idea on the type of support.

Division I

Abutments on one side of the edentulous area are capable of rendering support (Cantilever FPD).

Division II

Abutments on both sides of the edentulous space are capable of giving support. (Conventional FPD).

Division III

A single tooth in the center with edentulous space on either side (Pier Abutments).

Sub-divisions

Denote the position of a prospective abutment tooth.
Sub-division I: Ideal abutments.
Sub-division II: Tilted abutments.
Subdivision III: Periodontally-weak abutments.
Subdivision IV: Extensively damaged coronal structure with good bone support.
Sub-division V: Implant abutment.

Groupings

Each of the subdivisions are further grouped into A and B.
Group A: A single abutment on one side of the edentulous space each is sufficient.
Group B: More than one abutment support is required from each side of the edentulous space.

Another classification based on site

Anterior Bridge—Unilateral (not crossing midline) or bilateral (involves both sides).
Posterior Bridge—Only in posterior region.
Complex Bridge—One of terminals beyond canine.

Classification based on type of connector

1. Rigid connector.
2. Semi-rigid connector.
3. Removable fixed partial denture.

Classification based on type of abutments

1. Ideal abutment.
2. Cantilever abutment.
3. Pier abutment.
4. Abutment receiving pin support from coronal structure.
5. Telescopic crown.
6. Endodontically-treated abutment with cast post or post and core support.
7. Resin-bonded bridges.

Classification based on retention

Simple and compound.

Simple

Fixed-Fixed—Fixed at both ends.

Fixed-Movable—Nonrigid connector at one terminal (limited movement).

Cantilever—Free end bridge.

Spring cantilever—Pontic at the end of resilient curved arm with support from a distant abutment.

Resin bonded—Presently a single wing is commonly used.

Compound bridge/Hybrid

When more than one type of simple bridges are employed.

Classification based on materials used

Metallic, nonmetallic and combined

Metallic

- Precious (gold alloy)
- Semi precious
- Nonprecious (base-metal alloy).

Nonmetallic

Resin/Ceramic.

Combined

- Metal with labial/buccal ceramic veneer
- Metal with fullveneer
- Metal-reinforced bridges.

Classification based on temporary and permanent nature of bridges

Provisional

Temporary—After preparation till, a definitive prosthesis is given.

Immediate—Made before extraction and placed immediately after extraction.

Interim prosthesis, splints.

Definitive/Permanent

Fixed partial dentures (single, complex and pier-abutment prosthesis).

Implant abutments.

Classification based on span length

Short span—One missing tooth

Medium span—Two missing tooth

Long span—More than two missing tooth.

Types of Retainers

Complete crowns

1. All-metal crowns.
2. All-ceramic crowns.

3. Metal–ceramic crown.
4. Acrylic-fused-to-metal crowns.
5. Metal-free (fiber-reinforced composites) crowns.

Partial crowns

Posterior tooth

1. Mesial one-half crown.
2. Three-quarter crown.
3. Modified three-quarter crown.
4. Seven-eight crown.

Anterior tooth

1. Three-quarter crown.
2. Variations of three-quarter crown (Selberg crown).

Complete crowns

All-metal fixed partial dentures

- They are used for replacing maxillary and mandibular posterior teeth
- They also provide proper guide planes for removable partial denture
- Aids in occlusal plane modifications.

Advantages

- They have the maximum strength and durability
- Less tooth structure is reduced as compared to all porcelain (chamfer margin).

Disadvantage

They are not esthetic.

Indications

- For posterior tooth with short clinical crowns
- For grossly caries or fractured tooth.

Preparation steps

1. Occlusal reduction: Using round-end tapered diamond.
2. Functional cusp bevel: Round-end tapered diamond.
3. Buccal, lingual, axial reduction: Chamfer diamond.
4. Proximal reduction: Short thin and chamfer diamond.
5. Seating groove: No. 170 bur.

Metals that can be used

Gold

Base-metal alloys.

All ceramic fixed partial dentures

- All ceramic partial dentures are brittle and less fracture resistant compared to all metal partial dentures
- Castable and alumina-reinforced porcelains have more strength compared to conventional porcelains.

Advantages
- Can duplicate tooth color exactly
- Good translucency
- Different shades of luting agent give the retainer a natural appearance
- Good as anterior retainers.

Disadvantages
- Reduced strength
- Brittle
- More expensive
- Cannot be used on extensively-damaged teeth
- More amount of tooth structure need to be removed compared to other restorations
- Large connectors cause impingement of inter-dental papilla
- Wear of opposing natural teeth
- Two opposing retainers in porcelain can cause a clicking sound
- Not advisable in posterior tooth if heavy loads have to be applied.

Preparation steps
- After placing depth orientation grooves approximately 1.0 mm on labial surface and 2.0 mm deep on incisal half is reduced
- Incisal reduction: 1.5–2.0 mm with flat-end tapered diamond
- Labial and lingual axial reduction: With flat-end tapered diamond
- Lingual reduction: Small wheel diamond
- Axial reduction: Flat-end tapered diamond (aids in retention, resistance and structural durability)
- Shoulder margin: Helps in resistance and marginal integrity.

Types of ceramics
1. Conventional platinum matrix ceramics.
2. Alumina-reinforced ceramics.
3. Slip cast alumina (Inceram).
4. Castable ceramics (Dicor).
5. Mica glass ceramic (Machinable ceramic: CAD CAM).
6. Heat-pressed ceramics: Leucite crystals dispersed ceramics (Optec HSP, IPS empress).
7. Resin-bonded ceramics.

Metal–Ceramic fixed partial dentures
This retainer consists of a core of metal with a ceramic external surface.

Two types
1. Metal is fused with porcelain on all the surfaces.
2. Only the lingual and occlusal surface is of metal, whereas the labial and gingival surface is formed by porcelain.

Advantages
- Esthetic and also incorporates the strength of metal
- Characterization can be done by internal and external stains.

Disadvantages:

- Not conservative preparation
- For better esthetics, the facial margin needs to be extended subgingivally. This can cause gingival destruction
- Failure at the metal–ceramic junction can occur.

Preparation steps:

- For type one with a complete metal and porcelain, preparation is same as for all porcelain
- For type two in which the lingual surface is of metal, a chamfer margin is sufficient, with a shoulder margin on labial aspect to accommodate for the bulk of porcelain.

Acrylic fused to metal

- Poor wear resistance
- Easy to fabricate and adjust
- Esthetically pleasing
- Less expensive.

Fiber-reinforced composite resin bridges

Materials used

Polymer or resin matrices reinforced with glass, polyethylene or carbon fibers. The reinforcing fibers may be unidirectional (long, continuous and parallel), braided or woven.

Classification

- Pre-impregnated with resin (e.g. Fiberkor)
- Impregnation required with fiber (e.g. Ribbond).

Contraindications

- Cannot be used in long-span bridges
- Patients with parafunctional habits
- When opposing tooth is unglazed porcelain.

Advantages

- Optimal esthetics
- Metal free
- Decreased wear of opposing teeth.

Tooth Preparation

- Lingual reduction: Flat end-tapered diamond
- Groove preparation on the palatal surface of the edentulous side
- A shoulder or chamfer margin can be prepared.

Partial crowns

Posterior tooth

1. Mesial halves

For tilted molar abutments to obtain a parallel path of insertion and to alter the occlusal plane.

2. Three quarter crowns

- Only the lingual aspect is prepared extending till mesiolingual and distolingual transitional line angles
- Proximal grooves are prepared perpendicular to the prepared surface and the buccal wall is flared with tapered carbide bur
- In case of additional retention offset is prepared extending from proximal grooves along the buccal cusp.

3. Modified three quarter

Done on premolars with the preparation extending buccally.

4. Seven-eights

Includes lingual, occlusal and distal half of buccal surface.

Anterior tooth

Three quarter

Refer to posterior tooth three quarter crown preparation.

Pin ledges

Indications

- When large amount of tooth structure is lost with intact buccal walls
- For restoration and alteration of occlusal surface.

Contraindications

- In short clinical crowns
- In long-span FPD
- In endodontically treated tooth
- In patients with active caries
- In malaligned abutment tooth.

Advantages

- Conservation of tooth structure
- Supragingival preparation
- Better visibility of seating and cementation.

Disadvantages

Less retentive

Not esthetic if metal is displayed.

5. **Define and classify retainers. List the advantages and disadvantages of partial veneer crown over other types of retainers. What are the factors that come into play in the selection of retainers?**

Retainer

Definition

Any type of device used for stabilization or retention of prosthesis—GPT.

Function

Is to support and connect the body of the bridge with the abutment. It also restores the form, function and esthetics of the abutment.

Classification of Retainers for Fixed Partial Denture

Class I—Extracoronal restorations

A. Full-coverage crowns
1. All-metal crowns.
2. All-ceramic crown.
3. Metal–ceramic crown.
4. Acrylic-fused-to-metal crown.
5. Metal-free composites.

B. Partial-coverage crowns
1. Posterior tooth
   - Mesial one-half crown
   - Three-quarter crown
   - Reverse three-quarter crown
   - Seven-eight crown.
2. Anterior tooth
   - Three-quarter crown
   - Variations of three-quarter crown (Selberg crown).

Class II—Intracoronal restorations
1. Inlays.
2. Onlays.
3. Pin ledge.
4. Combinations.

Class III—Radicular retainers
1. Cast core.
2. Blue island posts.
3. Para post techniques.
4. Kurer technique.

Class I—Extracoronal restorations
- The preparation of the tooth and its cast retainer lies externally to the body of the coronal portion of the prepared tooth and restores a tissue-compatible contour for the crown
- The retention and resistance to displacement is developed between the inner walls of the casting and the external walls of the prepared tooth (complete crowns).

Class II—Intracoronal restorations
- The prepared cavity and its cast retainer lie within the body of the coronal portion of the tooth

- Retention and resistance are developed between the casting and the internal walls of the prepared cavity.

Class III—Radicular retainers

- The dowel type of retention is confined to the root portion
- Retention and resistance to displacement is developed by the extension of an attached metal dowel into the radicular portion of the tooth.

Partial Veneer Crowns

- A partial veneer crown is a restoration covering two or more surfaces of a tooth
- The surfaces usually covered are the lingual, proximal, occlusal, or incisal
- The retention and resistance to displacement depend on the internal surfaces and the auxiliary retentive means, such as grooves, boxing, and pins.

Types of partial veneer

Three-quarter crowns

Covers three fourths of the gingival circumference of the tooth, leaving the facial surface intact.

Advantages

- Esthetically pleasing
- Can serve as a single unit or as an FPD retainer
- Can be used on anterior and posterior teeth as retainers.

Reverse three-quarter crown

- Is when the preparation is done on the buccal aspect leaving the lingual surface of a mandibular posterior tooth intact
- Commonly done on mandibular molars with severe lingual inclination.

Seven-eighths partial veneer crown:

Covers seven eighths of the gingival circumference of the tooth leaving the mesial aspect of the buccal surface intact.

Indications

- For maxillary molars and premolars with extensive carious involvement or restoration on the distal surface with intact mesial surface
- Used on a mandibular premolar with the preparation extending from the distal finish line to the mid-facial surface.

Mesial half crown

Is a three-quarter crown rotated 90 degrees, preserving the distal surface of the tooth while covering the remaining surfaces.

Indications

- In tilted mandibular molar abutment
- Used as a single retainer in drifted or tipped mandibular molar to alter the occlusal plane.

Contraindication

If distal surface of the tooth is damaged by caries or large restoration.

Advantages of partial veneer crowns over complete crowns

- Conservative tooth reduction
- Good esthetics compared to complete veneer cast crown
- Better biocompatibility with supportive tissues as there is less gingival involvement than with complete coverage
- Due to supragingival finish line margin, accessibility for finishing and cleaning is good compared to complete crowns
- Easy verification of complete seating of the casting
- Seating is complete compared to complete crowns as the luting agent has space to flow out (less hydraulic pressure)
- Electric pulp testing can be conveniently accomplished on the intact enamel surface
- Reduced pulpal and periodontal trauma during tooth preparation
- Access to supragingival margins is easy and hence, better for oral hygiene as compared to full crowns
- Due to direct visibility, cement removal is easy.

Disadvantages

- Less retentive than complete veneer crown
- If good preparation is not carried out, there will be display of metal with the partial veneer crown
- The partial veneer crown preparation can be done only on intact teeth with average crown lengths
- Less resistance form as compared to complete crowns
- The placement of grooves, boxes, and pinholes requires good skill otherwise difficulty occurs in seating of casting
- Not recommended in caries prone patients with poor oral hygiene
- Unseating is common if excessive loads are applied.

Indications

- Intact or minimally restored teeth with intact buccal wall
- To re-establish anterior guidance
- Used as retainers for a fixed partial denture when alteration of the occlusal plane is needed
- To splint teeth
- Can be prepared on teeth with average crown length
- Prepared when teeth have normal anatomic crown form
- Anterior teeth need to have adequate labiolingual thickness.

Contraindications

- High caries rate (More for partial veneers where both the un-veneered surface and the margin to finish line interface are susceptible to decay
- Teeth with extensive core restorations

- Deep cervical abrasion
- Short teeth
- Teeth that are severely constricted at the cervical require more axial reduction to provide adequate groove length
- In long-span FPD
- Should not be given on endodontically treated posterior teeth if the buccal cusps are weakened by the access cavity, or on teeth with an extensively damaged crown
- Should not be placed on teeth that are proximally bulbous
- Not recommended in thin teeth of restricted faciolingual dimension
- Not recommended in poorly-aligned teeth

In all of the above situations complete veneer crowns need to be given. When there is difficulty in establishing adequate retention and resistance form, complete veneer restorations are more suitable.

Selection of Types of Retainers

- The selection of the types of retainers depends on the oral-hygiene habits or the DMF rate of the patient, or both
- If caries index is low any type of retainer is safe provided other factors as periodontal status crown length are all present
- The length of the bridge span and the type of bridge determines the type of retainer selected
- Retainer selection for terminal abutments is a crucial decision.

Retainer selection is affected by the following factors
- Age
- DMF rate
- Edentulous span
- Periodontal support
- Arch position of the teeth
- Skeletal relationships
- Interocclusal and intraocclusal conditions, such as crown length
- Existing and projected oral hygiene of the patient
- Vitality of the potential abutment.

Ideal Retainers

- An ideal retainer needs to support and connect the body of the bridge with the abutment
- It should restore the form, function and esthetics of the abutment
- Should be biocompatible with tooth and its adjacent tissues
- Retainer should be constructed without injury to pulp and supporting structures
- Should protect and maintain the pulp against thermal and galvanic shock
- Should provide safety for the tooth during the lifetime of the restoration
- Should provide self-cleaning property
- Should be resistant to corrosion and tarnish
- Should be a conservative preparation with uniformity of reduction of the abutment tooth

- Load should be dispersed to the more receptive areas of the abutment
- There should be large surface contact between the abutment and a retainer
- Selection of an adequate luting agent is important.

6. Define retention and resistance form in fixed partial denture. What are the factors affecting retention and resistance in posterior tooth preparation?

Definitions

Retention

Retention prevents removal of the restoration along the path of insertion or along the path of the tooth preparation.

It is the quality of a preparation that prevents the restoration from becoming dislodged by such forces parallel to the path of withdrawal.

Resistance

Prevents dislodgement of the restoration, by forces directed in an apical or oblique direction and prevents any movement of restoration under occlusal forces.

Factors Affecting Retention

- Magnitude of the dislodging forces
- Geometry of the tooth preparation
- Roughness of the fitting surface of the restoration
- Type of restorative materials being cemented
- Type of luting agent
- Film thickness of the luting agent.

Magnitude of the dislodging forces

Factors influencing dislodging forces:
- Stickiness of the food
- Surface area of the restoration
- Texture of the restoration being pulled.

Of all the type of forces sticky food exhibits large dislodging forces.

Geometry of the tooth preparation

Factors influencing geometry of tooth preparation:
- Taper
- Surface area
- Stress concentration
- Type of preparation.

Taper
- Maximum retention is obtained if a tooth preparation has parallel walls
- Smaller degrees of taper have more retention
- Two opposing surfaces each with a 3° taper provide a 6° taper for the preparation
- Ideal convergence between opposing walls is 6°. This amount of convergence is required to restrain the cemented restoration.

Factors decreasing retention in regard to taper:
- Less amount of taper will form an undercut causing divergence between opposing axial walls, in an occlusocervical direction
- An increased amount of taper increases free movement of the restoration and retention will be reduced (Experimented by Jorgensen in 1955).

Preparation rule:
A rotary instrument of the desired taper held at a constant angulation produces the amount of taper required.

The rotary instrument of ideal taper when moved through a cylindrical path during tooth preparation will produce the desired axial wall taper on the completed preparation.

Surface area
- The greater the length of the clinical crown, the more is the retention
- In short clinical crowns, the surface area needs to be increased with the help of grooves and box preparation
- The greater the width of the clinical crown, the better the retention
- A restoration with limited path of withdrawal is more retentive depending on the length of the surface area in sliding contact.

Stress concentration
- Round margins reduce stress concentrations, which in turn increases the retention of the restoration
- Stresses are generally concentrated around the junction of the axial and occlusal surfaces
- Changes in the geometry of the preparation (e.g. rounding the internal line angles) reduce stress concentrations and hence, increase the retention of the restoration.

Type of preparation
- Additional grooves and boxes to a preparation increase the retention as the surface area is increased
- Retention is double for complete crowns than for a partial crown
- Luting agent is only effective if the restoration has a single path of withdrawal
- The occluso-axial line angle of the tooth preparation should be a replica of the gingival margin geometry
- Fixed prostheses depend on the geometric form than on adhesion of the luting agents for retention.

Roughness of the surfaces
- Retention is increased if the restoration is roughened or grooved by air abrading the fitting surface with alumina
- A smooth internal surface of a restoration can cause retentive failure at the cement-restoration interface.

Materials being cemented
- The more reactive base-metal alloys have more adhesion with certain luting agents than less reactive high-gold content metals
- Cement adheres better to amalgam than to composite resin or cast gold.

Type of luting agent

Adhesive resin cements are the most retentive.

Factors Affecting Resistance Form

Lateral forces tending to displace the restoration by causing rotation around the gingival margin is prevented by areas of the tooth preparation that are placed in compression called resistance area.

Resistance depends on:
- Magnitude and direction of the dislodging forces
- Geometry of the tooth preparation
- Physical properties of the luting agent.

Magnitude and direction of the dislodging forces
- Patients with abnormal biting forces should be given a complete metal crown. A proper design and preparation can help to resist these displacing forces
- In patients with parafunctional habits and pipe smoking to prevent large oblique forces from being applied to a restoration, additional retentive grooves and the restoration should be luted with adhesive cements.

Geometry of the tooth preparation
- Increased preparation taper and rounding of axial angles tend to reduce resistance
- Short tooth preparations with large diameters have less resistance form
- A partial-coverage restoration has less resistance when compared to complete crown.

Resistance can be increased by:
- Preparation of boxes or grooves with walls that are perpendicular to the direction of the applied force
- U-shaped grooves and flared boxes provide more resistance than V-shaped ones
- Pinholes increase resistance as they prevent rotational movement and subject additional areas of the luting agent to compression. The buccal and lingual walls must meet the axial walls at 90° to resist rotational forces.

Physical properties of the luting agent.

Factors affecting resistance to deformation of luting agent are as follows:
- Compressive strength
- Modulus of elasticity.

Compressive strength
- Zinc phosphate cement should have compressive strength above 70 MPa at 24 hours
- Silico-phosphate cements have a higher compressive strength
- Glass ionomer, resin, polycarboxylate and reinforced zinc oxide-eugenol have lower values
- Increase in temperature during manipulation, decreases the strength of the luting agent.

Modulus of elasticity

Zinc phosphate cements have a higher modulus of elasticity than polycarboxylate cements, hence, polycarboxylate cement depends more on the taper of the preparation than zinc phosphate cement.

Conclusion[1]

- A prepared teeth should have the following charecteristics as 10–20 degrees of total occlusal convergence, an occlusocervical dimension of 4 mm and occlusocervical to faciolingual ratio greater than 0.4
- Facio- and lingoproximal line angles should be preserved if not auxillary features as box or grooves need to be added
- All line angles should be rounded and supragingival finish lines are more acceptable in case of esthetic requirements finish lines at gingival level or sometimes subgingival if restoration are present.

Reference

1. Goodacre CJ, et al. Tooth preparations for complete crowns: An art form based on scientific principles. J Prosthet Dent. 2001;85:363-76.

7. Classify finish lines. Enumerate the functions, indications, advantages and disadvantages of finish lines. Add a note on selection of type of finish line to be used.

Definition

Finish line/margin is the part of tooth preparation/restoration that is in close proximity to the periodontium and that forms the most important and weakest links in the success of full-coverage restorations.

It is the outer edge of a crown, inlay, onlay or other restoration.

Other names

Finish line, finish curve.

It is a line of demarcation, peripheral extension of tooth preparation and planned junction of restoration.

Classification Of Gingival Finish Lines

Basic types

1. Knife-edge/Chisel-edge/Shoulderless cervical finish line.
2. Chamfer.
3. Shoulder.

Variations

Variation in knife-edge/Chisel-edge/Shoulderless cervical finish line

Feather edge.

Variations in chamfer

- Hybrid
- Ski-sloped
- Round shoulder
- Heavy chamfer
- McEwen's chamferette.

Variations in shoulder

- Full shoulder with bevel

- Full shoulder with bevel and butt joint
- Radial shoulder.

Functions of Finish Lines

- Helps in evaluating the amount of tooth structure removed during tooth preparation
- To evaluate the accuracy of impression of the tooth preparation
- To evaluate quality of die
- To evaluate the marginal adaptation of wax pattern
- To check the seating of the final restoration
- To evaluate the marginal adaptation of the final restoration.

Characteristics of an ideal finish line has

- Good marginal adaptation
- Biocompatibility with supporting structures
- Adequate contour
- Sufficient strength.

Feather-edge/Chisel-edge Finish Line (Fig. 4)

Definition

Knife-edge preparation is a tapered preparation that has maximum tooth reduction at occlusal, incisal surfaces and tapers to zero cutting at the gingival termination.

Indications

- In young patients
- Pin ledge three fourth crowns
- In tipped teeth
- In long clinical crowns
- In inaccessible areas in the oral cavity
- When finish lines are on cementum
- As proximal finish line for inaccessible areas.

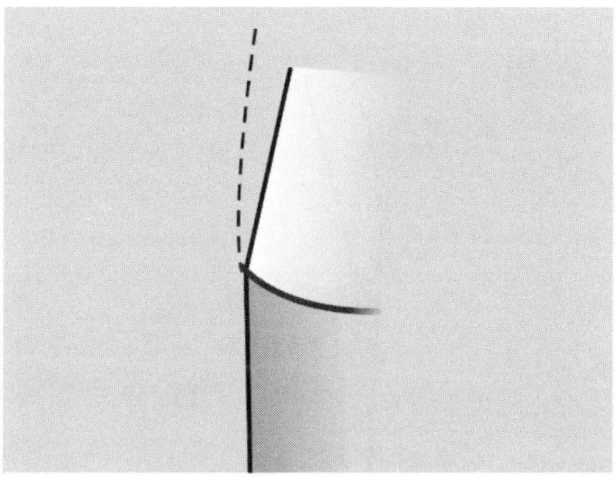

Fig. 4: Feather-edge finish line

Advantages

- Easy to prepare
- Conservative tooth preparation.

Disadvantages

- Location of margin difficult to detect
- Over contouring of restoration is possible
- Over or under extended crown due to difficulty in locating the finish line
- Decreased marginal adaptation.
- Decreased retention
- Wedging effect due to internal stresses
- Distortion of the margin is possible during lab procedures as it is thin
- Knife-edge finish line is not a recommended finish line.

Chamfer Finish Line

Definition

This is a marginal finish line either curved or formed by a plane at an obtuse angle to the external surface of a prepared tooth (Boucher).

It is a concave extracoronal finish line that possesses greater angulation than knife-edge with less width than shoulder finish line (Fig. 5).

Instrument used

Round-end tapered diamond.

Indications

- Ideal gingival finish line for cast-metal restorations
- Lingual finish line for metal–ceramic crowns
- For metal collars.

Advantages

- Provides a slip joint
- Provides gingival area with acceptable stress distribution, adequate seal and minimum uniform tooth reduction (El-Ebrashi et al)

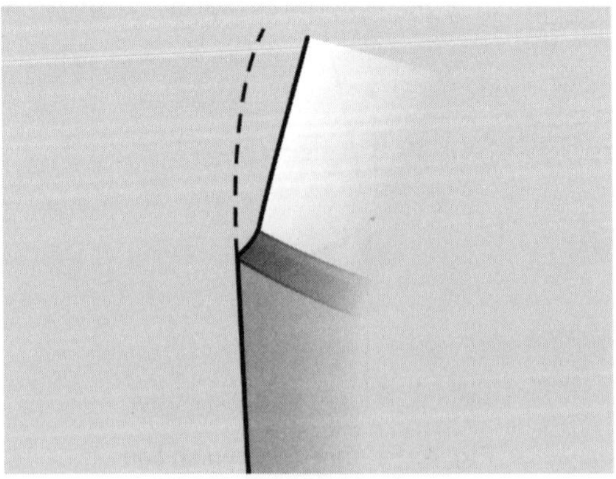

Fig. 5: Chamfer finish line

- Aids in accurate die trimming
- Can be terminated as subgingival preparation
- Adequate bulk and tooth contour
- Easy to prepare.

Disadvantages
- Marginal distortion during firing of porcelain
- Reverse lip can form if the entire diameter of instrument is used
- Less room cervically than shoulder preparation, therefore cannot be prepared with low-speed cutting instrument.

Variations

Hybrid
When the chamfer bur is inserted to one third of depth of stone a hybrid preparation results. It is a preparation between chamfer and knife-edge.

Ski-sloped
When the chamfer bur is inserted to half the depth of stone a Ski-sloped preparation results.

Rounded shoulder
When the entire depth of chamfer bur is used in preparation a rounded shoulder results.

Heavy chamfer
Used in restorations where more axial reduction is required due to caries or previous restoration. As heavy chamfer forms a butt joint, bevel is added to make it a slip joint.

McEwen's chamferette
Finish line between chamfer and feather edge.

Shoulder Finish Line

Definition
When the external line angle of the preparation is perpendicular to the long axis of the tooth, a shoulder finish line results (Fig. 6).

Instrument used
Flat-end tapered diamond and flame diamond for gingival bevel.

Indications
- Facial margins of metal–ceramic preparation
- Preparation margin for all ceramic restorations
- Margin for castable and injectable ceramics
- 135° shoulder can be used for long clinical crowns.

Advantages
- Least stress in cervical area compared to other margins
- Better resistance to occlusal forces
- Bulk of porcelain can be accommodated
- Esthetic

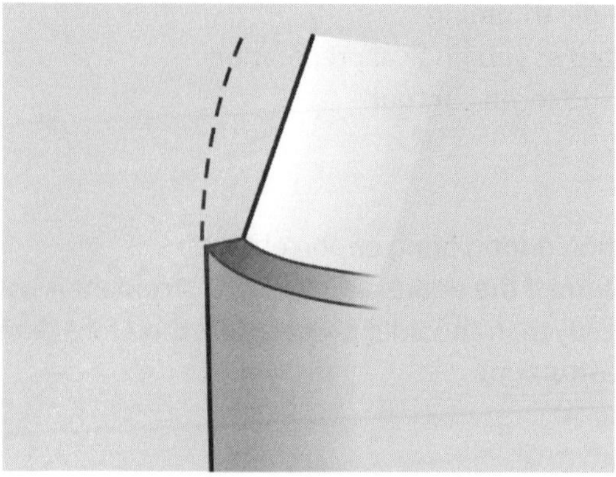

Fig. 6: Shoulder finish line

- Easy to identify margin and fabricate wax pattern
- Increased retention
- Good marginal adaptation
- Less marginal distortion
- For proper contouring of restoration with a straight emergence profile
- Easy to check seating of restoration.

Disadvantages

- Least conservative preparation of all the other preparations
- If a metal collar is not used labial porcelain butt fit is more difficult to achieve
- Difficult to prepare
- Can cause adverse pulpal involvement
- Difficult preparation.

Variations

Full shoulder with bevel

In erosion of tooth structure, gingival finish line for proximal boxes and for porcelain fused to metal restorations (Fig. 7).

Full shoulder with bevel and facial butt joint

Bevel on proximal and lingual surfaces and butt joint on facial surfaces to avoid metal display on labial side.

Radial shoulder

Shoulder with internal line angle rounded.

Complete shoulders

Finish lines for all porcelain crowns and injectable ceramic restorations.

Bevelled shoulders

Used for veneers and selected posterior teeth.

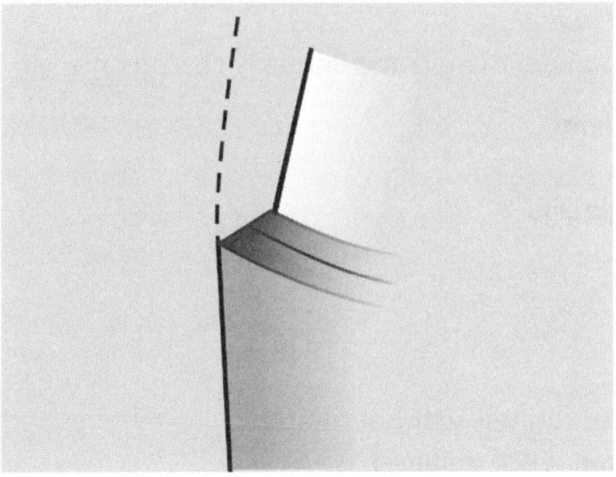

Fig. 7: Bevelled shoulder

Functions of the bevel:

- Seals restoration against cement leakage and subsequent bacterial invasion
- Easy finishing and burnishing on die or tooth
- Provide circumferential rigidity
- Iinitiate reproduction of the contour and provide control of the emergence profile during framework try-in.

Chamfer margin

For posterior crowns and the lingual surface of anterior metal ceramic crowns.

Knife-edge finish lines

Used for younger patients, pin ledge three-quarter crowns, inaccessible areas of the oral cavity, and finish lines on the cementum.

Principles in Determining Type of Finish Lines

1. Type of restorative materials.
2. Location of finish lines.
3. Configuration.
4. Marginal Fit.

Type of restorative materials

Gold alloys

- Good burnishability.
- Chamfer margin.

Base-metal alloys

- Lack of burnishability
- Chamfer margin.

Porcelain

Shoulder margin.

Metal–ceramic materials

Buccally/labially-shoulder margin and lingually chamfer margin.

Location of finish lines

- Supragingival
- At the crest of gingiva
- Subgingival.

Supragingival

Advantages

- Easy to prepare accurately without trauma
- Gingival retraction is not required
- Seating of the restoration can be evaluated
- Can place finish line on enamel
- More biocompatible with surrounding tissues
- Good contour can be achieved
- Easy oral hygiene maintenance
- Easy evaluation of margins during recall
- Can clean luting agent after luting easily.

Subgingival

Indications

- Extensive restorations, caries, cervical erosion extending subgingivally
- Proximal contact area extending to gingival crest
- In short clinical crowns
- For esthetics when labial metal collar needs to be hidden
- In root sensitivity, fracture subgingivally
- When axial contour modification is indicated
- In young patients with high-risk caries
- For additional retention and resistance form.

Disadvantages

- Difficult to access and finish
- Difficult to evaluate fit and cementation procedure
- Periodontal health can be affected if oral hygiene is not maintained.

Configuration

- Ease of preparation without overextension
- Should be able to identify finish line in the impression and on the die
- A good and clear boundary to which the wax pattern can be finished
- For wax pattern to be handled without distortion and for strength of restoration
- Conservation of tooth structure
- Studies by El-Ebrashi[1] showed that shoulder with rounded internal line angle and chamfer showed less stress concentrations. Shoulder with bevel and featheredge showed the maximum stress concentration.

Marginal Fit

- An ideal marginal fit is smooth and even
- A sliding joint has better marginal fit.

Mathematical equation (Cosine rule) (Rosner 1963)

- To calculate the marginal gaps
- The closer the hypotenuse of the right triangle approaches the adjacent leg of the triangle, the smaller the gap between the bevel of the wall of the cavity and the casting. This relation is in the un-cemented state
- When a luting agent is used, the fit depends on the film thickness of the luting agent used.

Reference

1. El-Ebrashi MK, Craig RG, Peyton FA. Experimental stress analysis of dental restorations. Part III. The concept of geometry of proximal margins. J Prosthet Dent. 1969;22:333.

8. Illustrate with diagrams, the tooth preparation on right upper central incisor for receiving porcelain jacket crown. Add a note on the advantages, indications and contraindications of all-porcelain jacket crown.

Steps in Tooth Preparation for All-ceramic Restorations

1. Placement of depth-orientation grooves.
2. Incisal reduction.
3. Facial reduction.
4. Lingual reduction.
5. Axial reduction.
6. Lingual axial reduction.
7. Marginal development and refinement.

Armamentarium

1. Mouth mirror.
2. Periodontal probe.
3. Explorer.
4. Chisels and hatchets.
5. High- and low-speed handpieces.
6. Thin tapering fissure diamonds.
7. Narrow round-tipped tapered diamonds, regular and coarse grit.
8. Flat-end tapered diamond, regular grit.
9. Football-shaped diamond.
10. Finishing stones and carbides.

Placing of depth orientation grooves (Fig. 8)

1. Three depth orientation grooves, 1.0 mm deep, are placed:
   One in the middle of the facial wall and one each in the mesiofacial and distofacial transitional line angles in the incisal edge.

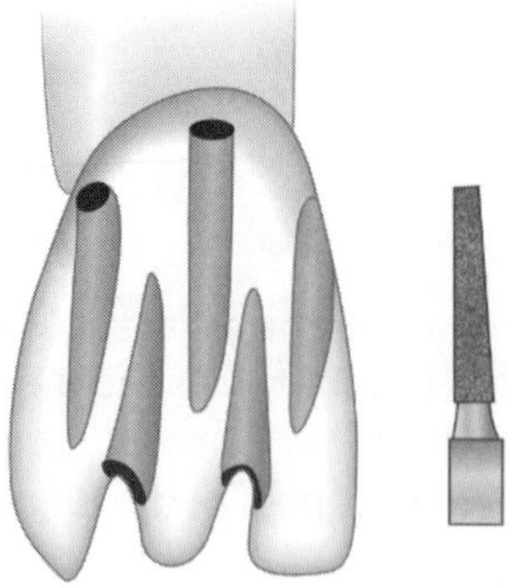

Fig. 8: Placing of depth orientation grooves

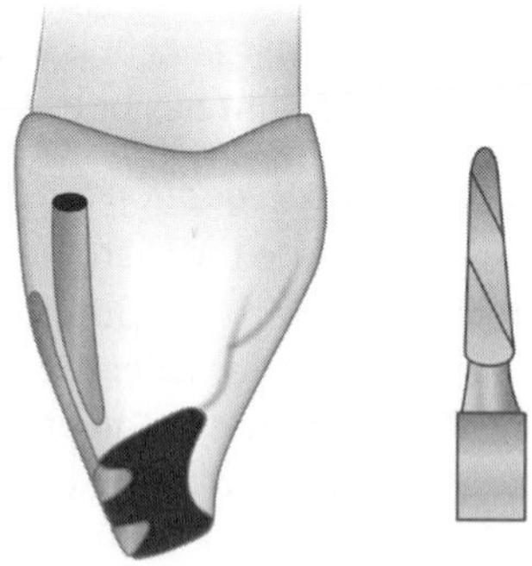

Fig. 9: Incisal reduction

2. Two more depth orientation grooves of 2.0 mm depth are placed on the incisal half.
3. 2 mm deep grooves are placed on the incisal edge for incisal reduction.

Incisal reduction

Instrument used

Flat-end tapered diamond.

The completed incisal reduction should provide 1.5–2 mm of clearance for porcelain in all excursive movements of the mandible (Fig. 9).

Facial reduction

Done in two stages:

First step: Incisal half reduction (Fig. 10)

1. A coarse, flat-ended diamond or No. 700 carbide bur is used to plane away tooth structure between the depth of orientation grooves, on the incisal half, at a 45° angle to the long axis of the tooth in a normal occlusal relationship.
2. The reduction is done parallel to the original contour of the tooth to provide uniform porcelain thickness and good esthetics.

Second step

1. Gingival portion of the labial surface is reduced with a flat-end tapered diamond in a flat plane perpendicular to the long axis of the tooth to a depth of 1.0 mm (Fig. 11).
2. The reduction is carried out with cervical component parallel to the proposed path of withdrawal.
3. This reduction extends till the labioproximal line angles.
4. The reduction is done on half of the facial surface at a time.

Lingual reduction (Fig. 12)

Depth orientation grooves of 0.8 mm depth are placed.

Football-shaped diamond/Small wheel-diamond is used for lingual reduction.

Reduction is carried out until a clearance of 1 mm in all mandibular excursive movements are obtained.

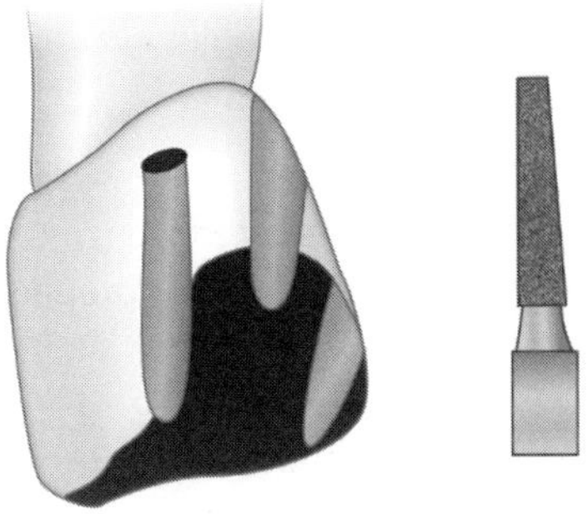

Fig. 10: Incisal half reduction

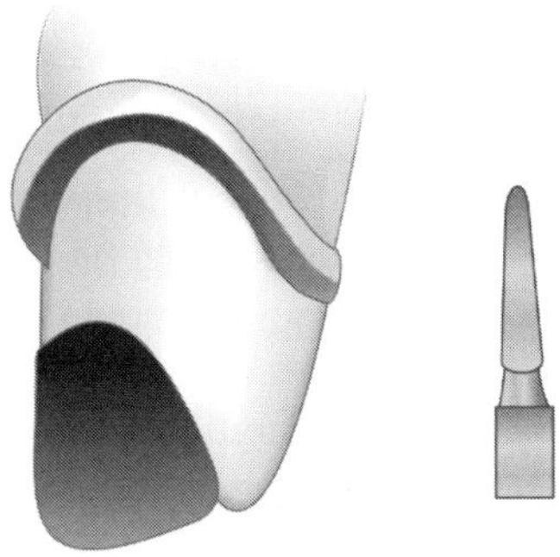

Fig. 11: Labial surface reduction

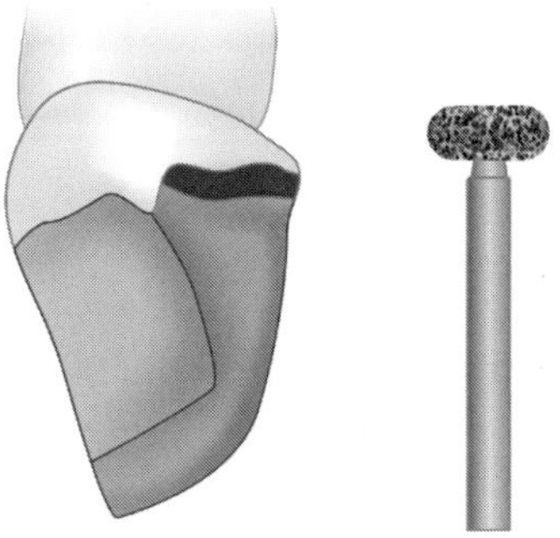

Fig. 12: Lingual reduction

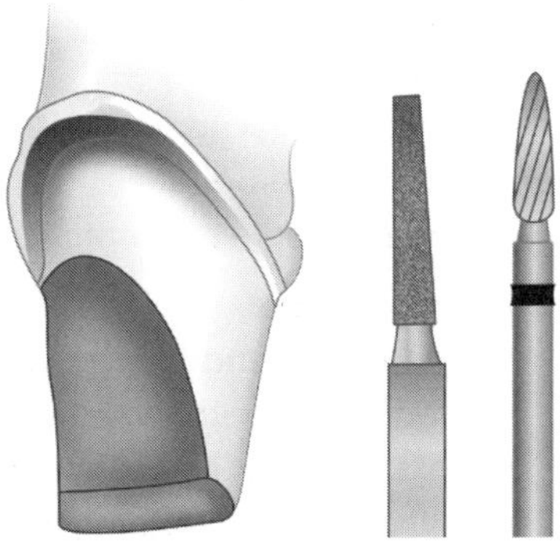

Fig. 13: Lingual axial reduction

Axial reduction

A thin tapered fissure diamond is used to break the contact point with the adjacent tooth. While breaking the contact point, the adjacent tooth should not be abraded.
The mesial and distal areas are first reduced to a 2°–5° taper without establishing a shoulder at this time.

Lingual–axial reduction (Fig. 13)

Instrument used

- Flat-end tapered diamond
- The same path of withdrawal as that of the facial preparation is followed with lingual axial reduction
- A depth groove is placed in the middle of the cingulum wall
- The preparation of 2°–5° taper is done from the centre of the cingulum wall until the lingual shoulder meets the facial shoulder
- A 0.75 mm cingulum shoulder is placed with a flat-ended tapered diamond.

Marginal development and refinement

Instruments used

- An end-cutting bur held perpendicular to the shoulder can be used for lowering margins

- A sharp chisel is used to remove undermined enamel and finishing the shoulder
- The axial walls are smoothed and all the sharp line angles and point angles are rounded. An acceptable emergence profile needs to be created for good esthetics.

Variation in margin preparation

- Instead of shoulder preparation an heavy chamfer can also be prepared
- For subgingival margin placement, a gingival retraction is done before the preparation for good access and less trauma to gingival tissue
- Initial preparation is followed by refinement with chisels
- The completed shoulder should be 1 mm wide, smooth, continuous and without any irregularities.

All-ceramic Crowns

Advantages

- Superior esthetics
- Good translucency as to that of natural tooth
- Good biocompatibility
- Can select the appropriate shade for luting agent.

Disadvantages

- Reduced strength of the restoration if metal reinforcing substructure is not given
- Significant tooth reduction on proximal and lingual aspects
- Less conservative than metal-ceramic crown
- Difficulties in obtaining a well-fitting margin
- The success of the restoration depends on proper preparation design
- An extensively damaged tooth cannot be restored with an all-ceramic crown
- Cannot be used as retainers in long-span FPD
- Large cross-sectional dimension connectors need to be incorporated for all-ceramic restorations to have bulk of material
- Due to large connectors, impingement on the interdental papilla can lead to periodontal failure
- Wear on the functional surfaces of opposing natural teeth.

Indication

Where a high-esthetic requirement exists with sound tooth structure present.

Contraindications

- Where a more conservative restoration can be used
- Not recommended for molar teeth
- Where increased occlusal loads are present
- When adequate support cannot be provided
- When an even shoulder width cannot be prepared.

9. Define a crown and mention the advantages, disadvantages and indications of a full metal crown. Describe in detail, with diagrams, the step-by-step procedure in the preparation of a full-metal crown on a mandibular first molar.

Definition

An artificial crown is a fixed restoration of the entire coronal part of a natural tooth that restores anatomy, function and esthetics, usually of metal, porcelain, synthetic resin, or combinations.

Full-metal Crowns

Advantages

- Good strength
- Better retention
- Greater resistance form than a partial-coverage restoration
- Conservative tooth preparation
- Less chance of pulpal injury
- Can easily modify axial tooth contour
- Convenient development of contact areas
- Can be given for caries damaged tooth after core build up
- Can be given for endodontically treated teeth
- Ideal retainer for restoring craniofacial anomalies
- Can withstand occlusal loads
- Occlusal plane modifications are easily facilitated with supraerupted teeth
- Ideal retainer for long-span FPD and short clinical crowns
- Embrasure areas can be enhanced in periodontally compromised dentitions
- Buccal flutes developed for preferred contours
- Provide desirable guide planes for RPDs
- Only restoration that permits modifications to shape survey lines, guide planes and occlusal rests.

Disadvantages

- Not esthetic
- Cannot be used as anterior retainers
- Not as biocompatible as ceramic restorations
- Chances of over contouring the restoration (overcountering can result in periodontal problem)
- Distortion of metal margins is common
- Uniform gingival finish lines are difficult to achieve
- Postcementation gingival caries is difficult to detect
- Good laboratory implementation is required for good fit of the restoration
- Margins are difficult to locate in the die
- After cementation, electric vitality testing of the abutment tooth cannot be done
- Restricted to maxillary molars, mandibular molars and premolars.

Indications

- For restored posterior tooth in nonesthetic zone unable to withstand normal occlusal loads

- For a retainer requiring maximum retention
- For short clinical crowns
- For extensively damaged or fractured teeth
- Complete gold veneer crowns can be prepared on both vital and pulpless teeth
- Ideal retainer for long-span FPD
- For endodontically treated teeth
- Retainers for RPD.

Preparation of a Full-metal-crown on a Mandibular First Molar

Metals that can be used

- Gold alloys
- Base-metal alloys.

Armamentarium

- High- and low-speed contra-angles
- Tapered carbide bur used for occlusal guiding grooves, additional retentive features
- Round-end tapered diamond regular (0.8 mm) used for occlusal reduction, axial reduction and chamfer preparation
- Round-end tapered diamond fine grit for finishing
- Utility wax and wax caliper for verification of occlusal clearance.

Steps in full metal crown preparation

1. Placement of occlusal guiding grooves.
2. Occlusal reduction.
3. Placement of functional cusp bevel.
4. Placement of axial alignment grooves.
5. Axial reduction.
6. Margin placement.
7. Finishing of preparation.

Placement of occlusal guiding grooves

1. A tapered carbide bur is used to place the guiding grooves of approximately 1 mm depth in the central, mesial, and distal fossae.
2. These grooves are connected along the length of the central groove extending into the mesial and distal marginal ridge for occlusal reduction.
3. Guiding grooves are also placed in the buccal and lingual grooves and in each triangular ridge extending from the cusp tip to the centre of its base.

Occlusal reduction

1. One half is reduced and then the other half is reduced.
2. Occlusal reduction should follow the anatomic configuration for a conservative tooth preparation.
3. The occlusal reduction follows the depth orientation grooves (Fig. 14).
4. Functional cusps (buccal cusps) on mandibular molars are "stamp cusps' and require a "two-plane" reduction with minimum clearance of 1.5 mm.

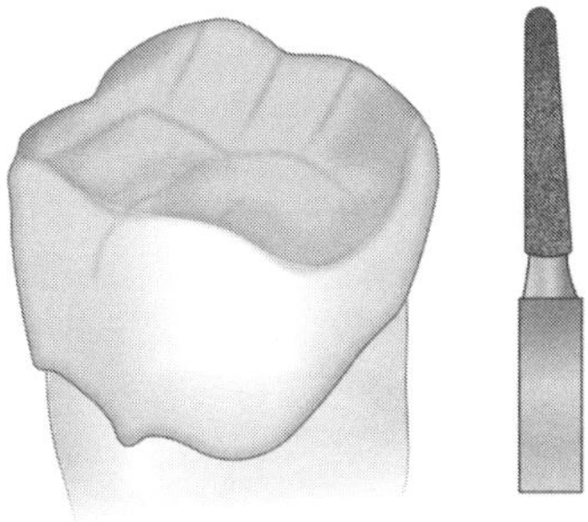

Fig. 14: Occlusal reduction

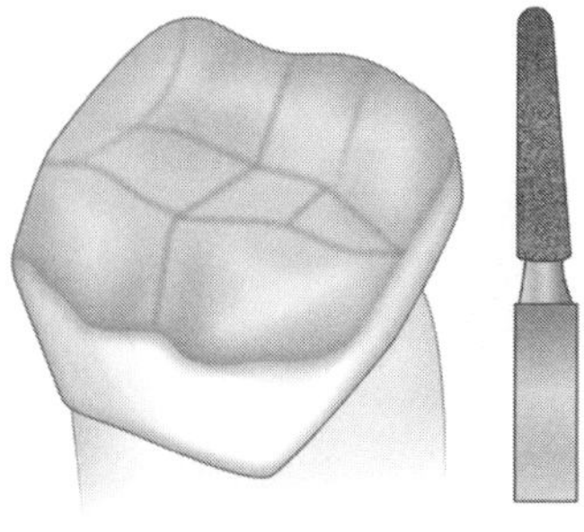

Fig. 15: Placement of functional cusp bevel

5. For non-functional cusp a minimum of 0.6–1 mm reduction is required.
6. Reduce the inclined planes between the depth guides in the developmental grooves and those along the triangular ridges.
7. Reduce the marginal ridge by 1.5 mm.
8. The occlusal surface is smoothened to duplicate the tooth anatomy.
9. Occlusal reduction is completed when necessary clearance during excursions of the mandible, especially at the ceramic/metal junction is achieved.
10. Evaluate occlusal clearance with wax bite and measure with wax gauge.

Placement of functional cusp bevel (Fig. 15)

1. A functional cusp bevel is placed to protect tooth during function by ensuring adequate thickness of metal, as this area contacts with the opposing tooth.
2. Functional cusp bevel ensures ideal restoration contour, maximum durability and conservation of tooth structure.
3. A functional cusp bevel is placed 45° to the long axis of teeth on the functional palatal cusp for maxillary molar and buccal cusp for mandibular molar.

Placement of axial alignment grooves

1. Three depth orientation grooves are placed:
   - On each buccal and lingual wall with round end tapered diamond
   - In the centre of the wall
   - On each mesial and distal transitional line angles.
2. A round end tapered diamond with a taper of 6° forms an identical taper on the preparation wall.
3. Gingivally:
   Only one half of the tip of diamond should penetrate.
4. Facial and lingual reduction (Fig. 16):
   - The facial and lingual surface reduction is done with taper of 2°–5°. For maxillary molar a two-plane reduction is common on the facial surface
   - During the facial and lingual reduction, the taper established is in relation to the path of insertion

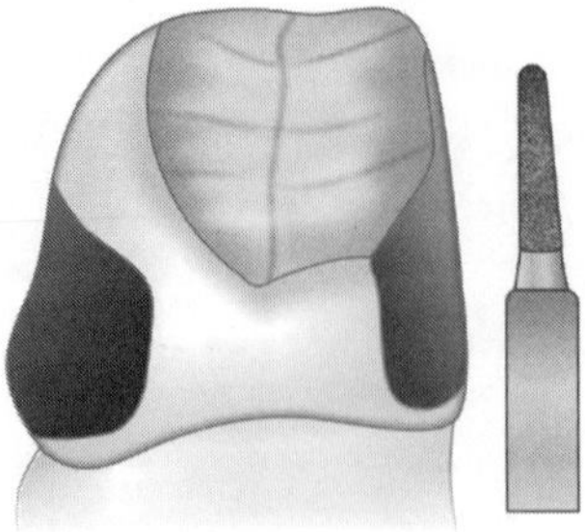

Fig. 16: Facial and lingual reduction

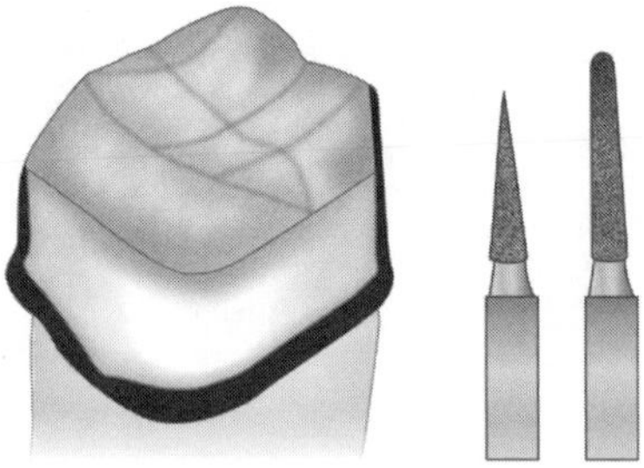

Fig. 17: Axial reduction

- The sharp line angles created after the proximal, facial, and lingual surfaces are rounded
- Vertical seating grooves on the buccal cusp fossa for mandibular and palatal cusp fossa for maxillary, improve retention.

Axial reduction (Fig. 17)

1. Break the contact points with a thin tapering fissure bur without abrading the adjacent tooth.
2. In tight contact point areas a metal matrix band can be placed.
3. Axial reduction forms the retention and resistance form.
4. The islands of tooth structure between the alignment grooves are removed while the chamfer margin is placed with a round end tapered diamond.
5. The preparation is done on one half at a time.
6. A 5° convergence on the mesial surface of the tooth is required. Gingival finish line is not made at this time.
7. The distal surface is prepared next.

Margin placement

1. The width of the chamfer margin should be 0.5 mm.
2. Chamfer margin must be smooth and continuous mesiodistally and ideally located supragingivally.
3. Unsupported enamel should be removed with chisel.
4. The tip of the bur should not exceed the depth of one-half the diameter of the bur.

Finishing the preparation (Fig. 18)

Finish the preparation by refining the line angles and point angles.

Smoothen sharp angles or surface irregularities with the diamond and, finally with a cuttle fish disc.

10. Describe in detail, with diagrams, the step-by-step preparation of a maxillary canine to receive a three quarter crown. Explain and justify different impression techniques for fixed partial denture.

Definition

Partial veneer crown is an extracoronal metal restoration that covers only part of the clinical crown. Partial veneer crowns include all tooth surfaces except the buccal or labial wall in the preparation.

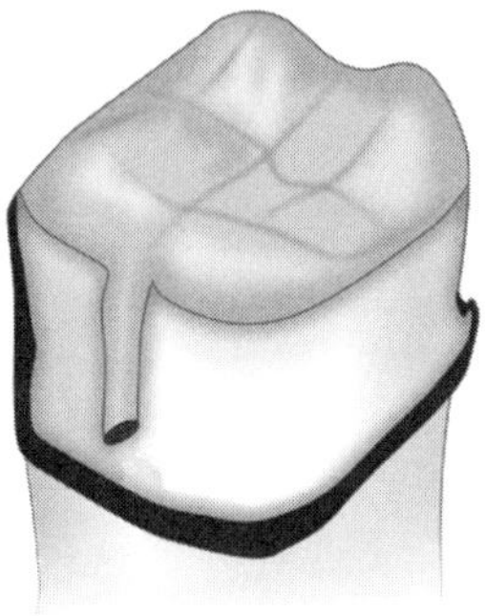

Fig. 18: Finishing the preparation

Steps in Preparation of Partial Veneer Crowns are

1. Incisal reduction.
2. Lingual reduction.
3. Interproximal reduction.
4. Proximal box or groove placement.
5. Incisal offset placement.
6. Facial bevel.
7. Finishing the preparation.

Armamentarium

1. High- and low-speed contra-angle handpiece.
2. Burs as listed below (Table 1).
3. Utility wax and wax gauge to evaluate lingual reduction.

Table 1: Uses of various burs in preparation of partial veneer crown

Burs used	Used for
• Round-ended tapered diamond	• Incisal reduction, axial reduction
• Football-shaped diamond	• Lingual reduction
• 169L carbide bur	• Interproximal reduction
• Narrow chamfer diamond	• Chamfer margin
• 167 carbide bur	• Proximal groove
• Flame-shaped diamond	• Flare for proximal extensions
• Inverted cone carbide bur	• Incisal groove
• Fine, flame-shaped diamond bur	• Facial bevel
• Carbide finishing bur	• Finishing preparation
• No. 1/2 round bur	• Pilot hole
• Hatchet instrument	• For contact breaking

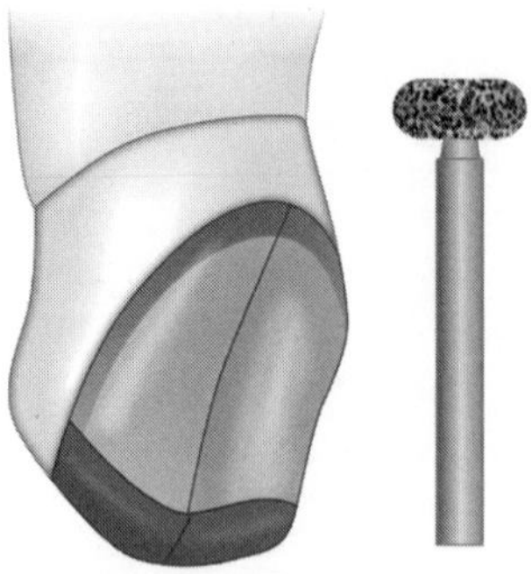

Fig. 19: Lingual reduction

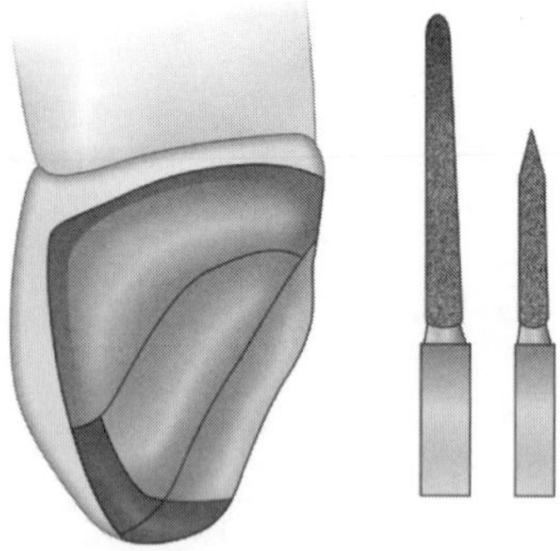

Fig. 20: Interproximal reduction

Incisal reduction

- Round-ended tapered diamond is used
- Reduce the incisal edge 1 mm at a 45° angle to the long axis of the tooth. Remove 1.0–1.5 mm following the facial contour of the tooth.

Lingual reduction (Fig. 19)

Done in two steps.

1. Lingual surface reduction

   A football-shaped diamond is used to reduce the lingual surface in two planes, with a slight ridge along the centre of the lingual surface incisogingivally. A clearance of at least 0.7–1 mm is required with the opposing tooth.
2. Lingual–gingival reduction

   A round-ended tapered diamond is used to achieve a chamfer of 0.5 mm deep at the cervical finish line. The chamfer is extended to include the lingual line angles.

Interproximal reduction (Fig. 20)

Done in three steps.

1. The proximal surface is reduced with a 169L carbide bur from the lingual to the facial surface with the contact point intact. The facial line angles must remain intact for good esthetic results.
2. A light chamfer finish line is made on the proximal surface with a narrow chamfer diamond. This chamfer should merge with the lingual chamfer.
3. The contact with adjacent tooth is broken with a hatchet instrument from the facial surface, to form labial proximal extensions. The flare of proximal extensions is finished with a flame-shaped diamond.

Proximal grooves (Fig. 21)

A 167 carbide bur is used for groove placement at the proper alignment. The proximal grooves are placed parallel to the incisal two thirds of the facial surface (169L carbide bur).

These grooves resist lingual displacement and should be a minimum of 3 mm long with 0.5 mm of the gingival finish line. The facial and lingual walls of the grooves should have a 2–5 degree incisal divergence.

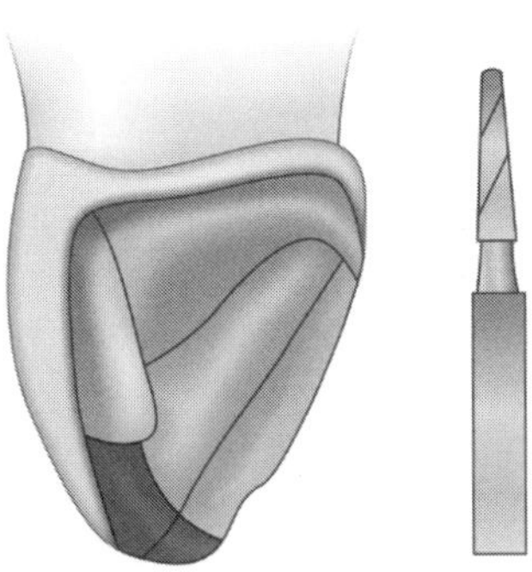

Fig. 21: Proximal grooves

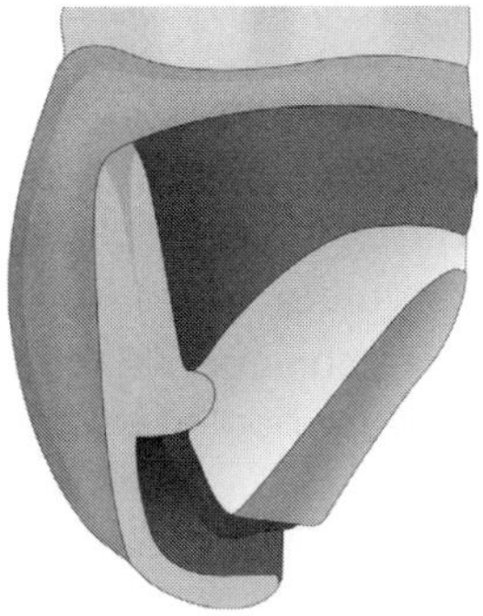

Fig. 22: Incisal groove and facial bevel

The lingual wall of the proximal grooves should have a 2–5 degree incisal convergence with the lingual gingival wall.

The facial wall of the groove should be continuous with the proximal flare to add bulk to the facial margin.

Incisal groove (Fig. 22)

Inverted cone carbide bur is used.

A 0.5–1 mm groove is prepared within the dentin and is made parallel to the DEJ connecting the proximal grooves. The groove is not placed at the expense of the incisal edge.

Facial bevel

Fine, flame-shaped diamond bur is used.

A narrow bevel <0.5 mm is prepared on the labioincisal finish line at right angles to the incisal two thirds of the facial surface.

Finishing the preparation

A carbide finishing bur is used.

All the sharp and point angles are rounded to ensure continuity of all finish lines.

Cingulum modification if needed for additional retention

1. After paralleling a 170 bur to the long axis on the proximal grooves, a ledge is prepared in the cingulum.
2. A pilot hole is cut in the ledge with a No. 1/2 round bur.

Different Impression Techniques

1. Stock Tray/Putty wash (single mix and double mix).
2. Custom tray (single mix).
3. Closed bite/Double arch/Dual quad tray/Triple arch.
4. Copper band.
5. Reversible hydrocolloid (laminate and wet field technique).
6. Matrix system.

Stock Tray/Putty wash

Polyvinyl siloxane is used.

Materials used

Reversible, irreversible hydrocolloids and elastomeric impression materials.

For accuracy, elastomeric impression materials are the commonly used.

In this technique, a single impression with polyvinyl siloxanes or a double mix with medium and heavy-bodied elastomers can be done.

Single mix technique

Advantages of single mix

- Less time required
- No need to fabricate a custom tray
- Metal stock trays are rigid and chances of distortion are less.

Disadvantages

- Each time the tray is used it needs to be sterilized
- More impression material is required.

Technique

1. After adjusting the chair position, a proper stock tray with the correct border extensions, and tray shape and size depending on the patient's arch shape and size is selected.
2. Apply tray adhesive on the inside and rim of the stock tray.
3. Manipulation of impression material:
   Mix the high-viscosity putty impression material and roll putty into elongated cylinder.
   Place the putty in the stock tray and cover with polyethylene sheet.
4. Seating of tray:
   Insert and seat the tray with a rocking type motion.
   Seat the tray in the mouth without movement till initial set occurs (approximately 2 minutes).
   For stock tray (putty wash) single mixing technique, the unset high-viscosity impression material should already be in the tray, and the preparations syringed with low-viscosity impression material.
5. Setting of material and tray removal:
   Remove from the mouth with minimal sideward movement and ensure the material is set using a fingernail test (material rebounds completely).
6. Trimming the impression:
   After removing the spacer, the excess impression material is removed with a sharp knife.

Double mix technique (PVS PS CS)

1. After a stock tray is selected, tray adhesive is applied; the impression putty is mixed and placed in tray.
2. A polyethylene sheet is used to cover the putty material and impression is seated in the patient's mouth.

3. After the complete set of the impression is ensured by fingernail testing, the tray is removed.
4. Relieving the tray:
   A sharp hand instrument is used to remove uniform amount of impression material from the tissue surface.
5. After gingival retraction evaluate tissue displacement, check the finish line area(s), and leave cord(s) in place for 8–12 minutes.
6. Manipulation of light-body material:
   After measuring the arch length of tray, one times the length of the tray low-viscosity elastomer is dispensed, after trimming the tip of the syringe.
7. Making final impression:
   - A mixing pad, (6 by 8 inches) or an automatic gun dispensing system is used
   - The low-viscosity impression material is mixed with a circular motion combining the two strands, then a figure eight motion to blend and flatten the mixture onto the mixing pad (approximate mixing time less than 1 minute).
8. Loading the impression material:
   - The syringe is loaded by holding it at a slight angle while scraping the pad
   - Screw on the tip, and insert the plunger
   - While the plunger is inserted into the syringe, the cord is removed
   - After evaluating retraction site for seepage, hemorrhage, or debris, first syringe inaccessible areas. (E.g., distal lingual finish line)
   - The syringe is positioned so the elastomer is ahead of the tip's orifice.
9. Tray Insertion:
   - Insert the low-viscosity impression material into the tray slightly less than the depth of the external borders
   - Seat the tray from posterior to anterior, allowing the excess to extrude anteriorly
   - Seat the tray firmly in position
   - The tray should not be moved while the material is setting.
10. Final impression:
    - After the final set is over, tray is removed
    - Rinse impression with ambient water, and dry with short, small bursts of compressed air
    - Retraction cord (s) remaining in the impression material are removed carefully.
11. Evaluate set impression:
    - The area 0.5 mm beyond visible finish line should be visible. There should be no show-through in any areas of the impression, except at tissue stops
    - There should be no shiny smooth areas, no voids present
    - Review for tears. There should be no thin areas leaving the finish line unsupported.

Custom Tray: PVS PE PS, CS

Advantages

- Less impression material required compared to stock tray
- Sterilization is not a problem

- Less chances of impression material getting distorted due to curing shrinkage
- Precuring of the tray material is not required.

Disadvantages

- Time consuming due to tray fabrication
- The tray must be used after complete curing to prevent further distortion
- Monomer sensitivity during tray fabrication for some personnel.

Technique

Fabrication of tray

(Wax adaptation.)

- The diagnostic cast is soaked in slurry water for 10 minutes and then painted with a layer of tinfoil substitute to prevent the resin from adhering to the cast
- Outline of the tray extensions is marked on the cast and two sheets of base plate wax are adapted to the cast
- Excess wax is trimmed and a thin tinfoil (or polyethylene) sheet is placed over the wax to protect resin from wax during the exothermic cure.

Placement of tissue stops

Four widely spaced hard tissue stops of 3 mm/2 mm are placed on non-functional cusps.

Manipulation of tray material

- The right proportion of monomer (liquid) and polymer (powder) are mixed and in dough stage, it is flattened to approximately 4 mm thick
- The flattened putty is adapted to the tin-foiled cast; excess material is trimmed off and handle is formed with excess resin.

Removal of tray from the cast

After the resin material sets (approximately 15 minutes), the tray is lifted from the cast.
The wax spacer is removed (all wax needs to be removed).

Finishing the tray

Tray is trimmed and polished. Gingival retraction is carried out and tray adhesive is applied.

Making final impression

- A mixing pad, (6 by 8 inches) or an automatic gun dispensing system is used
- The low-viscosity impression material is mixed with a circular motion combining the two strands, and then it is blended and flattened onto the mixing pad. (In less than I minute).

Loading the impression material

- The syringe is loaded by holding it at a slight angle while scraping the pad
- Screw on the tip, and insert the plunger
- While the plunger is inserted into the syringe, the cord is removed
- After evaluating retraction site for seepage, hemorrhage, or debris, first syringe inaccessible areas (e.g., distal–ingual finish line)
- The syringe is positioned so the elastomer is ahead of the tip's orifice.

Tray Insertion

The low-viscosity impression material is placed into the tray and the tray is seated firmly in position until the material sets.

Final impression

After the final set is over, tray is removed; the impression is rinsed with water and dried with compressed air.

Closed–bite Double–arch Method

Synonyms: Dual quad tray, double arch, triple tray, Accu-bite, closed-mouth impression. Materials used are polyvinyl siloxane and polyether.

Minimum conditions

1. The articulator must have a vertical dimension holding stop, such as an incisal pin to maintain vertical dimension.
2. There should be sufficient space distal to the terminal tooth for tray approximation.

Advantages

- A functional impression is achieved
- Less elastomeric impression material is needed
- The physical deformation of the mandible during opening is minimized
- Less gagging may occur.

Disadvantages

- Tray is not rigid
- It is not a functionally generated technique, so it is limited to one casting per quadrant
- The distribution of the impression material is not uniform.

Procedure

- After evaluating the fit of the tray in patient's mouth, the tray is positioned accurately with the trays crossbar distal to last tooth in arch
- The patient is asked to close mouth to observe the complete bilateral closure and the patient's comfort.

Making final impression

- A mixing pad, (6 by 8 inches) or an automatic gun dispensing system is used
- The low-viscosity impression material is mixed with a circular motion combining the two strands then a figure of eight motion to blend and flatten the mixture onto the mixing pad (in less than 1 minute).

Loading the impression material

- The syringe is loaded by holding it at a slight angle while scraping the pad
- Screw on the tip and insert the plunger
- While the plunger is inserted into the syringe, the cord is removed
- After evaluating retraction site for seepage, hemorrhage, or debris, first syringe inaccessible areas (e.g., distal-lingual finish line).

Tray insertion

- Insert the low-viscosity impression material into the tray slightly less than the depth of the external borders
- Seat the tray from posterior to anterior, allowing the excess to extrude anteriorly
- Seat the tray firmly in position
- For quadrant trays, position the crossbar distal to the last tooth in that arch.

Closed-mouth technique

Instruct patient to slowly close mouth and evaluate the interdigitation on the opposite arch.

Tray removal

- When the patient opens the mouth, the impression adheres to one arch
- Tray is removed by placing a finger on either side of the tray
- The handle is not used to remove tray
- Residual impression material in sulcus or interproximal areas is removed
- Rinse impression with water, and dry with small bursts of compressed air
- Retraction cord(s) remaining in the impression material are removed carefully.

Copper Band

Copper tube impressions are made when there are multiple preparations with vague margins.

Fitting copper band to preparation

- A copper band of adequate diameter is adapted to the prepared tooth
- This adapted band is annealed by heating in flame and quenching in alcohol
- The finish line area is marked with a sharp explorer tip
- The marked area is cut with scissors and smoothened with carborundum stone.

Checking the fit

- The copper band should extend at least 1 mm beyond finish line with a slight gap between finish line and copper band
- Orientation holes are placed in top one-fifth of facial surface of tube.

Making of compound plug

- Red stick compound is heated over a Bunsen burner flame
- Once the appropriate temperature is reached the warm compound mass is inserted on top one-third of copper tube
- The copper band is oriented and seated till the compound touches the occlusal surface of band.

Removing the impression

- The impression is cooled in water
- A towel clamp is used to remove copper band from mouth.

Relieving for final impression

- A slow-speed hand piece with No. 6 or 8 carbide bur is used to remove 0.2 mm of compound from the impressed occlusal surface creating a space for the heavy body polyvinyl siloxane
- A relief vent is placed with a long shank No. 6 round carbide bur, through the center of the compound plug.

Making impression (PVS)

- More relief vents are placed with a sharp No 4 or No 6 round carbide 2–3 mm above the bottom of the copper tube. These holes help to retain the polyvinyl siloxane impression material and provide a suitable space at the finish line area
- Some areas in the internal surface are mildly coated with adhesive
- The prepared tooth is cleaned and isolated.

Final impression

- Either a automatic gun or a syringe loaded with heavy-viscosity, polyvinyl-siloxane impression is injected into the copper band, filling the space completely from the compound to copper band edge
- After loading the impression material in the copper band the band is positioned and seated properly.

Removing the final impression

After the final set is completed a towel clamp is used to remove impression by grasping on top one-fifth of impression.

Laminate technique/Agar–alginate combination technique

- The agar material is syringed around the prepared tooth area and the alginate is used as tray material for the rest of the arch
- Alginate sets by chemical reaction and agar sets when it comes in contact with cool alginate.

Wet Technique

Area to be recorded are flooded with warm water and immediately syringe material is injected and while still the syringe material is liquid the tray material is loaded and seated. The pressure of the viscous tray material pushes fluid syringe material around areas to be recorded.

Matrix System[1]

Uses three types of impression consistencies as initially a quick setting matrix forming material is used in a clear tray. This matrix impression is retrieved and trimmed to hold a high-viscosity polyether to record the prepared teeth surfaces and then a third less viscous tray material is used which encloses the matrix with light-body material and rest of the arch.

Reference

1. Livaditis GJ. The matrix impression system for fixed prosthodontics. J Prosthot Dent. 1998;79(2): 208-16.

11. Name the component parts of a bridge. Define and classify pontics. Add a note on selection of pontic design in anterior and posterior teeth. What are the requirements of a pontic?

Parts of a Bridge

- Retainers—Are attached to the prepared abutments
- Connectors—Pontic is connected to the retainer by a connector
- Pontic—Artificial tooth suspended from the abutment tooth.

Pontic

Definition

An artificial tooth in a fixed partial denture that replaces a missing natural tooth, restores its function and usually fills the space previously occupied by the clinical crown (GPT).

Classification

1. According to the shape of the surface contacting the ridge.
2. According to the material used in construction of pontic.
3. According to the type of fabrication.
4. According to mucosal-contacting or non-mucosal-contacting.

According to the shape of the surface contacting the ridge

1. Spheroidal/Egg shaped/Bullet shaped.
2. Conical.
3. Saddle.
4. Modified ridge lap.
5. Sanitary/Hygienic.
6. Modified sanitary.

According to the material used in construction of pontic

1. Metal pontics.
2. Metal–ceramic pontics.
3. Aluminous core-porcelains.
4. Resin-veneered porcelain.

According to the type of fabrication:

1. Prefabricated:
   - Trupontic
   - Pin facing
   - Interchangeable
   - Modified pin facing
   - Reverse pin facing
   - Harmony facing.
2. Custom made.

According to mucosal-contacting or non-mucosal-contacting

1. Mucosal contacting:
   - Saddle
   - Modified saddle
   - Ridge lap

- Modified ridge lap
- Conical
- Ovate.

2. Nonmucosal contacting
   - Sanitary/hygienic/perel
   - Modified sanitary.
3. According to materials used
   - All metal
   - Metal porcelain
   - Resin/facings.

Requirements of A Pontic

- To provide good esthetics
- To restore function
- Should preserve residual ridge
- Should be biocompatible
- Should be comfortable for the patient
- Should be able to maintain good oral hygiene
- It should stabilize adjacent and opposing teeth.

Pontic Design

Saddle/Ridge lap design (Fig. 23)

Definition

A ridge lap is one in which contact extends beyond the midline of the edentulous ridge or that forms a sharp angle at the lingogingival aspect of the tissue contact. It forms a large concave contact with the ridge obliterating the facial, lingual and proximal embrasures.

Disadvantages

- Difficult to maintain oral hygiene
- Can cause tissue inflammation.

Modified ridge lap (Fig. 24)

Lingual surface: Slight deflective contour.
Facial surface: Slight faciolingual concavity.
Ridge contact: Only on crest of ridge facially (contacting area of pontic is convex).
Used: In maxillary and mandibular esthetic zone areas.

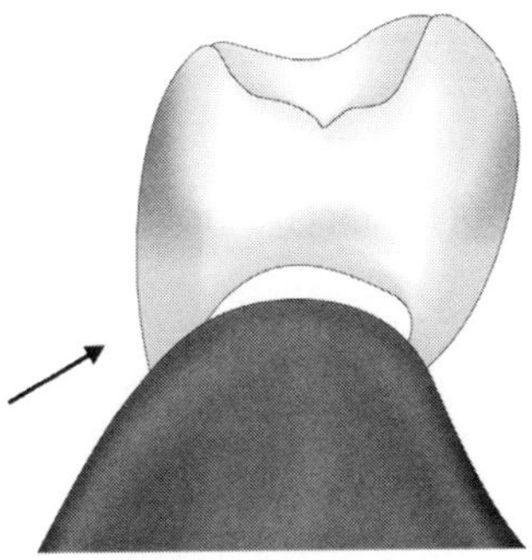

Fig. 23: Saddle/Ridge lap design

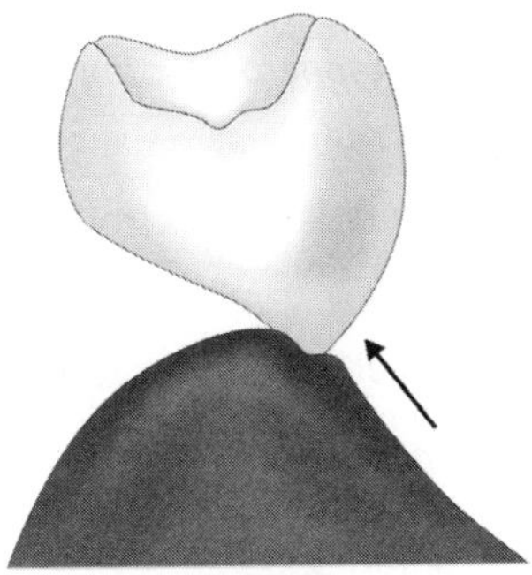

Fig. 24: Modified ridge lap

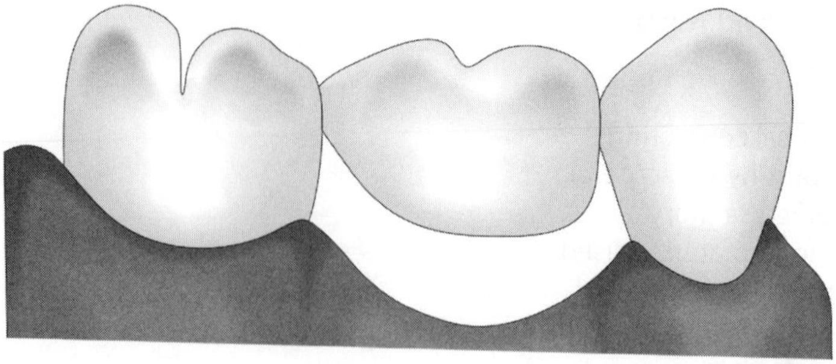

Fig. 25: Hygienic pontic

Hygienic pontic (Fig. 25)

No contact with ridge, easily cleansable.

Uses

Mandibular molar and nonesthetic zones.

Design

- Occlusogingival thickness should be a minimum of 3 mm and with space between the pontic and ridge for easy cleaning
- Its an all convex design mesiodistally and faciolingually (Fish-belly design).

Modified sanitary pontic (Fig. 26)

Design

Concave mesiodistally and convex faciolingually (hyperbolic paraboloid design).
If in esthetic zone, visible area is veneered with porcelain.

Spheroidal/Egg-shaped/Bullet-shaped pontic (Fig. 27A)

Design

This pontic is convex from all directions with only one point of contact at the center of the ridge.

Use

Mandibular posterior tooth.

Modified spheroidal pontic (Fig. 27B)

Design

This pontic is convex from all directions with the only point of contact on the buccal surfaces.

Use

Mandibular posterior tooth.

Conical Pontic (Fig. 28)

Design

Rounded and cleansable with a small tip.

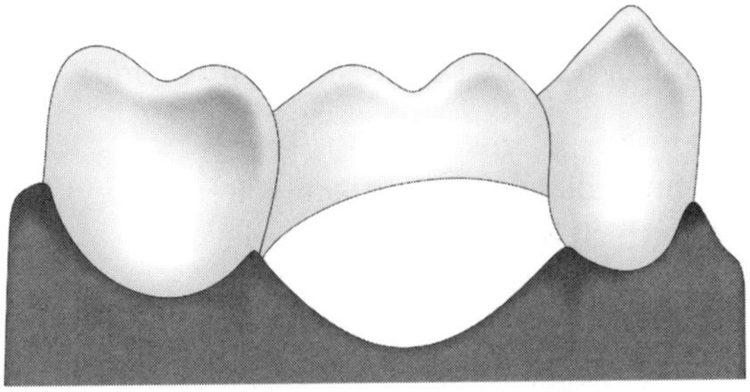

Fig. 26: Modified sanitary pontic

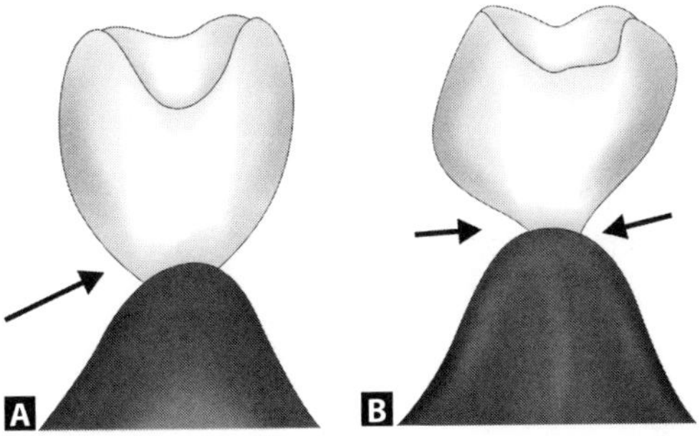

Figs 27A and B: (A) Spheroidal pontic; (B) Modified spheroidal pontic

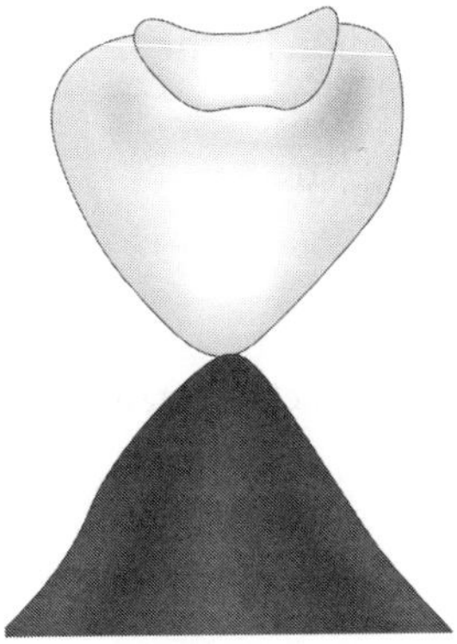

Fig. 28: Conical pontic

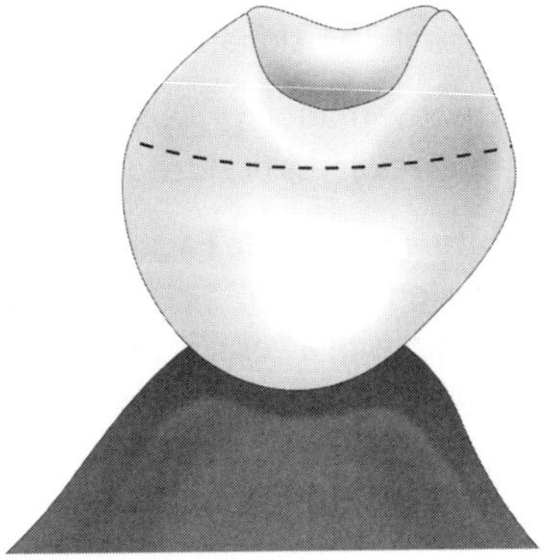

Fig. 29: Ovate pontic

Use

In nonesthetic zone in thin mandibular ridges.

Ovate pontic: Term coined by Dewey and Zugsmith in 1933 (Fig. 29).

Definition

A pontic that is shaped on its tissue surface like an egg in two dimensions, partially submerged in a surgically prepared soft tissue depression to enhance the illusion that a natural tooth is emerging from gingival tissues (GPT).

Design

The round tissue contacting area is set into concavity of ridge.

Indications

- For esthetic zone, immediately after extraction (temporary)
- In broad flat ridges which is surgically prepared.

Modified Ovate Pontic[1]

- Coined by Liu in 2003
- Modification include moving the height of contour at the tissue surface from the center of base more labially.

Advantages

- More esthetic
- Ease of cleaning
- Effective air seal
- Minimizes black triangle
- Little or no ridge augmentation.

Prefabricated pontics

Trupontic

Was widely used earlier.

Design

The facing consists of a horizontal tubular slot, which runs from the centre to the lingual aspect. This slot along with wide proximal bevels provides retention for the facing.

Disadvantage

In case of less occlusogingival, height fabrication of facing is difficult.

Interchangeable Facing (Fig. 30)

Design

Consists of a vertical slot running down the flat lingual surface, which is retained by a lug that engages the retention slot.

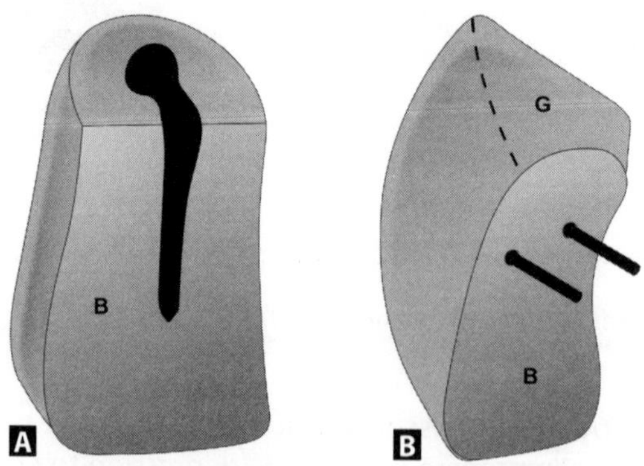

Figs 30A and B: Interchangeable facing

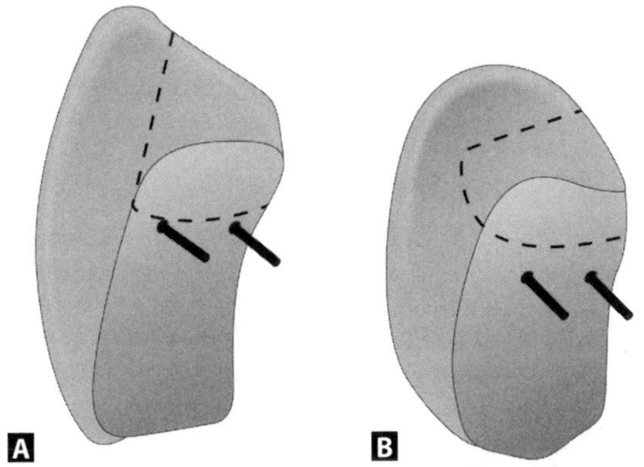

Figs 31A and B: Harmony Facing: (A) Anterior tooth; (B) Maxillary posterior tooth

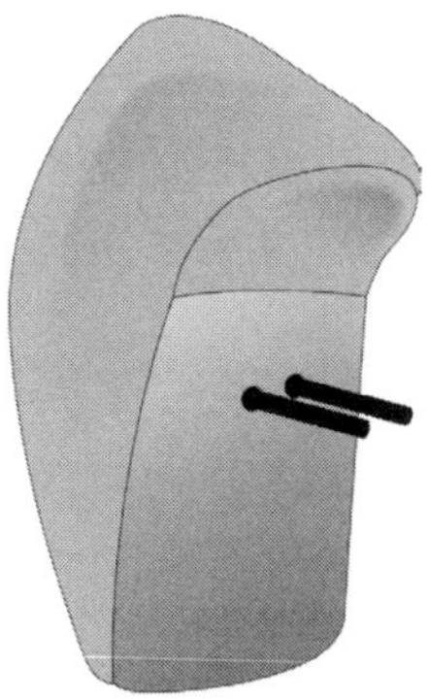

Fig. 32: Modified pin facing

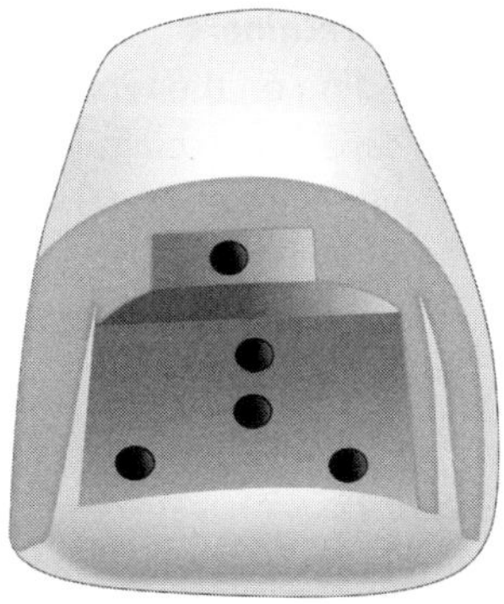

Fig. 33: Harmony reverse pin facing

January Pontic

Design

- It is a rounded blunt porcelain with a slot running out to one side, which is oriented towards the lingual during fabrication of the pontic
- After it is ground to fit into the edentulous space it is reglazed.

Harmony Facing (Fig. 31)

Design

This facing consist of an un-contoured porcelain gingival surface and two retentive pins.

Indication

For maximum esthetics in anterior tooth.

Modified Pin Facing (Fig. 32)

This facing is made by adding porcelain to the lingual gingival area of a pin facing.

Harmony Reverse Pin Facing (Fig. 33)

Design

- Porcelain denture teeth modified as pontic facings

- Multiple pinholes 2 mm deep are made with drill press in the lingual surface of reverse pin facing
- The pins come out of the backing providing retention.

Indication

Deep overbite situations.

Pontic Selection

Factors determining pontic selection

- Type of retainers
- Esthetics
- Occlusal gingival height
- Mesiodistal width of the edentulous area
- Ridge resorption and contour.

Type of retainers

Depending on the type of retainer used, the selection of pontic varies.

- In case of porcelain-bonded-to-metal retainers, the same type of pontics is used
- If partial veneer retainers are used, prefabricated facings with the same metal as for the retainer is used
- In maxillary anteriors and posteriors and mandibular anteriors—Modified ridge lap is pontic of choice
- In mandibular posterior region—Spheroidal or hygienic pontic is preferred.

Esthetics

For maxillary anterior tooth modified ridge lap is the design of choice. Depending on the location of pontic placement, the selection of pontic varies.

Occlusogingival height and mesiodistal width

The amount of space available for a pontic alters the choice of design. When there is limited space for a pontic an acrylic pontic with facing is the choice.

Ridge resorption and contour

Classification of ridge deformity (Siebert)

Class I Less faciolingual width, normal apicocoronal height.

Class II Decreased ridge height with normal faciolingual width.

Class III Loss of ridge height and width.

- Class I defects can be corrected by subepithelial or submucosal connective tissue grafts
- Class II defects and Class III defects can be corrected by onlay grafts
- If there is severe bone resorption, placement of fixed restoration will hamper esthetics
- In such cases, surgical ridge augmentation is done or a roll of soft tissue is created labial to the pontic site.

Reference

1. Chiun-Lin SL. Use of a modified ovate pontic in areas of ridge defects: a report of two cases. J Esthet Rests Dent. 2004;16(5):273–81.

12. What are the biological, mechanical and esthetic considerations in designing a pontic? Add a note on fabrication of pontics.

Pontic Design

Pontics are fixed partial denture components that replace missing teeth and restore function and appearance compatible with continued oral health and comfort.

Prerequisites

- Proper diagnosis and treatment planning phase
- Proper diagnostic waxing procedures
- Pontic space.

Biologic Considerations

Pontic design needs to maintain and preserve:

- Residual ridge
- Abutment
- Opposing teeth
- Supporting tissues.

Factors affecting biologic considerations are:

- Pontic ridge contact
- Removal of dental plaque
- Direction of occlusal forces
- Surfaces of pontic.

Pontic ridge contact

Pressure-free contact between the pontic and the underlying tissues is indicated to prevent ulceration and inflammation of the soft tissues. Passive contact should be present only on keratinized attached tissue.

Dental plaque

Dental plaque releases toxins that cause tissue inflammation and calculus formation.
This occurs in the area between the tissue surface of the pontic and ridge.
Non-mucosal contacts have better cleansing space than mucosal contacts—Spheroidal and sanitary design.
Factors influencing plaque accumulation:

- Design of the pontic
- Materials used in its fabrication
- Oral hygiene measures.

Design

Mandibular posteriors

- An egg-shaped or bullet-shaped pontic is easiest to keep clean
- It should be as convex as possible with one point contact at the center of the residual ridge.

Maxillary posterior and all anterior pontics

The lingual surface is still made convex and the embrasures are exaggerated on the lingual side to facilitate cleaning.

The tissue surface of the pontic must contact the ridge passively along the faciocervical line-angle and on attached keratinized tissue.

Pontic materials

Should possess good biocompatibility, rigidity, strength and longevity.
Materials which can be used include:

- Porcelain
- Metal
- Gold
- Glazed porcelain.

Occlusal contacts should not fall on the junction between metal and porcelain during centric or eccentric tooth contacts. Glazed porcelain is the most biocompatible of the above pontic materials. Well-polished gold is smoother, less prone to corrosion, and less retentive of plaque than an unpolished or porous casting.

Occlusal forces

- If the buccolingual width of the pontic is reduced by 30% the amount of occlusal forces transferred to the abutment teeth is reduced
- Other forces, such as biting on a hard object, parafunctional activities, load the abutment teeth even if the occlusal table is narrowed.

Pontic surfaces

- Tissue surface
- Occlusal surface
- Buccal surface
- Lingual surface
- Interproximal surface.

Tissue Surface

The tissue surface of the pontic should have only minimal passive contact with the ridge. Pontic should not be placed on movable mucosa and should not blanch the tissue.

Occlusal Surface

- The occlusal table should be reduced to limit forces transferred on to the abutment teeth
- It should be placed within the neutral zone concept and provide a stable vertical dimension support
- The maxillary buccal cusps and mandibular lingual cusps should not be altered. Altering of pontic is done when there is lack of space or to create a favorable occlusal relationship.

Buccal and Lingual Surfaces

- The pontic contours of these surfaces are determined by esthetic, functional and hygienic requirements
- Esthetically, the pontic needs to be contoured facially with proper axial alignment and length
- Embrasures on the lingual side are wider than the buccal or facial side.

Interproximal surface

Should be contoured physiologically to maintain oral hygiene. For proper contouring vertical clearance should be adequate.

Mechanical Considerations

Factors influencing mechanical aspects:

- Improper choice of materials
- Poor frame work design
- Poor tooth preparation
- Poor occlusion.

Pontic materials

- Metal
- Porcelain
- Metal and porcelain
- Resin-veneered pontics
- Bis-GMA resin.

Resin-veneered pontics

Resin-veneered pontics wear and discolor easily as water absorption and thermal fluctuations cause leakage at the metal–resin interface.

Advantages

- Easy to manipulate and repair
- Do not require high-melting range alloys.

Microfilled composites have better physical properties than resin veneers.

Prefabricated porcelain pontics

As slotted facings, long pin facings. Harmony facings and reverse pin facings were used earlier.

Metal–ceramic pontics

Metal–ceramic pontics are strong, easy to clean and natural appearing.

Causes of failure in metal-ceramic facings:

- Uniform thickness of porcelain is required for longer durability
- The metal surfaces to be veneered must be smooth and free of pits
- Sharp angles on the veneering surface increases stress concentrations causing mechanical failure
- Metal–porcelain junction must be placed at least 1.5 mm away from the centric contact junction.

Esthetic Considerations

Pontics should copy the form, contours, gingival margin, incisal edge, gingival and incisal embrasures and color of the adjacent teeth.

Factors affecting esthetics

- Alveolar bone resorption and remodelling
- Incorrect visual perception
- Abnormal mesiodistal width.

In excessive bone loss cases

- Recontouring the gingival half of the labial surface

- Pink porcelain to simulate the gingival tissues
- Ridge augmentation procedures using hydroxylapatite
- RPD is better than an FPD.

Abnormal mesiodistal width

- Can be corrected by orthodontic treatment
- Space can be adjusted between retainers.

Pontic Fabrication

Available materials

- Metal–ceramic pontics
- Resin-veneered
- All metal
- Unidirectional reinforced composite.

Metal–ceramic pontics

Steps in metal–ceramic pontics

1. Wax pattern formation.
2. Cut-back design.
3. Investing and casting.
4. Metal preparation.
5. Application of porcelain veneer.

Wax pattern formation

1. Inlay wax is softened and shaped to the desired pontic shape, by waxing up the internal, proximal, and axial surfaces of the retainers.

   The basic pontic shape can either be waxed up, or an impression of the provisional restoration can be made and duplicated in wax or a prefabricated pontic shape can be used.
2. After the pontic is waxed up it is connected to retainers.

Cut-back design

1. After outlining the area to be veneered with porcelain, make depth cuts in the wax pattern and complete the cut-back as far as access will allow with the units connected. The porcelain–metal junction should be placed as lingual as possible for good esthetics.
2. Separate each retainer and complete the cut back till there is a distinct 90° porcelain–metal junction.

After cutting back reflow and finalize the margins. Do each retainer one at a time and join the entire unit back.

Variation

In some cases the gingival surface of the pontic is cut back in the metal.

Investing and casting

Sprue the units and invest and cast.

Metal preparation

- The casting is recovered from the investment, the sprue is cut off and the remaining investment material in the casting is removed by sand blasting with aluminum oxide
- The gingival surface of the pontic is finished without over reducing.

Application of porcelain veneer

1. A separating agent needs to be applied on the residual ridge of the cast to prevent porcelain powder from sticking to the stone.
2. The metal is prepared and opaquer is applied.
3. Cervical porcelain is applied to the gingival surface of the pontic with the castings seated on the master cast.
4. Porcelain is built up layer-by-layer with the appropriate cervical body and incisal shades and condensed.
5. After condensing, section between the units with a thin razor blade to prevent porcelain from pulling away from the framework due to firing shrinkage.
6. A second application of porcelain is done to correct deficiencies caused by firing shrinkage (additions are needed proximally and gingivally on the pontic).

Contouring gingival surface

1. After application of a porcelain separating liquid to the stone ridge, the desired tissue contact is achieved and gingival surface is contoured (as convex as possible).
2. The porcelain on the tissue surface is made as smooth as possible.
3. Pontic is ready for try-in, staining, glazing, finishing and polishing.
4. The metal framework should be highly polished and gingival embrasures well contoured.

Alternate fabrication technique

In case of partial-coverage retainers made of conventional gold alloys, the retainers must be soldered to the pontic after porcelain application, final staining and glazing.

Resin-veneered pontics

- Resins have low abrasion resistance and bonding between the resin and the metal framework is poor
- New resins have better physical properties than the older ones.
  - Waxing and cut-back are similar to those for metal–ceramic restorations
  - Mechanical undercuts to retain acrylic resin can be formed by retention grooves, acrylic beads to the wax pattern, wax loops, or using an electrolytic etchant
  - Acrylic beads are placed on the entire metal surface to be veneered. The cast metal is also air abraded with an aluminum oxide
  - An opaquer is applied to the metal to mask the metal color and body shade of resin is added with a modelling instrument and polymerized under pressure in a heated water bath. A light-curing resin can be used as an alternative
  - The body resin core is ground to the desired shape, before adding the incisal shade
  - Incisal resin is applied and polymerized
  - The finished restoration is polished.

All-metal pontics

- A wax pattern is made of the desired contour
- The completed wax pattern is finished, sprued and casted
- Casting is retrieved, finished and polished.

Unidirectional reinforced composite

- An impression is made after tooth preparation, and a cast is poured
- After application of a special separating medium, glass fibers are placed on the groove in the cast
- The pontic is built in indirect composite resin, finished, polished and cemented on to the prepared teeth.

13. Describe different types of provisional restorations. Describe various techniques used for making provisional restoration for anterior and posterior tooth preparation.

Definition

A fixed or removable prosthesis designed to protect enhance esthetics, stabilization/or function for a limited period of time after which it is replaced by a definitive prosthesis.

Also known as interim, transitional, temporary and treatment restorations

Classification

- Custom made
- Prefabricated.

Custom made

- Cast metal (precious–gold scrap and nonprecious—Ni-Cr)
- Heat-polymerized resin treatment restorations (custom)
- Visible light-cure composite (Mortan et al. 1984).

Prefabricated

- Aluminum shell, (Brotman—1952) copper band temporization (Amesterdam—1950)
- Preformed metal crowns
- Cellulose acetate forms/Vinyl polyethyl methacrylate crowns (Snap and Trim—1960)
- Prefabricated polycarbonate forms (Charles et al. 1973)
- External surface forms include polycarbonate cellulose acetate, aluminum tin–silver and nickel–chromium.

Depending on the period of use as

- Short-term (up to 2 weeks, e.g.—polycarbonate or aluminum crowns)
- Medium-term (>2 weeks, e.g.—resin-based provisionals)
- Long-term (for months, e.g.—cast-metal crowns).

Cast-metal treatment restorations

Indications

- Patients with maladies difficult to diagnose
- Patients with gross maxillomandibular discrepancies

- As a healing matrix for medically compromised patients
- For maintenance of vertical dimension
- For duplication of the pretreatment canine function.

Variation

Preformed metal crowns can be modified at the gingival and then cast.

Heat-polymerized resins

- A wax pattern with the desired shape is made on the mounted casts
- Wax patters are flasked, dewaxed and packed with heat-cured acrylic resin and cured
- If the provisional restoration was fabricated on mock tooth preparations then the crown needs to be relined with resin before cementation.

Variation

Plastic denture teeth can be trimmed and lined with tooth-colored self-curing acrylic on the lingual aspect of the crown to fabricate esthetically pleasing, functional treatment restorations.

Visible light-cured resin

- Based on urethane dimethacrylate (Provipont DC, Kristall)
- Good mechanical properties
- More shades available
- No residual monomer.

Disadvantages

- Stains
- Expensive
- Lacks good marginal fit.

Aluminum shell crowns (aluminum and tin–silver)

Availability

In anatomic tooth forms and cylindrical shells resembling a tin can.

Indication

Only to be used in premolars and molars.

Technique

- A shell of suitable diameter is selected and festooned to adapt to the preparation and height of the gingival crest
- A resin mixture is placed within the shell for patients with a reduced interocclusal distance to enhance retention
- The shell is then removed, trimmed for adequate occlusal relationships, and seated with a sedative cementing media.

Disadvantages

- Less marginal strength and proximal contacts
- Copper band temporisation is not biocompatible and has poor occlusion.

Preformed metal crowns

- Nickel–chromium shells are used primarily for children with extensively damaged primary teeth
- Nickel–chromium shells are not lined with resin but are trimmed and adapted with contouring pliers and luted with a high-strength cement
- Nickel–chromium alloy is very hard and thus can be used for longer-term provisional restorations.

Indications

- For the posterior teeth
- In pedodontics for fractured teeth.

Advantages

- Improved occlusal and axial surfaces
- Better biocompatibility than aluminum shells.

Cellulose acetate crown forms

- Cellulose acetate is a thin (0.2–0.3 mm), soft, and transparent material available in all tooth types and sizes
- Shades are dependent on the autopolymerizing resin
- Mould guide for different sizes and shapes are available.

Procedure

1. A selected crown form is trimmed and festooned to fit the preparation.
2. The selected crown is filled with any of the resins (polymethyl methacrylate, vinyl polyethyl methacrylate or epimine).
3. Commonly used resin is polymethyl methacrylate.
4. The resin filled crown is gently pressed upon the lubricated preparation while the excess is removed.
5. The crown matrix is repeatedly removed and reseated to minimize distortion and to ensure removal after the resin is set.
6. The cellulose shell is peeled off after the material has set.
7. The occlusion is adjusted and the treatment restoration is trimmed and polished.

Prefabricated polycarbonate crowns

Indications

Can be used for anterior teeth (incisor, canine and premolar).

Requirements of provisional restoration

Biologic—Pulp protection, periodontal health, occlusal stability and prevent enamel fracture.

Mechanical—Resist functional load, resist removal and maintain interabutment alignment.

Esthetic—Restore tooth contour, color translucency and texture.

Techniques in Fabrication of Provisional Restorations

- Shells— custom, such as beaded acrylic and milled crown and proprietary, such as plastic shells—polycarbonate and metal shells, such as aluminium and stainless steel

- Matrices can be formed by impression, vacuum-formed thermoplastic and proprietary celluloid by either direct or indirect technique
- Direct syringing.

Provisional restorations can be done in the following modes
- Indirect
- Direct
- Indirect–direct.

Indirect procedure

In this technique, the provisional restoration is fabricated outside the mouth. Impression is made of the prepared teeth and is poured in quick-setting gypsum.

Advantages
- No contact of free monomer with the prepared tooth or gingiva
- Risk of pulpal damage to tooth is less
- The marginal fit is better for this technique than direct technique
- More comfortable for the patient with less chair side time.

Direct technique

Autopolymerizing resin–alginate impression technique
- An alginate impression of the teeth is made before tooth reduction and impression is stored in a damp environment
- After tooth preparations are completed, acrylic resin is mixed and placed in the corresponding section of the alginate impression
- A separating agent is applied on the tooth preparations and the alginate impression filled with the resin and is then replaced in the mouth
- Impression is removed when the resin reaches a doughy stage, and ones the rigid stage is almost reached the temporary crown is removed from the alginate impression
- After evaluating occlusion in the mouth crown is finished, polished and luted with an appropriate luting agent.

Vacuum-formed plastic template technique
- Transparent sheets in cellulose acetate or polypropylene in various sizes and thicknesses are available. Polypropylene or Omnivac is adapted over the unprepared cast using a thermal vacuum machine
- A suitable shade of autopolymerizing tooth-colored acrylic resin is selected and filled in the template and seated onto the lubricated tooth preparations
- The matrix is removed and reseated
- The restoration is copiously irrigated with cold water
- After the resin has completely set, the matrix is removed, the crown trimmed to the correct finish line with a convex tissue surface and luted with a temporary cement.

Disadvantage

Can cause pulpal injury if the polymerisation temperature is not controlled.

Post crown technique

- For endodontically treated teeth
- A wire (paper clip) or a nonprecious metal post is adapted to the canal
- The selected polycarbonate crown form is then filled with an acrylic resin and placed over the post, including a portion of the radicular surface of the tooth
- The crown form must be removed and reseated repeatedly to prevent resin from locking into undercuts
- After the resin has set, the crown is removed with the temporary post set within the resin
- The entire assembly of post extension and crown form is cemented with a weak adhesive.

Indirect–direct procedure

1. After selecting an appropriate preformed crown with the gingival margin adjusted to approximate the gingival termination, tooth-colored acrylic is mixed and placed inside the crown.
2. The filled polycarbonate crown is seated onto the lubricated tooth preparation on model; the seated crown is reseated repeatedly to prevent excess resin from setting into proximal undercuts.
3. After the resin has set, the excess resin is removed, the emergence profile and fit of the gingival margin is evaluated.
4. The crown is polished and is cemented with a temporary sedative luting agent.

Advantages

- Chairside time is reduced
- Less heat is generated in the mouth
- Contact between the resin monomer and soft tissues is minimized.

14. Describe ideal requirements of luting agents and various luting agents used in crown and bridge cementing. Explain the procedure and care to be taken to lute porcelain jacket crowns.

Ideal requirements of luting agents are as follows:

- Should be tissue compatible
- Should be resistant to disintegration in the oral cavity
- Should provide a durable bond between dissimilar materials
- Should possess favorable compressive and tensile strengths
- Should have sufficient fracture toughness
- Should be able to wet the tooth and the restoration
- Should form a complete seal
- Should demonstrate adequate working and setting times.

Various luting agents are as follows:

- Zinc phosphate cement
- Zinc polycarboxylate cement
- Glass ionomer cement
- Resin modified glass or hybrid ionomers

- Zinc oxide-eugenol with and without ortho ethoxybenzoic acid (EBA)
- Silico-phosphate cement
- Unfilled resins—hydroxyethyl methacrylates and 4 methacryl-ethyl trimellitic anhydride (4-META).

Zinc phosphate cement

Advantages

- Prolonged success rate
- Good compressive strength (9000–20000 psi)
- Adequate tensile strength (720 psi)
- It is a basic cement for comparison
- Reasonable working time
- Excess material is removed easily.

Composition

Powder

- Zinc oxide and magnesium oxide in the ratio of 9–1
- Water content is 33%.

Liquid

Phosphoric acid buffered by aluminum (50%) and zinc salts (traces).

Disadvantages

- Pulp irritation
- Solubility
- Poor seal between the cement and the dentin
- Not an ideal cement when preparation is close to pulp.

Manipulation

- A cooled thick glass slab is used for mixing
- Small increments of powder is incorporated into the cement liquid and mixed with a wide circular motion on about one-half of the glass slab
- When the mixture follows the spatula, it is ready for use as a luting medium.

Zinc polycarboxylate cement

(Introduced in 1968).

Advantages

- Good biocompatibility
- Adhesive to tooth structure
- Exhibit thinning with increased shear rate (less film thickness)
- Less pulpal irritation as polyacrylic acid molecules are large and cannot penetrate the dentinal tubule
- Cleaning the surfaces of metal with an airborne abrasive increases the adhesion of polycarboxylate cement to the metal.

Disadvantages
- Working time is short (2.5 minutes)
- Residual zinc polycarboxylate is more difficult to remove
- It provides less retention.

Indication

On retentive preparations (e.g. in children with large pulp chambers).

Properties
- The compressive strength is at least one-half that of zinc phosphate cement, whereas the tensile strength is similar to zinc phosphate cement
- Solubility of carboxylate cements is about the same as zinc phosphate
- The film thickness of the polycarboxylate cements is approximately ±20 um.

Glass ionomer cement

- Invented by Wilson and Kent
- Put to clinical use by McLean and Wilson.

Advantages
- Adhesive to enamel and dentin
- Good biocompatibility
- Anticariogenic effect (releases fluoride)
- Set cement is translucent, more esthetic when used with the porcelain labial margin technique
- The mechanical properties are almost similar to zinc phosphate.

Disadvantage

Is susceptible to moisture contamination.

Composition

Glass particles and polyacrylic or polymaleic acid—Polyhyrogel + Silica gel.

Reaction

When the powder and liquid are mixed, the aluminium and calcium are displaced forming a alumino-silicate network, which degrades to form hydrated siliceous gel.

Manipulation
- Measured powder is divided into two equal parts and mixed with a plastic spatula
- The first increment is rapidly incorporated in 10 seconds and the second increment incorporated and mixed for a further 10 seconds
- The mixing is completed when the cement can be lifted off the slab with the spatula.

To reduce belated sensitivity following can be done:
- Rapid incorporation of powder and liquid (10–20 seconds)
- Slight hydration of the tooth before cementation by placing a drop of water on the tooth during mixing, which is gently blown off just before placing the prosthesis on the tooth
- Allowing the cement to set hard to the touch, plus 1 minute before removing the excess

- Placing glass ionomer cement varnish on the margins of the restoration after removing the excess cement.

Resin modified glass or hybrid ionomers (Fuji II LC and Vitremer)[1]

Differences from conventional resin and glass ionomer cement (GIC) are as follows:

1. First reaction is an acid/base setting reaction as in GIC.
2. Second reaction is that the limited quantity of a monomer present will polymerize by light cure (as in resin-based luting agents).
3. Polymer content is very minimal which will not interfere with the normal acid/base setting reaction and ion exchange adhesion with tooth structure as in GIC.
4. A third setting reaction occurs in which the remaining monomer will still polymerize chemically.

Zinc oxide eugenol (ZOE) with and without orthoethoxybenzoic acid (EBA)

Quartz and alumina have also been substituted in the mix.

Zinc oxide-eugenol

Advantages

- Reinforced ZOE cement is extremely biocompatible
- Provides an excellent seal.

Disadvantages

- Physical properties (such as compressive strength, solubility and film thickness) are inferior to other cements
- Eugenol leakage can occur
- Can be only used in restorations with good retention form.

EBA cement

- The 2-ethoxybenzoic acid (EBA) replaces a portion of the eugenol in conventional ZOE cement, which improves compressive strength without affecting its resistance to deformation
- The EBA cement has a short working time and excess material is difficult to remove
- The compressive strength of the reinforced zinc oxide eugenol cements is approximately one-half that of zinc phosphate, whereas the tensile strength is nearly identical to zinc phosphate. The values are similar to the averages for polycarboxylate cements.

Advantages

- Palliative effect on the dental pulp
- Ease of placement in a moist environment.

Silico-phosphate cement

It is a mixture of zinc phosphate and silicate cements.

Advantages

- Physical properties in the range of zinc phosphate cement
- Exhibits lower solubility

- Set material is translucent, useful with porcelain margin crowns
- Some anti-cariogenic properties.

Disadvantage

Low pH and consequent potential for pulpal irritation.

Unfilled resins

- Used since1950s
- Less biocompatible than other cements.

Based on polymerisation method:

- Chemical-cure
- Light-cure or dual-cure.

Metal restorations	: Chemically cured system is used
Ceramics	: A light or dual-cure is used
Resin bonded	: Resin cement bonded onto etched enamel surfaces.

Indications

For luting:

- Porcelain veneers
- Porcelain inlays and on-lays
- Resin-bonded prostheses
- Post and core reinforcements (calcium hydroxide placed in deep preparation followed by etched glass ionomer liner, before placement of resin cement).

Advantages

- Insoluble in oral fluids
- Good strength properties
- Easy to use.

Disadvantages

- Bonds to tooth structure
- Is not cariostatic
- Leaks at dentinal margins
- Film thickness of resin cements is greater.

Recent development

- Organophosphonates, hydroxyethyl methacrylate (HEMA)
- 4 methacryl-ethyl trimellitic anhydride (4-META).

Other Cements

- Red and black copper cements: Excessively irritating to the pulp
- Zinc phosphate cement mixed by adding water: Is weaker and more soluble than conventional cements
- Cyanoacrylate cements: Just in the beginning stages.

Procedure to Lute Porcelain Jacket Crowns

Glass ionomer is the luting agent of choice. Other luting agents that can be used are resins and zinc phosphate.

Cleaning tooth surfaces

- All preparation surfaces are checked for any remaining provisional luting agent
- The luting agent shade is selected depending on the adjacent tooth shade.

Preparing restoration

- The casting is cleaned ultrasonically and any remnants of polishing agents are removed.

Preparation for cementation

- Isolate the area with cotton rolls and place the saliva evacuator.

Manipulation of glass ionomer

- Powder-liquid ratio: 1.25 part of powder to 1 part of liquid
- After shaking the powder bottle, 2 level scoops of powder and 8 drops of liquid are dispensed in a paper mixing pad
- Reduced temperature while mixing increases working time and allows addition of more powder
- The measured powder is divided into two equal parts and mixed with a plastic spatula. The first part is rapidly incorporated in 10 seconds and the second part incorporated and mixed for a further 10 seconds
- Mixing time: 45 seconds
- Working time: 3 minutes from start of mix
- Luting consistency:

The cement lifts off the slab with the spatula and can be pulled into a thread of 20 mm in length before snapping back onto the slab. The consistency is more viscous than zinc phosphate, but the material thins out with seating pressure.

Application of cement

- A thin coat is applied to the clean internal surface of the restoration
- Ask patient to bite on wooden stick
- Dry the tooth with a light blast of air and seat the restoration into place.

Seating the restoration

- Final seating is seated firmly with a rocking, dynamic seating force
- After the casting is seated, the margins are verified for complete seating.

Removing excess cement

- After the cement has set (7 minutes from start of mix) remove excess cement with an explorer
- Early removal of cement exposes margins to moisture, increasing its solubility
- A margin seal can be applied to prevent moisture contamination
- Dental floss can be used to remove residual cement interproximally and from the gingival sulcus.

Evaluation of occlusion

- An articulating paper or Mylar strip is used to check the occlusion once more.

Instructions to patient

- As the cements take at least 24 hours for their final set, patients are instructed not to chew on that side for a day or two
- Oral hygiene instructions are also given.

Resin luting agents

A light- or dual-cure can be used for porcelain jacket crowns when retention form is compromised.

Reference

1. Nicholson JW, Anstice M. The development of modified glass ionomer cements for dentistry. Trends in Polymer Science. 1994;2:272–6.

15. Classify adhesive bridges/resin-bonded bridges. Cite the advantages, disadvantages, indications, contraindications and preparation steps. Add a note on types of bonding to metal and tooth.

Definition

Resin-bonded bridges are fixed partial dentures, which are cemented onto the abutments using special resins.

First described by Rochette in 1973 (to splint mandibular anterior teethusing cast gold bar).[1]

Introduction

- Howe and Denehy introduced the first form of resin-bonded FPD (RBFPD)[2]
- Livaditis proposed preparation of proximal and lingual surfaces to create a path of insertion, along with occlusal rest seat preparation[3]
- Livaditis and Thompson later introduced the concept of electrolytically etched non-precious metal[4]
- Other developments happened in regard to bonding techniques and etching which in turn depended on factors, such as type of casting alloy, type, time and concentration of acid etchant, acid and electrical current density
- Silicoating improved the longevity and bonding of metal. This involves the fusion of a 0.5µ thin layer of silica to the metal fitting surface which bonds with a silane coupling agent.

Classification

1. Rochette bridge.
2. Maryland bridge.
3. Virginia bridge.
4. Cast-mesh fixed partial dentures.

Advantages

- Minimal tooth reduction—Conservation of tooth structure
- Preparation is confined to enamel
- No pulpal trauma
- Anesthesia not required

- More biocompatible
- Supragingival margin placement
- Less periodontal trauma
- Less chair side time
- Does not require cast alterations or removable die preparation
- Reduced cost.

Disadvantages

- Good patient selection is a must
- Technique sensitive
- Laboratory errors cannot be corrected easily
- Chances of over contouring leads to plaque accumulation
- Over contouring can result in patient discomfort
- Can only replace one tooth
- Cannot be prepared on thin tooth
- Debonding can occur due to faulty preparation or improper luting technique
- Difficulty in isolation during bonding procedures
- Cannot be done on tooth with small clinical crowns.

Indications

- For abutments with sufficient enamel
- Splinting periodontally compromised teeth
- For medically compromised patients
- As a temporary restoration
- Young patient
- Large pulp chambers
- Post ortho-retention.

Contraindications

- Sensitivity to base-metal alloys
- Insufficient occlusal clearance
- Deep vertical overbite
- Thin teeth
- Loss of tooth structure
- Parafunctional habits
- Short clinical crowns
- Narrow embrasures
- Mobile tooth
- Defective enamel
- In extensive restorations.

Rochette Bridge (1973) (Fig. 34)

- It is a wing-like retainer with six perforations to provide mechanical undercuts for resin cement
- Etched retainers are coated with pyrolized silane and bonded with resin cements.

Disadvantage

The resin is exposed to oral fluids and external stress, which leads to abrasion and marginal leakage.

Variation

Nonperforated retainers can be used.

Maryland Bridge (Fig. 35)

(Livaditis and Thompson from University of Maryland School of Dentistry)
Here a nonperforated retainer was etched for mechanical retention to form microporosities present and was bonded by resin cement.

Virginia Bridges

(Moon and Hudgins)

- Use particle-roughened retainers
- The retainer wax patterns are sprinkled with salt crystals prior to resin fabrication
- The salt crystals get incorporated onto the tissue surface of the resin pattern
- During dewaxing the salt crystals dissolve leaving voids in the resin pattern for mechanical retention
- Air abrasion with aluminium oxide improves retention.

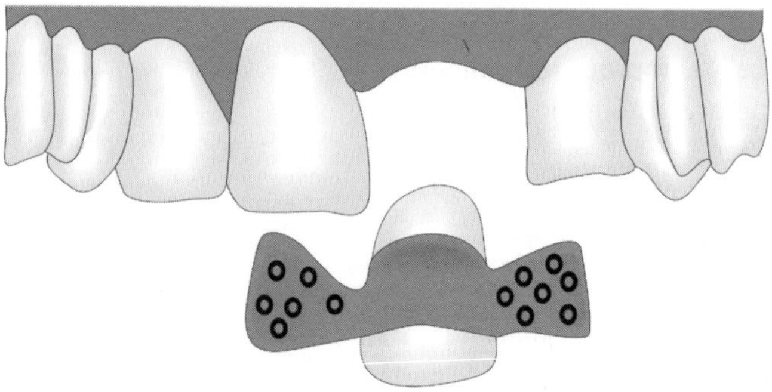

Fig. 34: Rochette bridge

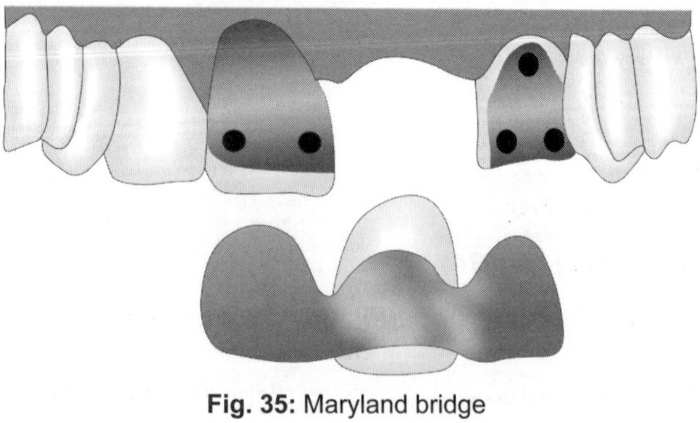

Fig. 35: Maryland bridge

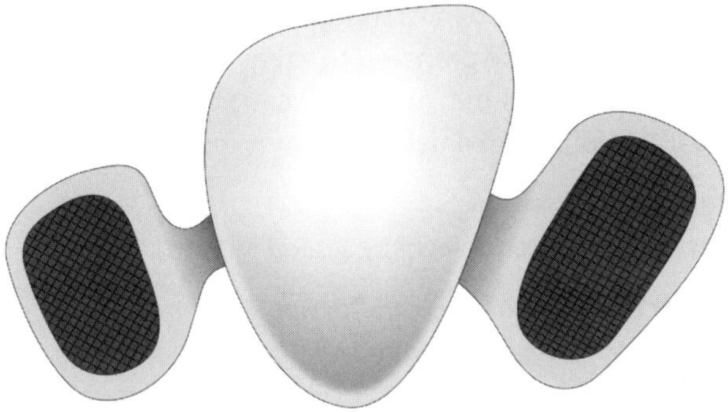

Fig. 36: Cast-mesh fixed partial denture

Advantages
- Surface treatment of the retainer is not necessary
- Noble metal alloys also can be used as retainers.

Cast-mesh Fixed Partial Denture (Fig. 36)

A nylon mesh is placed on the tissue surface of the retainer wax pattern before fabricating the wax pattern.

Disadvantages
- The nylon mesh adaptation to the cast is not good
- The wax may flow in between the mesh locking all the undercuts.

Steps in the Fabrication/Preparation of A Resin-bonded Fixed Partial Denture

1. Preparation of abutment teeth.
2. Fabricating the provisional restoration.
3. Design of the restoration.
4. Bonding.

Preparation of abutment teeth
- Single path of insertion
- The incisal finish line is kept 2 mm short of the incisal edge to avoid any esthetic impairment of incisal edge translucency
- A reduction of 0.5 mm palatally is ensured for adequate metal thickness
- The gingival finish line ends 1 mm supragingivally for optimal gingival health
- Proximal undercuts must be removed
- Interproximally, the finish line ends at the centre of the contact area or proximal grooves are given for maximum wrap effect
- Rest seats as cingulum rest should provide good resistance form and is prepared with flat-ended tapered diamond bur
- Definite and distinct margins should be present.

Design of Anterior Resin-bonded Fixed Partial Dentures
- A single path of insertion in the incisogingival direction along the proximal surface of the abutment

- Lingual clearance (0.8 mm–1.0 mm) should be provided
- Cingulum rest seat should be prepared to act as a vertical stop
- A supragingival finish line (1 mm above the crest of tissue)
- An additional retention in proximal facial extensions.

Cantilever Anterior Designs

Canine is used as abutment to replace the lateral incisor.

Design of Posterior Resin-bonded Fixed Partial Dentures

- The occlusal rest (for resistance to gingival displacement)
- The retentive surface (for resistance to occlusal displacement)
- The proximal wrap (for resistance to torquing forces).

Occlusal Rest Seat

Should be spoon-shaped and placed on the proximal marginal ridge of the abutment adjacent to the edentulous area.

Retentive Surface

Proximal and lingual axial walls should be reduced to about 1 mm above the gingival margin.

Proximal wrap:

The alloy framework should be designed to engage at least 180° of tooth structure with a knife-edge margin (1 mm supragingivally).

Types of material used

- Gold alloy earlier
- Presently Ni–Cr alloy
- Zirconium
- Fiber-reinforced composites.

Types of bonding to provide retention

- Mechanical
- Chemical.

Mechanical Bonding

Subtypes

Macroscopic retention

By mechanical locks as in Rochette's (six perforations in metal), mesh and water-soluble salt crystal.

Microscopic retention

By electrolytic etching (Maryland bridge).

Chemical bonding

Chemical bonding of resin:

1. Chemical etching.
2. Tin-plating.

Mechanical etching techniques

Electrochemical etching

Results in microscopic porosity.

Non-beryllium Nickel–chromium alloys

Two stages:

1. Retainer is immersed in 35% nitric acid under a current of 250 milliamps per square centimeter for 5 minutes.
2. Retainer is cleaned by immersing in 18% HCl in an ultrasonic cleaner for 10 minutes.

Beryllium-containing Nickel–chromium alloys

1. Retainer is immersed in 10% H_2SO_4 under a current of 300 milliamps per square centimeter.
2. Retainer is cleaned by immersing in 18% HCl in an ultrasonic cleaner for 10 minutes.

Other technique (Mc Laughlin technique)

1. Retainer is etched with a mixture of HCl and H_2SO_4 in a beaker.
2. The beaker with the retainer is directly placed in an ultrasonic cleanser for 99 seconds under an electrical field.

Nonelectrochemical

Roughening by aluminium oxide-air abrasion.

Chemical Bonding of Resin

Chemical etching

A gel consisting of nitric and hydrochloric acids is applied to the internal surface of the metal framework for approximately 25 minutes.

Tin plating

Precious alloys can be plated with tin and used as retainers to increase adhesiveness of resins thereby increasing bond strengths.

Conclusion

- Ketabi et al. observed a survival of 69% after 13 years of 74 RBFPDs. The fifteen failures were due to loss of retention, caries and fracture of porcelain[5]
- Djemal et al.[6] studied 832 RBFPDs and found survival of seven years and 10 months
- RBFPDs still debond frequently but showed an increase in survival rate after five years as 87.7%.

References

1. Rochette AL. Attachment of a splint to enamel of lower anterior teeth. J Prosthet Dent. 1973;30:418–23.
2. Howe DF, Denehy GE. Anterior fixed partial dentures utilising the acidetch technique and a cast metal framework. J Prosthet Dent. 1977;37:28-31.
3. Livaditis GJ. Cast metal resin-bonded retainers for posterior teeth. J Am Dent Assoc. 1980;101: 926-9.

4. Livaditis GJ, Thompson VP. Etched castings: an improved retentive mechanism for resin-bonded retainers. J Prosthet Dent. 1982;47:52-8.
5. Ketabi AR, Kaus T, Herdach F, Groten M, Axmann-Kromar D, Weber H. Thirteen-year follow-up study of resin-bonded fixed partial dentures. Quintessence Int. 2004;35:407-10.
6. Djemal S, Setchell D, King P, Wickens J. Long-term survival characteristics of 832 resin-retained bridges and splints provided in post-graduate teaching hospital between 1978 and 1993. J Oral Rehabil. 1999;26:302-20.

16. What are the requirements of dies? Describe materials used in preparation of dies and few techniques used for preparing dies?

Requirements of Dies

- It must reproduce all surfaces of the prepared teeth accurately without any bubbles or voids
- The remaining unprepared tooth structure 1 mm cervical to the finish line should be readily discernible on the die
- Should be dimensionally stable
- Strong and resistant to abrasion
- Should be easily sectionable and easy to trim
- Should be compatible with the separating agent used
- Should color contrasts with the wax used
- Should be easily wettable by the inlay wax
- Must be compatible with the impression material.

Classification

Metallic

- Amalgam
- Metal sprayed
- Electroplated.

Nonmetallic

- Gypsum
- Epoxy resin
- Silicophosphate cement
- Polymer
- Ceramic.

Others

- Divestment.

Gypsum (Type IV-Velmix die stone and Type V-Suprastone)

Disadvantages

- Decreased accuracy
- Decreased resistance to abrasion.

Advantages

- Inexpensive
- Easy to use
- Produces consistent results.

Variation of technique

Impregnate the surface of the die with a low-viscosity resin (cyano-acrylate) to improve abrasion resistance.

Epoxy Resin

Advantages

- Good strength
- Good abrasion resistance
- Can be cured at room temperature
- No complicated equipment required
- Dimensionally stable
- Retainers adapt better when made on epoxy dies
- Silicone and polyether are compatible with epoxy.

Disadvantages

- More expensive than gypsum
- Polymerization shrinkage
- Polysulfide and hydrocolloid are not compatible.

Variation

Epoxy resin, which is heat-treated after setting, is also available.

Electroplated die

Advantage

Good abrasion resistance.

Disadvantages

- Silicone and polyether impressions are difficult to electroplate
- Polysulfide can be silver plated, but cannot be copper plated
- Silver plating uses cyanide solution, which is extremely toxic.

Technique

- Finely powdered silver or graphite is brushed on to the impressions to make them conduct electricity
- The impression is than placed in the electroplating bath
- A layer of pure metal is deposited on the impression which is supported with type IV stone or resin.

Methods of Die Preparation

1. Working cast with separate die.
2. Divestment technique.
3. Working cast with a removable die.

Working cast with separate die

Impression

Two impressions are made, one for the sectional cast and another for full arch cast and poured in hard densite stones.

Pouring dental stone for full-arch impression

Dental stone is filled by gently vibrating, until the preparation area fills and then the entire area of impression. Additional base can be added after the initial set has occurred.

Pouring dental stone for sectional impression

The preparation area is filled without air entrapment and stone is built up to a height approximately 1 inch over the preparation for handle on the die.

Die preparation

After the cast is removed, separating agent is applied on the prepared teeth. A handle, larger in diameter than the preparation, octagonal in shape and parallel to the long axis of the tooth, is formed on the die. Finally prepared die should be smooth and free of ridges with the finish line highlighted with a sharp red pencil.

Divestment technique

A die is formed from a refractory material on which the restoration is waxed, kept for burnout and cast directly against the die.

Indications

For intricate patterns that are not readily removable from the die.

Disadvantages

- Does not perfectly fit as retainers made of other techniques
- The die is destroyed in the casting process and a second cast and die needs to be made for finishing purposes.

Working cast with removable dies (Fig. 37)

1. Dowel pin technique.
2. Curved dowel pin.
3. Di-lok tray.
4. Pindex system.

Requirements of removable dies

- Must return to their exact original positions
- Must remain stable when inverted
- Must be easily mountable on an articulator.

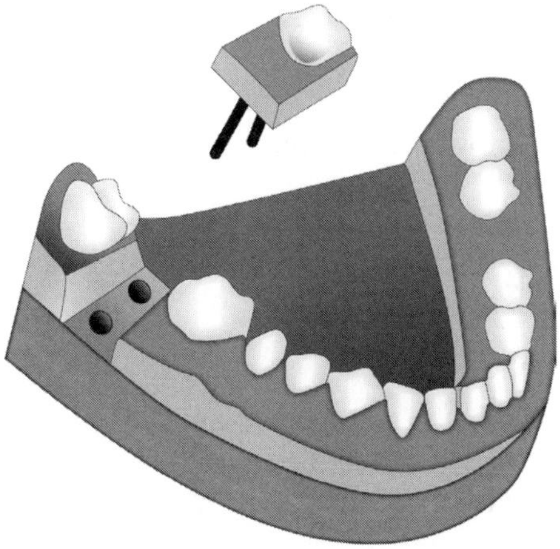

Fig. 37: Cast with removable die

Dowel Pin Technique

Synonyms
- Straight pin technique
- Tapered pin technique.

Advantages
- Least amount of inaccuracy in a horizontal direction
- Less vertical deviation.

Procedure
- An impression is made and the straight dowel pin is centred directly over the preparation
- Bobby pins are placed across the impression buccolingually with the dowel pins placed between the arms of a bobby pin and both are stabilised by straight pins with sticky wax.

Pouring the impression
- Die stone is poured in the impression by filling the prepared teeth and covering the knurled end of the dowel pin
- Paper clips are added to other areas to provide retention for the second pour of stone.

Removing bobby pins and straight pins
- After the first pour sets, the straight and bobby pins are removed
- The tip of each dowel is covered by soft wax
- A V-shaped buccolingual orientation groove is placed on each die
- The area around each die is lubricated.

Removing cast
- After the cast sets, its removed and trimmed

- The utility wax is uncovered and a jeweller's blade is used to cut through mesial and distal side of each die
- The die is loosened from the cast by gently tapping on the end of dowel
- The cuts should taper towards each other slightly from occlusal to gingival.

Mounting the casts

- After the die is removed and ditched, utility wax is placed back into the wells around the tips of the dowels
- The casts are mounted.

Curved dowel pin

Procedure

- A position bar is used to orient the curved dowel into the impression of the prepared tooth
- The position bar is oriented faciolingually till the dowel tip extends 1.1–2.0 mm into the impression with the tail pointing facially.

Pins placed

- One pin in the facial aspect—Straight pin
- Second pin in the lingual aspect
- Pins are placed for all prepared tooth and pontic region
- A dowel pin is also placed near the centre of each segment of unprepared tooth
- The dowel pin's head should be parallel to the long axis of the tooth.

Pouring of dental stone

Die stone is poured into the impression until it covers the heads, and 1.0–2.0 mm of the thicker hexagonal bodies of the dowels.

Removal of positional pins

- After the die stone has set the two straight pins and the positioning bar is slided off each dowel
- A 2.0 mm deep hole is cut on either side of each dowel
- Lubricate the exposed parts of the dowels
- Boxing wax is placed around the impression and dental stone is filled till the dowels are covered by at least 2.0 mm, except for the tips.

Sawing the cast

- After the stone sets, remove the boxing wax and place vertical saw cuts on either side of each die
- Separate each segment by gently tapping on the protruding tail of the dowel.

Preparing working cast

- A horseshoe-shaped working cast with the base trimmed flat is made
- Holes are drilled with drill press in the bottom of the cast directly under the center of each prepared tooth, pontic area and segment containing unprepared teeth
- A curved dowel is tried into the prepared holes till the head seats completely and luted with cyanoacrylate cement

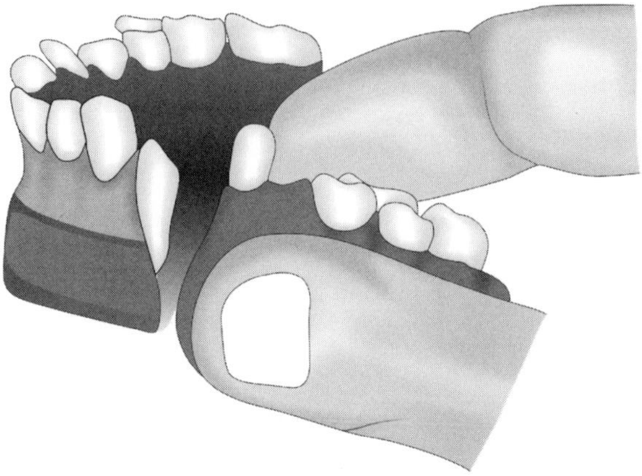

Fig. 38: Removable dies: Di-lok tray

- After the cement has hardened, a thin layer of petrolatum is applied and second pour is done.

Di-Lok tray (Fig. 38)

Requires a specially articulated tray with internal orienting grooves and notches to reassemble sectioned master cast accurately.

Procedure

- Evaluate the fit of the tray on articulator.

Pouring the impression

- The entire arch impression is poured with die stone to a height of approximately one inch. The U-shaped cast with an open lingual area must be trimmed to fit the di-lok tray
- After the cast is allowed to dry, trim the lingual side of the cast on an arbor band and try the cast in the di-lok tray.

Placing the cast in the tray

- After horizontal grooves are cut in the base of the cast, the tray is filled three quarter with dental stone
- Slurry water soaked cast is seated into the tray by jiggling it slightly till the cervical lines of the teeth are about 4 mm above the edge of the tray.

Removing cast from tray

- After the stone sets, the cast is removed from the tray by lifting back up, and then slide the buccal facing forward and tap on the base of the cast with a laboratory knife
- The removed cast is sawed with a taper between the prepared tooth and the adjacent tooth.

Preparation of removable die

- Remove all dies with finger pressure and trim the excess stone gingival to the finish line
- Mark the finish line with a red pencil.

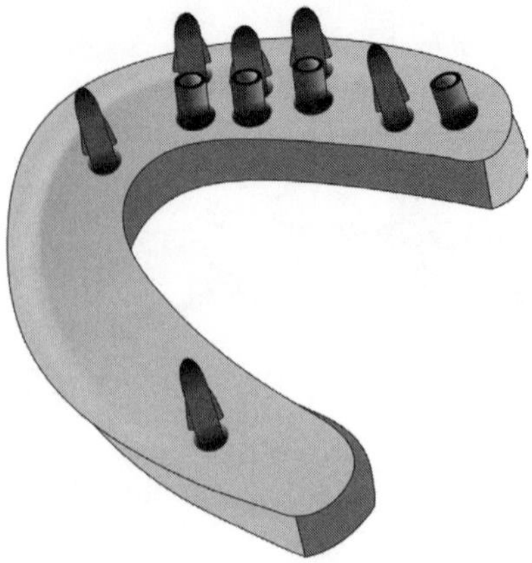

Fig. 39: Pindex system: Pin placement

Disadvantage

- Large size of the tray makes articulation difficult.

Pindex System (Fig. 39)

Preparing the master cast

- The final impression is poured in stone
- After the stone sets, the retrieved cast is trimmed to a horseshoe shaped form
- The buccolingual width of the base of the horseshoe is 13–18 mm, and thickness 15 mm between the gingival margins of the preparations and the inferior border.

Pin Placement

- After the under surface of the cast is trimmed perfectly flat, drill two holes for each removable section as far apart to provide space for the pins and sleeves
- The pins are cemented into holes using low viscosity cyanoacrylate cement
- The short index pins are cemented in the lingual holes
- Long pins cemented into the buccal holes
- The white sleeves are placed over the long pins and the gray sleeves over the short pins.

The Secondary Base

- A strip of carding wax is placed over the extensions of the long pins and the gray sleeves
- The master cast is boxed or placed in a rubber base former and a secondary base is poured with cast stone.

Removable Dies

- After the secondary base sets, remove the master cast and trim the secondary base on the model trimmer
- Dies are sectioned with a die saw and trimmed carefully to expose the finish line (Fig. 40)
- Clean the stone grindings from the dies, pins, base and pin holes
- Reseat the dies
- The master cast is mounted.

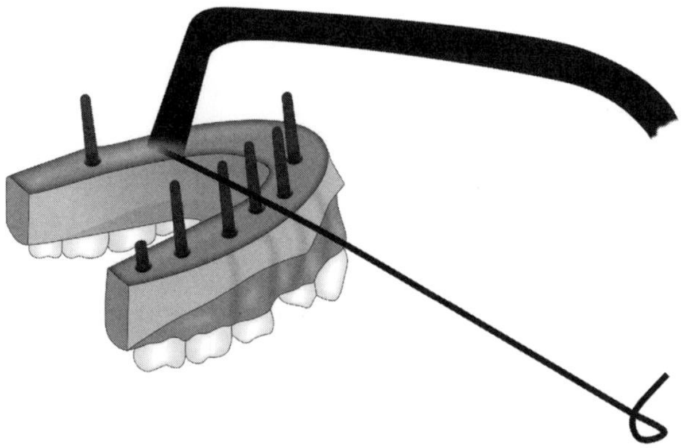

Fig. 40: Removable dies: Pindex system

17. Classify ceramics. Enumerate its advantages and disadvantages. Explain the mechanism of bonding and describe the laboratory steps involved in fabrication of different ceramics.

Classification

Depending on use

Type 1
For denture teeth
(Powders of feldspar, clay and quartz).

Type 2
For ceramometal applications
(Potassium feldspar and glass).

Type 3
- For all-porcelain restorations
- Porcelain jacket crowns, veneers and inlays
  (Feldspathic dental porcelain with increased amounts of aluminum oxide).

Depending on fusion temperature
- High fusing (1288–1371°C)
- Medium fusing (1093–1260°C)
- Low-fusing (871–1066°C)
- Ultra-low fusing (Below 850°C).

Based on application
- Core porcelain: The basis of porcelain jacket crown must have good mechanical properties.
- Dentine or body porcelain: More translucent than the above, this largely governs the shapes and color of the restoration. Enamel porcelain forms the outer part of the crown and is translucent.

All ceramic restorations

Types

- Conventional powder
  Slurry ceramics
  E.g.: Optec HSP, Duceram LFC.
- Castable ceramics
  E.g.: Picon, Dicor Plus.
- Machinable ceramics/Machined Densely Sintered Ceramics
  E.g.: Cerec vitablocs Mark I, Mark II, Dicor MGC, Celay.
- Pressable ceramics
  E.g.: IPS empress, OpTEC
- Infiltrated ceramics
  E.g.: INCERAM.

Advantages

- Highly esthetic, can match the tooth color in translucency, color and intensity
- Special types of porcelain are available that can simulate all colors including gingival tones
- Life-like porcelain is achieved by glazing porcelain
- Glazed porcelain in contact with tissue surface is more biocompatible than metal
- All ceramic restoration has less failure rates
- Porcelain fused to metal prepared from foil copings uses thin metal copings (0.2–0.3 mm), which can increase bulk of porcelain.

Disadvantages

- If there is difference in thermal matching between metal and porcelain, the porcelain fails at the margin
- More reduction of tooth structure to accommodate bulk of porcelain
- Brittle in nature and if surface glaze is removed cracks propagate leading to failure of porcelain
- Porcelain restorations do not give as close a marginal adaptation as metal marginal finish
- All Porcelain has less tensile and shear strength, hence ideal to make a metal coping
- Porcelain shrinks during firing and if porosities are present the overall strength and translucency diminishes
- Ceramics and glasses have tensile strengths that are much lower than their compressive strengths.
- Strength of ceramics reduces to 50% by sandblasting or by etching with hydrofluoric acid solution for 1 minute
- If tensile stresses or sub-microcracks are present on the surface, in presence of moisture may lead to stress corrosion
- Presence of a chemical environment decreases strength of porcelain.

Enamel–Metal Bond

1. Mechanical bond
   Porcelain wets the surface of metal.

2. Compressive stresses
   Compressive stresses set up during cooling of the sintered porcelain veneer, aid in bonding of porcelain.
3. Chemical Bonding.

Mechanical Bond

Microscopic irregularities on metal surface are filled with porcelain; retention of the porcelain veneer by mechanical interlocking is achieved.

Increasing mechanical bond strength

- Grinding or sand blasting
- Roughening by oxidation
- Electrochemical corrosion of the metal by molten glass
- Selective oxidation of grain boundaries
- Etching by acid in pre-treatment for fusing.

Compressive Stresses

- A very small degree of thermal mismatch between metal and porcelain leaves the porcelain in a state of compression
- This increases the bonding between metal and porcelain.

Chemical Bond

True chemical bonding results from electron transfer between the oxygen of the glassy phase of porcelain and an oxidised metal surface.

Increasing chemical bond

- By addition of tin, indium, iron to a noble metal casting alloy
- In nickel–chromium alloy there is an indirect bond between glass and metal through an undissolved oxide formed on the metal surface.

Fabrication of a Ceramic Restoration

Condensation

Fine porcelain powder is mixed with water and condensed into the desired form.

Dense condensation provides

- Lower firing shrinkage
- Less porosity in the fired porcelain.

Methods of condensation

1. Vibration:
   - Mild vibration to densely pack the wet powder upon the underlying framework
   - The excess water is blotted with a clean tissue.
2. Spatulation:
   - A small spatula is used to apply and smooth the wet porcelain.
3. Brush technique:
   - Dry porcelain powder is added to the surface with brush to absorb the water
   - Porcelain must never be allowed to dry out until condensation is complete.

Firing

- The thermochemical reaction is complete during fritting
- Firing is done to fuse the particles of powder together, a process called sintering.

Method

- The condensed porcelain mass is placed in a preheated furnace (approximately 650°C) for 5 minutes
- This removes the remaining water.

Stages in Firing

A low bisque (low biscuit) firing

In which the glass grains have softened and have started to flow.

A medium bisque (medium biscuit) firing

The glass grains have flowed to the extent that the powder particles exhibit complete cohesion.

In high bisque (high biscuit) firing

- The shrinkage is complete and the mass exhibits a smoother surface
- Lesser the firing cycles higher will be the strength and esthetics.

Glazing

Air-fired porcelain cannot be polished.

Application of over glaze/self glaze

- Self-glazing, which was previously fired to a high bisque, is heated rapidly (10–15 minutes) to its fusion temperature
- It is maintained at that temperature for approximately 5 minutes before it is cooled
- Glass grains flow over the surface to form a vitreous layer
- Glazed porcelain is much stronger and reduces crack propagation than the unglazed variety.

Cooling

- Because of the low thermal conductivity of the porcelain, the differential between the thermal dimensional change of the outside and inside can introduce stresses, which embrittle the porcelain
- The ideal cooling method for a porcelain restoration from its firing temperature to room temperature is controversial.

Other Types of Porcelain Fabrications

Cast coping

Requirements

- To be fusible to alloys, the porcelain has to be sufficiently low fusing
- It has to have a coefficient of thermal expansion that is considerably higher than ordinary porcelain
- The alloy should be sag resistant at the firing temperatures of porcelain

- It should be rigid to prevent fracture of porcelain
- There should be no pigmentation reaction produced between the porcelain and the alloy
- Further oxide formed should be soluble in porcelain and provide good wetting of the metal or metal oxide for attachment.

Bonded platinum foil coping

- Makes use of tin oxide coatings on platinum foil
- The esthetics is improved with a thin platinum foil, which allows more room for porcelain
- The bonded foil reduces subsurface porosity and micro cracks in the porcelain and increases the strength of the unit.

Swaged gold alloy foil coping

- Renaissance, by the Williams Gold refining company, is a laminated gold-alloy foil that is delivered to the use in a fluted shape
- This foil shape is swaged onto the die and flame sintered to form a coping
- An interfacial alloy powder is applied and fired, and then coping is veneered with porcelain.

All-ceramic Materials

Conventional powder–slurry ceramics

Available as

- Powders to which water is added to produce a slurry
- Available in various shades and translucencies, with characterizing stains and glazes.

Manufacturing

- Leucite crystals are dispersed in a glassy matrix by controlling their nucleation and crystal growth
- The leucite and glassy matrix fuse together during the baking process
- The build-up and contouring of the crown can be done by using the powder–slurry technique on semi permeable die material.

Advantages

- Greater strength than conventional feldspathic porcelain due its leucite content
- Does not require a core as with aluminous porcelain jacket crowns
- The body and incisal porcelains can be pigmented to provide desired shade and translucency
- Does not require special processing equipment
- These restorations fit accurately.

Disadvantage

Their high leucite content can cause increased wear to opposing teeth.

Other types

Duceram LF

- Hydrothermal low-fusing ceramic
- Composed of an amorphous glass containing hydroxyl ions.

Advantages

- Greater density, higher flexural strength, greater fracture resistance and lower hardness than feldspathic porcelain
- No special laboratory techniques or equipment required.

Uses

For fabrication of ceramic inlays, veneers and full-contour crowns.

Procedure

Base layer:

Duceram metal–ceramic (a leucite-containing porcelain) is placed on a refractory die using powder–slurry techniques and baked at 930°C.

Over base layer:

Duceram LFC is applied using the powder–slurry technique and baked at a relatively low temperature (660°C).

Castable ceramic systems

Available as

- Solid ceramic ingots, which are cast using lost-wax and centrifugal casting technique
- Only one shade is available
- Staining is done to obtain proper shading of the final restoration.

Picon

A polycrystalline glass–ceramic material, in which glass is heat-treated under controlled crystallization.

Procedure

- When solid ceramic ingots are cast at 1350°C, a transparent glass crown is obtained
- This crown is then heat-treated at 1075°C for 10 hours. "Ceramming" causes partial crystallization (55%) of tetra-silic-mica-like crystals.

Advantages

- Easier, as it is a lost wax technique
- The transparent crown after heat treatment at 1075°C for 10 hours forms an opaque crown, which increases fracture resistance and strength
- Less abrasive to opposing tooth structure
- For final restoration colorant, stains are baked on the surface of the glass–ceramic material.

Dicor Plus

It is a shaded feldspathic porcelain veneer applied to the Dicor substrate.

Disadvantages

- Abrasive to opposing teeth
- Requires a special high-temperature, electric-heated casting unit
- Fracture of the restorations is common.

Machinable ceramics

Available as

- Ceramic ingots in various shades
- Used in computer-aided design and computer-aided manufacturing (CAD-CAM) procedures
- The machined restoration are stained and glazed to the desired characterization.

Cerec vitablocs Mark I

- This is a feldspathic porcelain, used with the Cerec system
- Composition, and properties are the same as feldspathic porcelain used for porcelain-fused-to-metal restorations.

Cerec vitablocs Mark II

This is a feldspathic porcelain of increased strength with less abrasive wear of the opposing tooth structure.

Dicor MGC

- Contains fluoro-silicic mica crystals in a glass matrix
- It has greater flexural strength than the castable Dicor and Cerec
- Less abrasive wear of the opposing tooth structure than Cerec Mark I.

Celay

- Can be used for CAD-CAM and copy-milling technique
- Identical in physical properties to Cerec Vitablocs Mark II.

Disadvantage

Marginal fit is not good.

Pressable ceramics

Available as

- Ceramic ingots, which are melted at high temperatures and pressed into a mould created by lost-wax technique
- Can be made to full contour, or can be built up using feldspathic porcelain.

IPS Empress

- This is a feldspathic porcelain supplied in ingot form
- The ingots are heated and moulded under pressure to produce the restorations.

Procedure

1. The ceramic ingot is placed under the plunger, and heated to 1150°C.
2. The plunger presses the molten ceramic into the mould.
3. The final shade of the crown is done by staining or veneering (cut back technique of wax pattern).

Optec Pressable Ceramic

This is a type of feldspathic porcelain with increased leucite content, processed by moulding under pressure and heat.

Advantages of IPS and OPC

- Produce strong, translucent, dense and etchable ceramic restorations
- Useful in fabricating ceramic veneers.

Disadvantage

Require special equipment to fabricate the restorations.

Infiltrated ceramics

Available as

- Powder (aluminum oxide or spinel), which is fabricated into a porous substrate, and a glass, which is infiltrated at high temperature into the porous substrate
- The infiltrated ceramic is then veneered using conventional feldspathic porcelain technique.

In-Ceram

- The spinel cores are more translucent than the aluminum oxide cores
- The core is made from fine-grained particles that are mixed with water to form a suspension referred to as a "slip".

Procedure

- The slip is placed on a gypsum die and baked at 1120°C for 10 hours to produce the opaque, porous core
- An appropriate shade of glass powder is applied to the core, which is baked again at 1100°C for four hours
- During this process, the molten glass infiltrates the porous alumina core by capillary action.

Advantages

- Extremely high flexure strength
- The aluminum oxide or spinel crystals limit crack propagation and the glass infiltration reduces porosity
- Provide an accurate fit.

Disadvantages

- Cannot etch internal surface hence a resin cement, such as Panavia 21TC is recommended
- Not as esthetic as other systems
- Requires specialized equipment to fabricate a restoration.

Recent Advances in Metal–Ceramics

- Pure titanium can be used as a coping and framework metal for metal ceramic restorations because of its excellent biocompatibility
- Copy milling is used to prepare duplicate dies of graphite and to machine the outer form of a titanium crown. The graphite die is then used as a positive electrode in a spark erosion system to serve as the pattern for removal of interior portion of the crown
- Other titanium-based products, such as Tycast are melted in a specialized casting machine and cast using the conventional lost-wax technology. Ultra low fusing porcelain is used along with this.

18. What are the types of veneering materials? Describe their advantages, disadvantages and indications. Add a note on the recent advances in veneering materials used in fixed partial denture.

Veneers are thin facings of porcelain or resin affixed directly to teeth using a composite resin-bonding agent.

Types of Veneering Materials

1. Porcelain veneers (Cerinate, Porcelite and Chameleon).
2. Resin veneers by direct technique (Durafill, Heliosit, Silux).
3. Resin veneers indirect technique (Dentacolor, Isosit).
4. Composite veneers direct and indirect (Visio-Gem).
5. Composite reinforced with glass fibers (Targis/Vectris, Variolink II System).
6. Castable hydroxyapatite (Cast apatite).
7. Injectable ceramics (Dicor, Cerestore).

Comparison of Veneer Systems

Direct composite veneers

1. Require only one appointment.
2. The shade, contour and final form can be corrected to the dentist's and patient's satisfaction.
3. Less expensive when compared to porcelain and other laminate systems.
4. Direct veneers can be repaired easily.

Indirect resin veneers

The indirect resins have better bond strength than direct resins.

Porcelain veneers

1. Have good translucency.
2. Reduced plaque adherence.
3. They can be fabricated only by indirect technique.
4. Their advantages are that chair side time is reduced even for placement of multiple units.

Have optimum color stability, esthetics, wear resistance, and tissue compatibility.

Porcelain Laminates

- Porcelain laminates are thin facings constructed on refractory dies
- The porcelain veneer's inner surface is etched with hydrofluoric acid and bonded to tooth with composite resin cement.

Indications

- When patient demands high esthetics
- For mildly stained tooth
- Enamel defects and diastema.

Contraindications

- In dark stains
- Patients with parafunctional habits.

Advantages

- Highly esthetic
- Good bond strength
- Resistant to abrasion and fluid absorption
- Good periodontal health.

Disadvantages

- The fragile veneer can break
- Loss of glaze while finishing
- Technique sensitive
- Expensive and extensive tooth preparation.

Different technique

- Platinum foil is burnished onto the die on which porcelain is applied
- This prevents build up of heat during firing and increases surface area for etching.

Steps before bonding

1. Check for fit of veneer.
2. Color check:
   Place laminate on tooth with glycerine and compare it with shade tab. If laminate appears darker then select a lighter shade composite luting agent.
3. The actual composite is placed and trial checked.
4. Clean the veneers and isolate the tooth.
5. The etched surface of veneer is applied with silane coupling agent.
6. The tooth is cleaned and enamel etching is done with 30–37% phosphoric acid for 15–20 seconds.
7. The tooth is cleaned, isolated again and light activated dentin bonding agent is applied.
8. The veneer is seated with composite cement and cured.
9. Lingual finishing and occlusal equilibration is carried out.

Variations

Rochette's bridge with lingual retainers and interproximal retainers.

Resin Veneer Direct Technique

Indications

- For dark stains
- Patients with parafunctional habits.

Advantages

- Good esthetics, if color blending can be done
- The longevity is equally good for recent resins when compared to porcelain
- Easy to repair.

Disadvantages

- Can produce staining
- Less abrasion resistant.

Resin Veneer Indirect Technique

Indication

- Mildly stained or striated teeth
- For patients with parafunctional habits.

Advantages

- Can be used in patients with parafunctional habits
- Can be adjusted with ease.

Disadvantages

- Can produce staining
- Less abrasion resistant.

Indirect Composite Veneers

Indications

- Enamel defects
- Diastema closures.

Advantage

Easy preparation.

Disadvantage

Less bond strength.

Technique

1. Intra-enamel preparation or extra enamel preparation can be done.
2. Intra-enamel preparations are more accurate.
3. Shade selection of body and incisal shades is done and impression is made after gingival retraction.
4. Die is fabricated and veneer is made.
5. At the second appointment the seating is evaluated and the veneer is bonded with a mixture of Visi-fil (75%)/Visio-bond (25%) blend.

Recent Advances In Veneering Materials

Reinforced composites

Encore Bridge

- The composite superstructure is bonded with porcelain veneers
- It is composed of 81% filled composite with a glass fiber reinforcement (Sculpture/FiberKo, Jeneric/Pentron, Inc)
- The framework has sufficient flexure to attain a Class I mobility
- An all-porcelain bridge will not allow flexure.

Advantage

Tooth Preparation is minimal (only on lingual surface with a small proximal extension).

Technique

The preparation starts 1 mm from the most distal aspect of the lingual surface and extends into the proximal area.

Bonding the Framework

After verifying the fit, the framework was bonded into place with C&B-Metabond (Parkel I), after which the veneers are bonded onto the composite pontics with UltraBond (Den-Mat).

Targis/Vectris

A product from Ivoclar Williams.

Composition

It is a glass fiber-reinforced composite, with silanized glass fibers, a BIS-GMA matrix and an 85% ceramic-filled composite veneer.

Advantages

- Class I flexure attainable
- Good fracture resistance
- Esthetic properties comparable to metal-free ceramic restorations.

Variolink II System

A product from Ivoclar Vivadent.

Technique

1. After sandblasting the veneer under surfaces, they are silanated with Monobond-S.
2. The teeth are now isolated, and the preparations are etched.
3. The enamel is etched for 30 seconds and the dentin for 5 seconds.
4. The etchant is thoroughly washed away and the preparations dried.
5. Syntac dentin primer is applied for 15 seconds.
6. Teeth are dried.
7. Syntac dentin adhesive is then applied for 10 seconds and dried.
8. Heliobond (Ivoclar Vivadent) is applied to tooth and the under surface of the veneer inlays and luted with Variolink II cement (has different consistencies and shades) and cured.

Castable hydroxyapatite

Synonym: Cast apatite.

Hydroxyapatite mixed with composite fibers is slip cast by vibration.

Studies are yet to prove its clinical use.

Injectable ceramics/Castable ceramics

(Dicor, Cerestore)

Dicor (Tetrasilicic fluoromica)

It was earlier used for FPDs, inlays and onlays. Recently, it is used for laminate.

Indication

Laminates for periodontally compromised patients.

Contraindication
In short clinical crowns.

Advantages
- Good strength
- Good marginal adaptation
- Biocompatible
- Highly esthetic
- Low thermal conductivity.

Disadvantage
Tooth preparation is extensive.

Cerestore (shrink free ceramic system)

Indication
For periodontally compromised patients.

Advantages
- Good flexural strength
- Highly esthetic
- Good marginal fit.

19. Discuss in detail failures in fixed dental prosthesis.

Failure can occur as a result of an isolated incident, a progressive disease or bad planning or execution of the treatment plan.
Prevention is largely under the control of the patient assisted by the dentist in well made restorations.

Classification of failures (Flowchart 1)

Flowchart 1: Classification of failures[1,2]

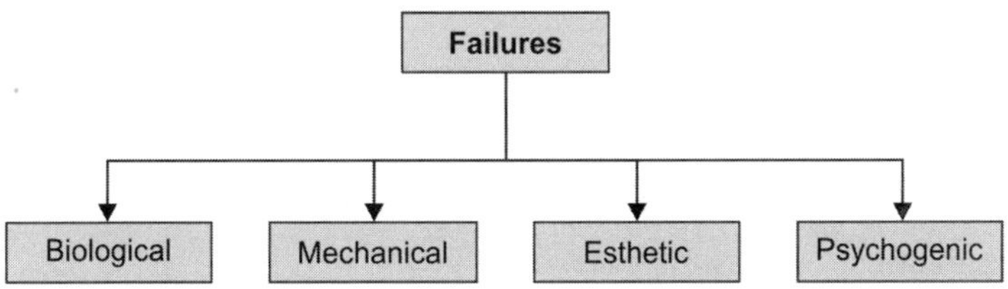

Biological failures
Some of the few biological failures include the following:
- Caries
- Pulpal degeneration
- Endodontic
- Periodontal
- Tooth perforation

- Sub-pontic inflammation
- Occlusal problems
- General pathosis
- Maintenance failure.

Caries

It is one of the commonest types of failure and can be due to secondary caries or caries in the abutment tooth.

Symptom

The patient may perceive this as pain, sensitivity to hot, cold or sweet substances.

Causes

Caries in teeth adjacent to fixed partial dentures due to poor proximal contact. Root caries in elderly patients or in patients undergoing radiotherapy.

Management

- Small carious lesions can be removed without removing the prosthesis and restored using amalgam, composite or glass ionomer
- Extensive caries require removal of the prosthesis followed by endodontic treatment and fabrication of new prosthesis.

Pulpal degeneration of abutment

Causes

Inadequate cooling during tooth preparation, abutments with old restoration, use of cements causing pulpal irritation, presence of occlusal forces.

Management

Access is made through the retainer and endodontic treatment is performed followed by post and core if required.

Endodontic failures

Causes

Inadequate endodontic treatment or an old root perforation.

Symptom

The patient perceives this as pain on biting or the presence of swelling.

Management

Endodontic retreatment if possible or as a last resort extraction. Generally retreatment must be done if required before the prosthesis fabrication itself.

Periodontal failures

Causes

Poor marginal adaptation, over contouring of retainer axial surfaces, large connectors, pontics contacting large tissue contact, prosthesis with rough surface, lack of abutment support, etc.

Management

Effective oral hygiene measures, periodontal therapy, or surgery Proper fabrication of prosthesis and proper maintenance can avoid this problem and prevent the failure.

Tooth perforation

Causes

Improper placement of pins, endodontic treatment, preparation of post and core.

Management

- If the defect occurs above the crest it can be covered up, below the crest it can be covered by periodontal surgery
- Defects in inaccessible areas can only be treated by extraction
- If pins or pinholes are the problems, only an endodontic treatment can save the tooth.

Subpontic inflammation

Causes

Excessive pressure by pontic due to improper pontic design or due to poor maintenance by the patient.

Symptom

Pain, swelling, bleeding gums or halitosis.

Management

Re-fabrication of the fixed prosthesis with modified pontic design. Reinforce hygiene instructions with stress on use of floss.

Occlusal problems

Causes

Interference in centric or eccentric contacts or an altered vertical dimension that can lead to pulpal damage and mobility causing unesthetic appearance.

Management

Refabrication of the prosthesis and if in a state of grade III mobility then extraction would be the only option.

General pathosis

Causes

Failure to diagnose a pathological change. More serious conditions must be treated before the treatment of missing teeth.

Maintenance failure

Causes

Failure of the dentist to prescribe a maintenance program, a recall system or inadequate motivation.

Mechanical failures

Loss of retention

Causes

Improper cementation, poor retention and resistance form, poor fit of casting, large span length and heavy occlusal forces. This in turn can cause marginal leakage and caries.

Management

If improper cementation is the cause then recementation needs to be done. If the design is the cause then a modification of design must be done and for repeated failure of long span bridges, removable prosthesis is the only option.

Connector failure

Causes

Supraeruption of opposing teeth, internal porosity, incomplete casting or soldering/welding.

Management

If the cause is supraeruption, then offending tooth must be contoured to provide adequate clearance. If severe, endodontic treatment may be required. If a casting defect is detected a new prosthesis must be made.

Occlusal wear

Causes

Insufficient thickness of restoration which can be due to inadequate preparation of occlusal surface. Bruxism, rough porcelain surface also can cause wear of occlusal surface.

Management

Modifying the preparation followed by new prosthesis, use of night guards; If bruxism is anticipated a metal occluding surface must be given.

Tooth fracture

Can be crown or root fracture.

Causes

- Crown fracture can occur due to excessive tooth preparation, endodontic treatment without post, interfering eccentric contacts, and unseating of cemented bridge
- Root fracture can be due to a poorly fitting post, post endodontic root fracture or increased load on endodontically treated teeth.

Management

- Small coronal fracture can be treated by a restoration
- Extensive fractures are treated with post and cores
- Root fractures must be extracted.

Metal–ceramic fracture

Causes

Improper framework design, heavy occlusal force, distorted impression, perforation in metal, unsupported porcelain and metal porcelain incompatibility.

Management

Resin repair using composite resin or the facing can be repaired with porcelain by attaching the portion with pins. If fracture is extensive redo the prosthesis.

All ceramic fracture

Causes

Inadequate finish line, sharp area on prepared tooth, round preparation without resistance forms, over prepared tooth, opposing tooth contact located incisal to prepared tooth and inadequate lingual tooth preparation.

Management

Remaking the prosthesis.

Esthetic failure

Causes

- Immediate esthetic failure can be due to poor shade match, poor tooth and gingival contour, poor marginal placement, framework displaying the metal and unrealistic expectations of the patients
- Delayed esthetic failure can occur due to gingival recession, sub pontic tissue shrinkage following extraction, after periodontal surgery, unglazed porcelain can lead to black specks overtime.

Psychogenic failure

Causes

Frequent complaints can be attributed to stress and behavioral changes in the individual. These patients require counseling and should be identified in the diagnostic phase itself.

Conclusion

Finally to resolve the failure in an effective and economical manner, ascertain the cause and re-evaluate the treatment plan and all the factors associated with failure.

References

1. Smith BGN, Howe LC. Planning and making crowns and bridges, ed4. Informa Healthcare; 2007.
2. Rangarajan V, Padmanabhan TV. Text book of prosthodontics. Elsevier; 2013.

IMPLANT DENTISTRY

20. Classify and discuss on various impression procedures involved in implant-supported prosthesis.

Definition

An impression is defined as the negative replica of teeth and the oral tissues.

Criteria for good impression

- Must accurately record the soft tissue and supporting areas
- Able to record the positioning of the implant components
- The resiliency difference between the implant and the mucosa should also be considered in the impression technique used
- Inaccuracies in impression can cause misfit of the prosthesis, uneven force distribution, abutment screw loosening and occlusal inaccuracies.

Classification

General classification[1,2]

- Direct transfer (open-tray impression technique)
- Indirect transfer (closed-tray impression technique).

Other systems

Virtual impression system

Other classifications

Are modifications of above two techniques by utilizing different—

- Impression materials
- Tray
- Type of transfer—Abutment or implant level
- In the type of derived support.

Techniques[3-5]

- Direct impression transfer (open-tray impression technique)
- It is the most accurate type of implant impression transfer in which impression transfer copings are picked with the impression. The transfer coping are disengaged through the impression trays opening after polymerization of impression and removed along with the impression (Fig. 41).

Armamentarium

1. Custom tray/stock-tray.
2. Tray adhesive.
3. Modelling wax.
4. Medium-bodied and light-bodied polyvinyl siloxane impression material.
5. Essential implant components alike transfer coping, lab analogues, abutments, hex drivers.

Procedure

- A custom acrylic resin tray is fabricated from the primary cast with openings in the area where the implants are located or a stock tray is perforated in the region of implant

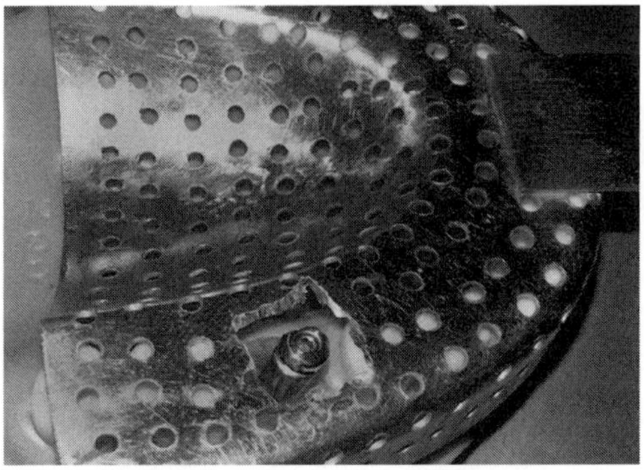

Fig. 41: Open tray for impression

- The healing abutments are removed and implant impression copings are placed. The approximation of components is verified with radiographs
- The impression tray is evaluated for good adaptation, uniform impression material space and for adequate clearances for the impression coping to protrude through the openings of the tray
- The excessive openings are sealed with the modelling wax
- Adequate amount of tray adhesive is coated on the tissue surface of impression tray
- Impression is made with medium body or monophase polysiloxane impression material. The tray is seated intraorally with all the impression coping pins protruding through the opening of tray
- After complete polymerization of the impression material the excess wax or impression material on the guide pins are removed from the impression pins for the drivers to gain acces
- The impression copings are disengaged from the implants and impression is removed from the patient's mouth (Fig. 42)
- The impression is evaluated, disinfected and components are replaced with suitable laboratory analogues
- Master cast is made with type IV gypsum product.

Advantages of Open Tray Technique

- Accurate
- The best technique for angulated implants
- Ideal for multiple implant restorations.

Disadvantages

- Accurate only with the use of custom trays hence, additional steps in the fabrication procedure of custom trays
- Not suitable in patients with restricted mouth opening and in posterior edentulous regions with reduced access.

Closed Tray Technique

In this technique the impression copings remain in the mouth on the removal of the set impressions. After removing the set impression from the mouth the copings are transferred or oriented to the set impressions.

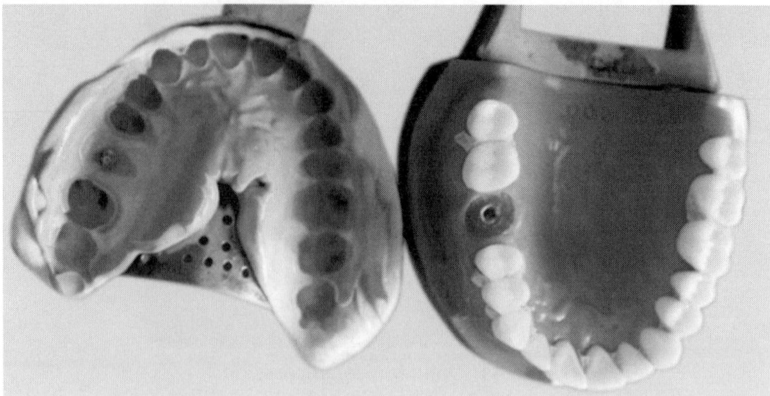

Fig. 42: Direct impression transfer technique

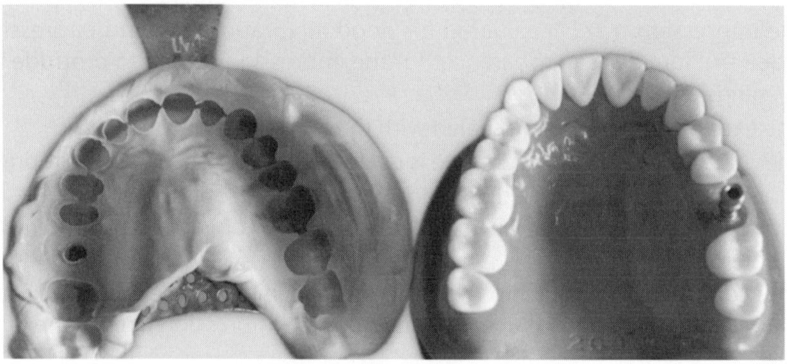

Fig. 43: Indirect transfer technique

Procedure
- The transfer coping is fixed to the implant after removing the healing abutments
- The screw of transfer coping are blocked with cotton balls or modelling wax
- Radiographs are made for verification of approximation of coping and implant
- Suitable stock or custom tray is selected
- A regular precaution of tray selection and adhesive application is followed
- Light-body viscosity material is injected around the implant and the tray is loaded with putty viscosity impression material and seated intraorally
- The set impression material is removed from the mouth and the components are approximated extra orally (Fig. 43)
- The evaluated impression is disinfected and type IV gypsum cast is made.

Advantages
- Simple and easy to follow
- May not require custom tray
- Is ideal in case of restricted mouth opening

- Employed for simple implant prosthesis as single crowns and small span FPD with parallel implant abutments.

Disadvantages

Reorientation of copings can incorporate errors that can lead to inaccuracy and poor fit of the prosthesis.

Virtual Impression System

- This is a CAD–CAM system
- Eliminates the inaccuracies possible in direct and indirect transfer impressions.

Procedure

- An optical scanner reads and translates the codes embedded in the healing abutments
- This data is transferred to the CAD software, the implant abutments are virtually designed and the CAM milling apparatus produces the final titanium abutments
- The completed abutments are returned to the laboratory for the completion of definitive prosthesis using conventional technique or by CAD–CAM procedure.

Advantages

- Offer options of both stock and custom abutments without their associated disadvantages
- Are custom made for each patient and hence possess the optimal peri-implant soft tissue support
- Require no manipulation after they are machined resulting in a more precise fit.

Modification in techniques by type of impression materials used[6]

- The most ideal materials for the implant prosthetic use (in the order of preference) are addition silicone, polyether and condensation silicone (Tables 2 and 3)
- The putty and light-body materials are used in combination
- Ideally auto mixing devices are preferred for better material properties.

Table 2: Summary of the merits and demerits of elastomeric impression materials

Material	Merits	Demerits
Polysulfide	Long working time High tear resistance Modest cost	To pour impression immediately Stretching leads to distortion Stains clothing Obnoxious odor
Condensation Silicon	Good working time Clean and pleasant	High polymerization shrinkage due to volatile by product Low tear strength Immediate pour for accuracy
Addition silicone	Clean and pleasant Ideally elastic Repeated pour can be done Stable dimensionally	Low tear strength High cost
Polyether	Good stability Delay pour Shelf life: 2 year	Bitter taste Leaches components High cost

Table 3: Comparison of properties of elastic impression materials

Property	Polysulfide	Condensation	Addition	Polyether
Tear resistance	+++	++	++	++
Elasticity	+++	++++	++++	++
Accuracy	+++	++	++++	+++
Dimensional stability	++	++	++++	++++

++ -Adequate, +++ - Good, ++++ - Very good

Impression trays

- Both stock and custom trays can be used
- Conventional method of evaluating the extension of tray is followed
- In order to accommodate the transfer copings the tray materials must be easier to modify
- Tray material needs to be rigid.

Tray Adhesive

Composition—Silicone adhesive (styrene acrylonitrate) dissolved in solvent, such as ketone, ethyl acetate or chloroform and colorant.

Significance

- The adhesive ensures that the impression remains firmly attached to the tray upon removal from the mouth
- Inadvertent tray separation while removing impression from mouth can lead to distortion errors.

Procedure

- A thin layer of tray adhesive is applied onto the inner surface of tray and allowed to air dry for at least five minutes, but no more than 30 minutes
- Mix and place desired tray viscosity impression material directly into coated impression tray in accordance to the manufacturer instructions.

Gingival Retraction

Before impression making gingival retraction need to be done.

Procedure

- Fix the desired abutment to the implant
- Fit the appropriate retractor impression cap over the abutments and on the exposed portion of the dental implant
- Move and verify the retractor cap to verify the snap fit without impinging adjacent teeth
- Inject the light body material into the impression cap and place heavy-body material, in the tray, over the impression caps
- Remove impression from the patient and inspect for accuracy. Secure the impression cap so that it has not been dislodged or so that its position has not been distorted
- Snap the shoulder analog on the white nylon gingival retractor impression cap in the final impression. Ensure that no change of portion or distortion has occurred when snapping shoulder analog in the cap

- Pour the impression in type IV die stone. Place the reinforcement pin in the assembly as the impression cap/shoulder analog is filled with stone.

Disinfection of Impression

On intra oral removal of impression immediately rinse with tap water, dry with an air syringe and disinfect with suitable disinfectants (Table 4).

Table 4: Recommended disinfectants for elastomers

Disinfectant	Polysulfide	Silicones	Polyether
Glutaraldehyde 2% (10 minutes soak time)	Yes	No	No
Iodophors	Yes	Yes	No
Chlorine compounds	Yes	Yes	Yes
Complex phenols	Yes	Yes	No
Phenolic glutaraldehyde	Yes	Yes	No

Repeat impression

Impression must be repeated if:
- Visible streaks of base or catalyst material is evident
- The tray exposure in vital areas. This can be due to inaccurate seating of the tray
- Occurrence of voids, folds or creases in critical areas
- Separation of the impression material from the impression tray.

Cast making

- There should be no impression material present between the critical implant components, impression coping and abutment
- The corresponding abutment or analogues is carefully threaded onto the impression
- The soft tissue mask is injected around the implant region to simulate soft tissue. The impression is trimmed, boxed and poured with type IV gypsum
- Once the stone has set completely, the transfer copings or corresponding analogues are removed.

References

1. Misch CE. Dental Implant Prosthetics. St Louis: Elsevier Mosby; 2004.
2. Misch, CE. 2nd. ed. Contemporary Implant Dentistry. St. Louis: Mosby.
3. Lee H, So JS, Hochstedler JL, Ercoli C. The accuracy of implant impressions: a systematic review. J Prosthet Dent. 2008 Oct; 100(4):285-91.
4. Burns J, Palmer R, Howe L, Wilson R. Accuracy of open tray implant impressions: an in vitro comparison of stock versus custom trays. J Prosthet Dent. 2003 Mar;89(3):250-5.
5. Bambini F, Ginnetti L, Memè L, Pellecchia M, Selvaggio R. Comparative analysis of direct and indirect implant impression techniques an in vitro study. An in vitro study. Minerva Stomatol. 2005 Jun;54(6):395-402.
6. Donovan TE, Chee WW. A review of contemporary impression materials and techniques. Dent Clin North Am. 2004 Apr;48(2):vi-vii, 445-70. Review.

21. Discuss on implants for fixed prosthesis work.

Definition

Dental implant prosthesis is defined as any prosthesis that utilizes dental implants in part or whole for retention, support and stability.

Advantages of implants over conventional prosthesis (Table 5):[1]

- Esthetics and functions are better
- The bone resorption is reduced by keeping the bone functionally active
- Occlusal and muscle functions are improved
- Improved proprioception, increase in success rate, and enhanced function has better psychological impact on the patient
- Prosthesis design is simpler even in distal extension situations with implant-supported FPD improving function and patient acceptance
- Caries, periodontal break down, teeth fracture are not associated with implant-supported FPD.

Table 5: Differences between implant and conventional FPD[2,3]

Implant-supported FPD	Tooth-supported FPD
Implants take support from adjoining bone	Support derived from adjacent teeth
Bone resorption in partially edentulous region is reduced	Bone resorption in partially edentulous region is more than implant-supported FPD
Better psychological impact on the patient.	Tooth preparation of adjacent teeth can affect patient psychologically
Prosthesis design is possible and simpler even in distal extension situations	Prosthesis design is complicated in distal extension situations
No postoperative complaints of teeth like caries, periodontal breakdown is expected	Caries, periodontal breakdown are expected if not properly maintained
Patient comfort and ease of maintenance is more	Patient comfort and ease of maintenance is less.
Involves surgical procedure	Simplified intraoperatory procedure

Types of Fixed Prosthesis supported by Implants

Based on implant type

- Subperiosteal implants
  - Unilateral
  - Interdental
  - Total
  - Circumferential.
- Transosteal implant/mandibular staple/transmandibur
- Endosteal implant.

Based on implant macro surface

- Threaded, non-threaded
- Tapered, parallel

- With vent holes, without vent holes
- Hollow cylinder, solid screws
- Root form, blade form.

Based on implant material

- Metallic implants commercially pure titanium
  - Titanium alloy
  - Cobalt chromium molybdenum alloy.
- Nonmetallic implants
  - Ceramics
  - Carbon.

Based on implant surface

- Turned surface/machined surface
- Titanium plasma spraying
- Hydroxyappetite coating
- Blasting
- Acid etching
- Combination—etching and blasting
- Electrochemical oxidation surface
- Ion implementation
- Doped surface
- Other surface modifications.

Based on type of prosthesis

- Single crown
- Cantilever prosthesis
- Three-unit FPD
- Multiple-unit FPD
- Segmental or full-arch prosthesis
- Over dentures.

Based on type of prosthesis materials

- Ceramic FPD
- Metal ceramic FPD
- Metal FPD
- Acrylic FPD
- Reinforced acrylic FPD.

Based on prosthesis movement

- PM0: Rigid no movement—O ring with bar
- PM2: Hinge movement—Dolder bar
- PM3: Apical and hinge movement—Dolder bar with spacer and clip
- PM4: Moves in all directions
- PM6: All range of movement—Resilient ERA.

Misch classification of implant prosthesis

- FP1
- FP2
- FP3
- RP4
- RP5.

Misch implant prosthesis classification

Misch classified five possible combinations of implant prosthesis which enlist three types for FPD and two for RPD. They are as follows:

FP 1

Fixed prosthesis that replaces the anatomic crown of missing natural teeth.

Criteria

- The residual bone quality and quantity should be good
- It is more seen in maxillary anterior situations
- The material of choice is all ceramic or noble materials because of less corrosive action of noble metal when compared to base-metals
- Soft tissue augmentation might be needed as interdental papilla might be missing in majority of the situations
- To regenerate or improve inter-proximal position for ideal esthetics and function.

FP 2

It restores crown and a portion of the root similar to the situations exhibiting gingival recession or periodontal pockets.

- The restoration fabricated is similar to position of adjacent teeth on occlusal or incisal surface but the margins extend towards gingival surface both facially and palatally
- The restoration has to be fabricated with metal ceramic or all ceramic. The extended cervical borders have to be matched to gingival color.

FP 3

FPD restores crown, gingiva and a portion of soft tissue of edentulous site.

- This situation arises due to greater bone loss or lesser availability of bone in the partially edentulous area
- All precautions have to be followed during restoration to check for cantilever action, function and esthetics.

RP 4

Removable prosthesis where the over denture is completely supported by implant

- Ideally 5 implants for mandible and 8 implants for maxilla are placed for supporting the restoration
- The superstructure additionally might have attachments and majority of the prosthesis is fabricated with acrylic teeth and supported by acrylic denture base.

RP 5

Removable prosthesis in which over-denture is supported by both soft tissue and implant.

- The prosthesis is supported with lesser implants

- The movement of prosthesis is controlled by obtaining support from both implant and the soft tissues
- The major limitation of this design is bone resorption in partially edentulous area which might necessitate frequent relining of dentures (Table 6).

Table 6: Differences between screw-retained and cement-retained implants[4-6]

Cement-retained prosthesis	Screw-retained prosthesis
Surgical placement of implants for cement prosthesis is easier. Smaller angulations can be accommodated	Meticulous surgical planning is essential. Access hole for screw might be difficult to locate
Prosthesis fit is more passive	Less passive when compared to cement-retained prosthesis
Highly esthetic since no openings are displayed on the crown	Screw opening might be visible on crown which can alter the esthetic value
Retrievability of crown is slightly difficult when compared to screw-retained prosthesis	Retrievability of crown is easier
Retention is good but can be compromised in limited interocclusal space	Retention of prosthesis can be achieved even in minimal inter-occlusal space
Best occlusal form can be obtained	Occlusal form gets altered due to the screw access opening
Impression procedures are slightly complicated when compared to screw-retained prosthesis	Impression procedures are relatively easy
Repair of prosthesis is difficult	Repair of prosthesis is easy
Cement might extrude to mucosal tissue which might be difficult to remove	Inter proximation of machined parts, no issues of cement
Cement entering the surgical site can interfere with the healing site of immediate implants	No cement can be more ideal for healing of immediate loading implants
The expansion or alteration of peri-implant mucosa with cemented provisional is difficult	It is easy to expand the peri-implant mucosa

Types of restoration[7,8]

Types include single crown, multiple-unit FPD and fixed removable prosthesis (FRP-Hybrid prosthesis).

The biomechanical factors that can influence the treatment plan are as follows:

Prosthesis forces on implant—Utmost care is taken to avoid deflective contacts.

Angulated abutment—Greater than 25 degrees generates more nonaxial forces and crestal bone loss hence, use of straight abutments are preferred.

Cantilever prosthesis—Advocated in lower denture than maxillary denture without deflective occlusal contacts.

Occlusal forces and pattern—All nonaxial forces have to be reduced in the prosthesis design by:

- Directing forces on occlusal contacts towards the central fossa
- Reducing the inclination of cusps of the restored teeth

- Reducing the size of occlusal table
- Any existences of parafunctional forces are relieved by protecting restorations in the form of night guards or splints.

Design of Superstructure—

- A maximum of 4–6 μm is the permissible space between the prosthesis and abutment
- Very minor numerical differences in force transmission exist between acrylic, metal and ceramic hence, the prosthesis design matters more
- In case an implant and tooth are joined, a rigid connection is preferred.

Risk factors involved in the FPD designing can arise due to the following:

- Design geometry
- Supporting structures
- Prosthetic factors.

Design Geometry

The risk factors that influence the design geometry are the number of implant, type of platform, positioning and connection of implants. The number of implants to be placed depends on the number of roots of the teeth rather than number of teeth[9] (e.g. it is preferential to have two implants for mandibular molar).

The other factors that reduces risk factors in design geometry are as follows:

- The wider implant platform to be used
- Cantilevering of implant prosthesis to be avoided
- Implants to be placed near to prosthesis aids in transmitting more of axial forces
- Proper crown: implant ratio to be maintained.

Supporting structures

Structures are the bone support, primary stability of implant during postsurgical stage and implant dimension.

Prosthetic factors

Prosthetic risk factor can be reduced by the following:

- Passive and accurate fit of the prosthesis
- Following more established and accepted procedures for prosthesis fabrication
- Premachined prosthetic components are more scientific and easier to use
- Proper use and applications of implant armamentarium. Standardized instruments with a stable and predefined tightening torque aids in reducing the future hazards
- Good overall treatment planning assessment to prevent bone component failures, ceramic fracture, screw loosening and bone resorption.

Conclusion

Extreme care in diagnosing, designing, surgical planning, fabrication and maintenance of restoration for good prognosis.

References

1. Layton D. A critical appraisal of the survival and complication rates of tooth-supported all-ceramic and metal-ceramic fixed dental prostheses: The application of evidence-based dentistry. Int J Prosthodont. 2011;24(5):417-27. Review.
2. Abt E, Carr AB, Worthington HV. Interventions for replacing missing teeth: Partially absent dentition. Cochrane Database Syst Rev. 2012;2:CD003814.
3. Salvi GE, Brägger U. Mechanical and technical risks in implant therapy. Int J Oral Maxillofac Implants. 2009;24 Suppl:69-85. Review.
4. Shadid R, Sadaqa N. A comparison between screw- and cement-retained implant prostheses. A literature review. J Oral Implantol. 2012;38(3):298-307.
5. Chaar MS, Att W, Strub JR. Prosthetic outcome of cement-retained implant-supported fixed dental restorations: A systematic review. J Oral Rehabil. 2011;38(9):697-711.
6. Wittneben JG, Millen C, Brägger U. Clinical performance of screw- versus cement-retained fixed implant-supported reconstructions--a systematic review. Int J Oral Maxillofac Implants. 2014;29 Suppl:84-98.
7. Pjetursson BE, Lang NP. Prosthetic treatment planning on the basis of scientific evidence. J Oral Rehabil. 2008;35 Suppl 1:72-9.
8. Mamalis A, Markopoulou K, Kaloumenos K, Analitis A. Splinting osseointegrated implants and natural teeth in partially edentulous patients: A systematic review of the literature. J Oral Implantol. 2012;38(4):424-34.
9. Hoffmann O, Zafiropoulos GG. Tooth-implant connection: A review. J Oral Implantol. 2012; 38(2):194-200.

22. Classify types of implants and discuss the role of surface topography of implants in osseointegration.

Definitions

The dental implant is defined as a prosthetic device made of alloplastic material(s) implanted into the oral tissues beneath the mucosal or periosteal layer on or within the bone to provide retention and support for a fixed or removable dental prosthesis; a substance that is placed upon the jaw bone to support a fixed or removable dental prosthesis.

Osseointegration—The process and resultant apparent direct connection of an exogenous material's surface and the host bone tissues, without intervening fibrous connective tissue present.

Classification of implants

The implants are classified on the basis of tissue placement, materials, based upon bone attachment, shape, surgical stage, upon angle of insertion and tissue - systemic responses[1] (Table 7).

Classified according to the tissue engagement as:

- **Subperiosteal implants**: An implant that is placed beneath the periosteum of the bone, it receives its primary bone support by resting on it (unilateral, interdental, total and circumferential)
- **Transosteal implant/mandibular staple/transmandibur**: A dental implant that penetrates both cortical plates and passes through the entire thickness of the alveolar bone

Table 7: Classification of implants based on different parameters	
Based upon	**Types**
Placement within the tissue	1. Subperiosteal implants – Unilateral – Interdental – Total – Circumferential 2. Transosteal implant/mandibular staple/transmandibur 3. Endosteal implant
Based upon materials used	1. Metallic implants, commercially pure titanium – Titanium alloy – Cobalt–chromium–molybdenum alloy – Non metallic implants – Ceramics – Carbon
Based upon the attachment mechanism	1. Osseointegration 2. Fibro osseous integration
Based upon the macro-design	1. Thread, nonthreaded 2. Tapered, parallel 3. With vent holes, without vent holes 4. Hollow cylinder, solid screws 5. Root form, blade form
Based upon the surgical stage	1. One-stage implant 2. Two-stage implant
Based upon mode of insertion	1. Axillary inserted (crestal approach) 2. Laterally inserted (basal approach)
Based upon tissue response and systemic toxicity effect of implants	1. Biotolerant materials—Polymethyl methacrylate 2. Bioinert materials—Titanium and aluminium oxide 3. Bioactive materials—Glass and calcium phosphate ceramic

- **Endosteal implant**: An implant that is present within the bone extending into basal bone for support (screw form, cylinder form and blade form).

Classification based on the degree of roughness, surface treatment and manufacturing process (Table 8).

Significance of implant surface and osseointegration[2,3]

- Enhances cellular activity and bone apposition
- The bone-to-implant contact (BIC) is enhanced with improved effects on cell migration, proliferation, biomaterial–tissue interaction
- In the early healing stages the implant surface properties provides ideal biological and chemical properties
- The implant surface chemistry can modify the interactions, protein adsorption and cellular activity
- Surface morphology with defined microstructures enhance stable anchorage, increases the wettability and osteoblast activity

Table 8: Classification of various implant surfaces	
Based on	**Types**
1. Degree of roughness	1. Isotropic 2. Anisotropic
2. Surface treatment	1. Additive surface 2. Subtractive surface 3. Modifications
3. Manufacturing process	1. Turned surface/machined surface 2. Titantium plasma spraying 3. Hydroxyapatite coating 4. Blasting 5. Acid etching 6. Combination—etching and blasting 7. Electrochemical oxidation surface 8. Ion implementation 9. Doped surface 10. Other surface modifications

- The expressions of bone-specific differentiation factors for osteoblasts are higher and blood coagulation is better on hydrophilic surfaces.

Implant surfaces[4]

Implant surface roughness is divided, depending on the dimension of the measured surface features into macro, micro- and nano-roughness.

Macro roughness

- Range of millimeters to tens of microns
- Directly relates to implant geometry, with threaded screw and macro porous surface treatments
- The primary implant fixation and long-term mechanical stability can be improved by an appropriate macro-roughness
- The macro-roughness enhances the mechanical interlocking between the implant surface and the surrounding bone.

Micro-roughness

Defined as being in the range of 1–10 µm. This range of roughness maximizes the interlocking between mineralized bone and implant surface.

Nano-roughness

Composed of nano-sized materials with a size range between 1 and 100 nm. They increase the process of bone growth, turnover and remodeling.

Various surface treatments[5]

Additive surface

The implant surfaces are modified with an addition of material that increases the implant surface area and enhances osseointegration. E.g. titanium plasma spraying (TPS) technique and hydroxyapatite coating (HA) technique.

Subtractive surface

Indents the implant surfaces with a suitable medium and thus, increases the implant surface area. E.g. blasting with titanium oxide/aluminum oxide and acid etching.

Based on manufacturing process

Turned surface/machined surface

When the titanium rod is loaded to the machine which turns titanium into screw or cylinder.

Titanium plasma spraying (TPS)

Titanium powder particles are plasma sprayed through a nozzle at a temperatures of around 1500 degrees centigrade under argon gas atmosphere at a velocity 600 m/s that results in 0.04–0.06 mm diameter projections.

Advantage

Primary stability is enhanced and surface area is increased to 5–6 times.

Hydroxyapatite coating (HA)

HA-coated implant has a bioactive surface with increased primary stability due to the greater bone to implant contact area.

Indication

Type IV bone, fresh extraction sites and newly grafted sites.

Blasting with titanium oxide/aluminum oxide

The implant surface is bombarded with particles of aluminum oxide (Al_2O_3) or titanium oxide (TiO_2) to produce a rough surface with irregular pits and depressions.
Blasting with $Al2O_3$ particles of 25–75 µm produces surfaces with roughness values of 1.16–1.20 µm, respectively.

Limitations

Embedded remaining particles interferes with osseointegration hence, resorbable blast medium (RBM), such as hydroxyapatite and calcium phosphate are substituted.

Acid etching

- A mixture of acids like HCL and H_2SO_4 is used. Other acids used for etching are HF, HNO_3 and H_2O_2
- The acid concentration, type of acids, temperature and duration of contact are determining factors in creating ideal surface microstructure.

Combination (SLA)

- The combination of two subtractive techniques, such as sand-blasted large-grit acid-etched technique (SLA) is the commonest example of this category
- This surface is produced by a large grit (250–500 µm) blasting process followed by etching with hydrochloric–sulfuric acid.

Objectives

Sand blasting creates surface roughness and acid etching cleans the surfaces producing a micro surface.

Electrochemical oxidized surface

A 3–10 nm coating is made on the implant by electrochemical process which improves the corrosion, wear resistance and increases osseointegration.

Ion implantation

High-energy nitrogen ion or calcium ion are added on to the implant surface using higher surface energy. These treatments are usually done in medical grade instruments to increase hardness, corrosion resistance and wear resistance.

Doped surface

Coating surfaces through sol–gel technique with various types of bone growth factors or other bone-stimulating agents enhance growth of bone and osseointegration.

Disadvantages

Include disintegration of coating during implant placement, plaque retention, greater chances of failure and increased cost.

Other surface coatings

Nanosized hydroxyapatite coated on nanotubular Ti surface promotes osteoblast cell adhesion and deposition of osteoblast.

Oxidation of implant surfaces with chemicals and laser roughening are the other methods.

References

1. Dohan Ehrenfest DM, Coelho PG, Kang BS, Sul YT, Albrektsson T. Classification of osseointegrated implant surfaces: Materials, chemistry and topography. Trends Biotechnol. 2010;28(4):198-206.
2. Gaviria L, Salcido JP, Guda T, Ong JL. Current trends in dental implants. J Korean Assoc Oral Maxillofac Surg. 2014;40(2):50-60.
3. Gittens RA, Scheideler L, Rupp F, Hyzy SL, Geis-Gerstorfer J, Schwartz Z, Boyan BD. A review on the wettability of dental implant surfaces II: Biological and clinical aspects. Acta Biomater. 2014;10(7):2907-18.
4. Novaes AB Jr, de Souza SL, de Barros RR, Pereira KK, Iezzi G, Piattelli A. Influence of implant surfaces on osseointegration. Braz Dent J. 2010;21(6):471-81. Review.
5. Anil S, Anand PS, Alghamdi H, Jansen JA (2011). Dental implant surface enhancement and osseointegration, implant dentistry–A rapidly evolving practice, Prof. Ilser Turkyilmaz (Ed.), ISBN: 978-953- 307-658-4.

23. Explain procedural options for single-tooth implant prosthesis.

Single-tooth partially edentulous space is the most frequently encountered clinical situations. The success rate of single-tooth implant depends on selection of patients, vigilant clinical procedures and follow-up protocol.

Indications

- Loss of teeth due to caries
- Endodontic failure
- Trauma
- Infection
- Fracture
- Repeated restorative failure.

Contraindications

- Reduced intertooth space—can alter the contour and form of the restoration leading to overcontouring of crown
- Insufficient bone width, height and volume—A minimum width of 5 mm of labiopalatal thickness and 10 mm of height is essential
- Poor periodontal health of adjacent teeth—can affect the bone density, volume and resorption of the adjacent edentulous area.

Advantages of single-tooth implant compared to fixed partial denture

- It is more conservative option
- Success of single-tooth implant restoration is greater
- Bone resorption is controlled in edentulous region and the bone health is maintained for longer period of time when compared to the conventional prosthesis
- It reduces the failure of abutment teeth which is commonly seen in tooth-supported prosthesis
- Post restorative complaints of sensitivity, tooth failure, need of endodontic treatment and poor gingival health are reduced with single-implant restoration
- Improve psychological comfort for patients.

Disadvantages

- The time spent both by the dentist and the patient on the treatment is more
- Expensive when compared to the conventional treatment modalities
- The problems associated with implant failure can affect the patient psychology and future decisions on the treatment modalities.

Factors affecting Treatment plan:[1,2]

- Patient age—Young patients
- Patient need—all treatment options need to be discussed
- Duration of treatment—3–6 months in delayed loading procedure
- Cost—Expensive
- Provisional restorations—In majority of situations, transitional removable partial denture is given to the patient
- Periodontal health—The patient has to be motivated to improve and maintain the periodontal heath
- Inter-tooth space—An implant should be placed at least 1.5–2 mm away from the adjacent teeth and should possess a minimum of 6.5 mm of mesiodistal space to achieve good esthetics and ideal function
- Bone dimensions and tissue support—if limitations exist in sufficient bone dimensions then augmentation, grafts and other options of enhancing the dimensions have to be verified before implant placement.

Treatment planning

A comprehensive data on medical history, dental history, radiographs, study casts, photographs are essential for the treatment planning.[3]

The dimensions of the implants are determined from diagnostic records, radiographs and in some cases the scans. The width of the implant can also be determined by bone mapping.

Procedure

- Determine the implant dimensions with suitable radiographs and bone mapping
- Make a surgical stent that guides in implant placement
- Disinfect and prepare the surgical site for implant placement
- Surgical incision is made along the crest of the edentulous area (palatal crestal line angle). A relief labial incision is placed involving interdental papilla. Full-thickness mucoperiosteoum flap is raised
- The surgical round bur is used to perforate the center of the bone cortex and that will facilitate the guiding of other drills
- Sequential drilling with different osteotomes is done in accordance to implant dimensions. One width shorter than width of implant dimension at same height of implant is preferred (osteotomy method for tapered-screw implants)
- Torque the implant on to the prepared osteotomy site
- In case of insufficient labial bone, subsequent bone grafting procedure have to done
- Place the cover screw and close the surgical site with interrupted sutures
- Sutures are removed after a week and evaluated for postoperative complications.

Second stage surgery

- Access for the cover screw either by surgical incision or punch technique
- Remove the cover screw and fix the gingival former. Wait for a period of 4–6 weeks for tissue cover or gingival cuff to be formed
- The gingival former is removed after a period of 4 weeks and subsequent procedures for fabricating the restoration is done.

Impression transfer

- The impression transfer can be done by direct or indirect method. The direct method is done with the impression post transfer, lab analogues are fixed to the impression post and cast is made. In indirect technique, implant abutment alterations are made intraorally and impression made like tooth-supported FPD
- The restorations are fabricated on the cast, try-in done on patients, milled abutments are torqued to 30N and restoration cemented.

Cementation of restoration

Cementation is done after checking for occlusal contacts and if any deflective contacts are present they are removed.

Additional care in single restorations

1. A proper chamfer or if the implant angulation and coping are placed labially, shoulder finish line is preferred.
2. Chosing a proper abutment platform depending on the clinical situation
3. Soft mask simulating gingiva provides the technician information of gingival margin that aids in designing the restoration.
4. The implant body has to be placed 4–5 mm below the CE junction of adjacent teeth predicting the labial bone resorption.

Evidence-based Study reports[4-6]

- Based on the meta-analysis of Jung et al, the survival rate of single crown implants are 97.2% for 5 years and 95.2% for 10 years
- The biological complications for a 5-year cumulative soft tissue complication rate of 7.1% and a cumulative complication rate for implants with bone loss >2 mm of 5.2% were calculated
- Technical complications reached a cumulative incidence of 8.8% for screw-loosening, 4.1% for loss of retention, and 3.5% for veneer fracture after 5 years
- The cumulative 5-year esthetic complication rate amounted to 7.1%
- The outcomes of the meta-analysis demonstrated high implant survival rates for both the single-tooth implants and the respective single crowns after 5 and 10 years.

References

1. Atieh MA, Atieh AH, Payne AG, Duncan WJ. Immediate loading with single implant crowns: A systematic review and meta-analysis. Int J Prosthodont. 2009;22(4):378-87. Review.
2. Lewis MB, Klineberg I. Prosthodontic considerations designed to optimize outcomes for single-tooth implants. A review of the literature. Aust Dent J. 2011;56(2):181-92.
3. Shah KC, Lum MG. Treatment planning for the single-tooth implant restoration--general considerations and the pretreatment evaluation. J Calif Dent Assoc. 2008;36(11):827-34.
4. Benic GI, Mir-Mari J, Hämmerle CH. Loading protocols for single-implant crowns: A systematic review and meta-analysis. Int J Oral Maxillofac Implants. 2014;29 Suppl:222-38.
5. Annibali S, Bignozzi I, Iacovazzi L, La Monaca G, Cristalli MP. Immediate, early, and late implant placement in first-molar sites: A retrospective case series. Int J Oral Maxillofac Implants. 2011;26(5):1108-22.
6. Jung RE, Zembic A, Pjetursson BE, Zwahlen M, Thoma DS. Systematic review of the survival rate and the incidence of biological, technical, and aesthetic complications of single crowns on implants reported in longitudinal studies with a mean follow-up of 5 years. Clin Oral Implants Res. 2012;23 Suppl 6:2-21.

24. Discuss the immediate loading and progressive loading of endosseous implants.

Definitions

Immediate loading

The prosthesis is attached to the implant within 24 hours of the implant being placed.

Early loading

The prosthesis is attached to the implant within days/weeks of the implant being placed.

Delayed loading

The prosthesis is attached to implant after a healing period of 3–6 months (Table 9).

Conventional or delayed loading protocol

Was initially proposed by Brånemark where a waiting period is essential for the implant to osseointegrate and the prosthesis is fabricated after the delayed waiting time after complete integration.

Advantages of the delayed protocol

- It can be used on weaker bone in both quality and quantity. The procedure provides sufficient time for the bone to heal and implant to integrate
- The stimulatory forces of bone metabolism aid in improving the bone density and enhance osseointegration
- Improved bone architecture and bone forming factors around implant is achieved better with delayed loading protocol
- Extensively documented data available on its success
- Increased predictability of osseointegration.

The prosthodontic loading time in delayed protocol varies with the type of bone, jaw and span of the restoration. The maxilla has increased waiting time than mandible because of lesser quality of bone. The universal waiting period for different bone type are listed below:

Table 9: Type of bone and waiting period before implant loading

Type of bone	D1	D2	D3	D4
Maxilla	6 months	6 months	6–8 months	6–8 months
Mandible	3 months	3 months	4–6 months	4–6 months

Disadvantages of progressive loading

- Time taken to fabricate the restoration. It can vary between 3 and 6 months depending on type of bone and prosthesis
- Patient psychology can be affected due to the delay in the implant loading.

The advancement in implant surfaces and improved understanding of bone science, prosthesis and occlusion has lead to development of improved implantology protocol of immediate loading which reduces the limitations of delayed implant loading.

Immediate loading

Immediate loading is loading the implant immediately. This occlusal loading can be with a provisional restoration or with a definitive prosthesis. The type of loading and prosthesis depends on the clinical situations (Table 10).

Indications

- Adequate bone quality and dimensions
- Psychology needs and patient who dislike temporary removable partial denture either due to prosthesis movement or due to its supporting mechanism.

Contraindications

- Inadequate bone architecture, poor bone quality and density (Type IV bone)
- Parafunctional habits
- Poor systemic health
- Inadequate bone height (≥12 mm) and bone width ≥5 mm
- Inability to achieve an adequate AP spread
- Contraindication factors associated with generalized implantology procedures.

Advantages of immediate loading

- Minimise the requirement of angle abutments since the implants can be placed in the same position as the extracted tooth or in extraction sites
- Immediate restoration improves patient satisfaction and psychology
- Osseointegration is more favorable when implants are placed immediately following an extraction
- The recession of tissue, bony receptors and the crestal bone are preserved better with immediate loading of implants
- Stage 2 surgery of conventional protocol is eliminated
- Countersinking of implants done in delayed protocol is avoided which reduces the chance of crestal bone loss
- Splinting of implants aids in early healing and improves biomechanical advantages
- The primary healing time of bone and tissues are reduced coupled with implant surgical healing in immediate loading.

Disadvantages of immediate loading

- If the primary stability of implant is reduced it affects the success rate of procedure
- The micro movements of implants increase chances of bone micro fracture
- Parafunctional habits like tongue thrusting can disturb the implant site and can cause crestal bone loss eventually leading to failure
- Entrapment of impression or surgical material can interfere in healing process.

Factors that influence the immediate-loading protocol[1,2]

Surface area

The implant surface area is enhanced with increase in the number, dimension, design and surface area of implants.

Nonaxial forces

The nonaxial forces are less endured by the supporting structures and it can enhance bone resorption in immediate loaded implants. The possibility of nonaxial forces is observed significantly in parafunction, cantilever and inappropriate crown/implant ration.

Occlusal consideration—Implant protected occlusal scheme reduces the damaging forces transmitted to the implants.

Implant position

Mandible is divided into three segment and maxilla into four segments.

The three mandible segments are bilateral canine region, canine and two posterior segments on either side.

In maxilla, there are four segments midline to canine on either side or posterior bilateral space present behind canine to molar on either side. An implant is also necessitated in the midline to improve the supporting mechanism.

Table 10: Different steps in delayed and immediate-loading protocol		
	Delayed-loading protocol	**Immediate-loading protocol**
1	Diagnosis and treatment planning	Diagnosis and treatment planning
2	Selection of implant dimensions	Selection of implant dimensions
3	Stage I—Implant surgery	Implant surgery
4	Waiting period between 3 and 6 months	Subsequent prosthodontic procedures followed
5	Stage 2 surgery—Removal of cover screw, gingival former placement	Implant loaded with provisional/final restorations
6	After 4 weeks of stage 2 surgery, gingival formers removed. Implant and soft tissues reevaluated for esthetics and function	
7	Choice of abutment in accordance to angulation, type of prosthesis is selected and try in done. If intraoral adjustments required, abutment is prepared	
8	Impression made by direct/indirect technique and subsequent laboratory procedures done	
9	The time, procedures of provisional and final restoration can slightly vary with the type of restoration, such as single crown, FPD, over denture and complete denture	

Immediate loading protocol for different kinds of prosthesis designs[3-5]

Single tooth replacements

- Ideal soft tissue, bone and implant conditions
- Threaded- or screw-type implant design with highest pitch and depth that increases the implant surface area
- Implant-protected occlusal scheme
- Definitive cement is used for luting the restoration.

Partially edentulous area (missing 2 or more teeth)

- Each missing tooth has to be preferentially restored with one implant
- Maximum dimension of implant that can be accommodated with minimum dimension is 10 × 3.75 mm
- Threaded- or screw-type implant design with highest pitch and depth that increases the implant surface area
- No cantilever load
- Implant-supported occlusal scheme.

Fixed prosthodontics in completely edentulous situations

- Necessitates minimum of 8 implants in maxilla and 5 in mandible
- Maximum implant dimension that can be accommodated should be used with of minimum 3.75 mm in width and 10 mm in length

- Threaded- or screw-type implant design with highest pitch and depth that increases the implant surface area
- No cantilevers
- Implant-supported occlusal scheme.

Overdenture
- Adequate residual bone height is essential
- Interarch space should be minimum of 12 mm
- Minimum of four implants to be placed between two mental foramen and widely distributed in maxilla (two bilateral canine and molar regions)
- Implants have to be splinted with bar for force distribution
- Acrylic denture with metal framework engaging the bar will be more ideal prosthesis.

Conclusion

The immediate loading of implants has become more a standardized protocol of acceptance. The choice between immediate- and delayed-loading protocol depends on the clinical situation.

References

1. De Bruyn H, Raes S, Ostman PO, Cosyn J. Immediate loading in partially and completely edentulous jaws: A review of the literature with clinical guidelines. Periodontol 2000. 2014;66(1):153-87.
2. Atieh MA, Payne AG, Duncan WJ, de Silva RK, Cullinan MP. Immediate placement or immediate restoration/loading of single implants for molar tooth replacement: a systematic review and meta-analysis. Int J Oral Maxillofac Implants. 2010;25(2):401-15. Review.
3. Del Fabbro M, Ceresoli V, Taschieri S, Ceci C, Testori T. Immediate loading of postextraction implants in the esthetic area: Systematic review of the literature. Clin Implant Dent Relat Res. 2013 Apr 22.
4. Esposito M, Grusovin MG, Polyzos IP, Felice P, Worthington HV. Interventions for replacing missing teeth: Dental implants in fresh extraction sockets (immediate, immediate-delayed and delayed implants). Cochrane Database Syst Rev. 2010;(9):CD005968.
5. Su M, Shi B, Zhu Y, Guo Y, Zhang Y, Xia H, Zhao L. Comparison of implant success rates with different loading protocols: A meta-analysis. Int J Oral Maxillofac Implants. 2014;29(2):344-52.

25. Occlusal consideration for implant-supported prosthesis.

Definition

Occlusion has been defined as the static relationship between the incising or masticating surfaces of the maxillary or mandibular teeth or tooth analogues.

Significance

- It determines the success of implant prosthesis
- The supporting structures of implant and the natural teeth are different, as natural teeth are suspended by periodontal ligament whereas the implant has a rigid connection to the bone (Table 11)
- An implant-protected occlusal scheme reduces the occlusal forces on implant thus, protecting and preserving the surrounding bone.

Table 11: Biomechanical differences between natural teeth and implant

	Tooth	Implant
Bone connection	Suspended by PDL	Rigid connection with bone
Proprioception	Mechanoreceptors of PDL	Osseoperception
Tactile sensitivity	High	Low
Axial mobility	25–100 µm	3–5 µm
Movement phases	Two phases Primary nonlinear and complex Secondary: Linear and elastic	One phase Linear and elastic
Fulcrum to lateral forces	Apical third of root	Crestal part of implant
Adjacent bone	More of cortical bone	More of trabecular bone
Load bearing characteristics	Shock absorption and stress distribution	Stress
Signs of overloading	PDL thickening, mobility, wear facets, fremitus, pain	Screw loosening or fracture, abutment or prosthesis fracture, bone loss and implant failure

Types of occlusion[1,2]

- Balanced occlusion
- Group function occlusion
- Monoplane occlusion
- Mutually-protected occlusion
- Lingualized occlusion
- Implant-protected occlusion.

Greater emphasis is placed on mutually-protected occlusion since most of the implant restorations are associated with the greater number of natural teeth.

Balanced occlusion

Definition

It is the bilateral, simultaneous, anterior and posterior occlusal contact of teeth in centric and eccentric positions.

Indication

Mostly preferred in complete dentures to enhance the stability of prosthesis.

Advantages

Uniform distribution of forces to all the occlusal units improves stability of the prosthesis.

Limitation

Lateral forces on the nonworking side of implants causes eccentric deflective contacts.

Group function occlusion

A variant of balance occlusal scheme is unilateral balance or group function occlusion. The teeth on the working side will be in contact and the balancing side teeth are not in contact. It can be a choice of occlusion when canine is replaced.

Monoplane occlusion

An occlusal scheme utilizing a zero degree or nonanatomic teeth commonly preferred in highly resorbed ridges. The flatter occlusal surfaces dampen the damaging forces transmitted to the resorbed and flat ridges.

Mutually-protected occlusion

The maxillary and mandibular anterior teeth disocclude the posterior teeth during protrusion and in lateral movement of mandible the canine on working side disocclude the other teeth. In centric, the posterior teeth prevent the anterior group of teeth from contacting.

Advantage

Distributes the forces.

Lingualized occlusion

The maxillary lingual cusp of posterior teeth is predominant teeth in contact during the movements rather than mandibular buccal cusp.

Advantage

This direction of arrangements helps in directing the occlusal forces towards the center of ridge and thus, reduces the lateral stress on the implants.

Implant-protected occlusion

Misch and Bidez in 1994 proposed the occlusal concept to reduce the force transmission to implant which lead to the better prognosis and success of implant restoration.

Factors to be considered in the implant-protected occlusion[3-6] are:
- Implant surface area
- Implant and abutment angulation
- Crown: implant ratio
- Implant crown contour
- Cusp inclination
- Occlusal contact and its timing
- Width of occlusal table
- Occlusal materials
- Protection of weaker component.

Implant surface area

An increase in surface area permits greater transmission of occlusal forces. This is done by increasing number of implants and splinting implants.

Implant and abutment angulation

The forces parallel to the long axis is better tolerated than the lateral forces.
- If the angulation is straight there are more of compressive forces which are more acceptable to biologic structures than the tensile force
- It is ideal to place the angulated abutment of same angulation rather than altering the angulation at the interface (e.g. for a 15° angulation of implant, better to use a 15°

angulated abutment) which makes the abutment –implant body interface straight and aids in transmitting the forces away from the crest
- If the angulation cannot be avoided then wider implant, ridge augmentation or additional implants can be placed.

Crown: implant ratio
- Ideal crown to root ratio is 1:2
- Any deviations from this generate cantilever and nonaxial forces to the crest of the implant.

Crown contour

Depends on:
- Bone contour and morphology in edentulous areas
- Bone resorption pattern
- Buccolingual dimension of the implant is lesser than that of natural teeth so it is essential to contour the crown which in turn will reduce the lateral forces to the bone crest.

Cusp inclination
- Increase in cuspal angulation increases the masticatory efficiency
- Broadening the angle and widening the cuspal angulation reduces the force concentration
- Recontouring of cusps with lesser angulation transmit lesser and favorable axial loads to the implant.

Occlusal contacts
- The occlusal contact of the prosthesis with opposing teeth determines the transmission of forces to the implant
- Occlusal contacts should exist within the diameter of the implant. Cusp fossa occlusal scheme is better than cusp marginal ridge contact which centralizes the forces of occlusion
- Occlusal contacts has to be matched to the difference in range of movements between natural tooth (27 µm) and implant (3–5 µm) with 28 µm articulating paper until an even contact is obtained
- Uniform occlusal contact ensures long-term success of the implant and also prevents fracture of the ceramic restorations.

Occlusal table

Narrow occlusal table reduces the forces and aids in easier maintenance.

Occlusal materials

The choice of material is metals, porcelain fused to metal (PFM), ceramics, composite and acrylics. Among these materials PFM are commonly used as permanent restorations and acrylic as provisional restorations.

Protection of weaker components

Weaker aspects as cantilever length, length of edentulous span, angulation of implants, poor labial or buccal bone have to be identified and the stress transmitted to these components should be reduced during prosthesis designing.

Occlusion schemes in different types of prosthesis

- The occlusal schemes vary with the type of implant prosthesis, number of teeth replacement, type of support and opposing dentition
- In full-mouth rehabilitation and if full-arch prosthesis opposes the natural dentition, mutually protected or group function is ideal
- Natural dentition opposing single complete denture a balance occlusal scheme is ideal
- For an over denture prosthesis, a balanced occlusal scheme with lingulaised occlusion is preferential choice
- In situations of highly resorbed ridges monoplane occlusal scheme is preferred
- For replacement of single teeth or fewer teeth, the already existing occlusal scheme (usually a mutually protected) is chosen
- When a segment of teeth are replaced or when the abutment teeth are periodontally compromised a group function occlusion is chosen for uniform force distribution.

Conclusion

The potential complications of decementation, screw loosening, abutment failure, fracture of restoration, crestal bone loss and implant failure can be avoided with an implant-protected occlusal scheme (Table 12).

Table 12: Occlusion determinants in implant-supported restoration
• Axial inclination to be parallel to the long axis of adjacent teeth or at right angles to the occlusal plane
• Minimum interimplant distance is 5 mm
• Increased number of implants reduces biomechanical risk
• Splinting of implant is preferable to reduce occlusal load
• Ideal crown/implant ratio is 2:1 or minimum of 1:1 is essential
• Minimum implant dimensions of 10 x 3.75 to reduce biomechanical risk
• Restore in centric relation
• Cusp fossa occlusal scheme in centric should be followed
• Constricted occlusal table
• Flatter cusps for improved implant biomechanics
• No cantilevers
• No heavy contacts or infra-occlusion in unavoidable cantilevered situations
• Reduced lateral or excursive guidance on restored teeth
• Group function or balance occlusion to reduce biomechanical risk
• Ceramic should be adequately reinforced with metal framework
• Use of night splint is recommended in bruxism

References

1. Ben-Gal G, Lipovetsky-Adler M, Haramaty O, Sharon E, Smidt A. Existing concepts and a search for evidence: a review on implant occlusion. Compend Contin Educ Dent. 2013;34 Spec No:26-31.
2. Koyano K, Esaki D. Occlusion on oral implants: current clinical guidelines. J Oral Rehabil. 2014 Oct 6.

3. Yuan JC, Sukotjo C. Occlusion for implant-supported fixed dental prostheses in partially edentulous patients: a literature review and current concepts. J Periodontal Implant Sci. 2013 Apr;43(2):51-7.
4. Kim Y, Oh T-J, Misch CE, Wang H-L. Occlusal considerations in implant therapy: clinical guidelines with biomechanical rationale. Clin Oral Impl Res. 2005;16(1):26-35.
5. Gross MD. Occlusion in implant dentistry. A review of the literature of prosthetic determinants and current concepts. Aust Dent J. 2008 Jun;53 Suppl 1:S60-8.
6. Chang M, Chronopoulos V, Mattheos N. Impact of excessive occlusal load on successfully-osseointegrated dental implants: a literature review. J Investig Clin Dent. 2013 Aug;4(3):142-50.

26. Recent advances in surgical techniques.

Introduction

- Placements of dental implants are by either one stage surgery or two stage surgery in ideal situation
- In limitations, such as bony defects, soft tissue defect, bony imperfections and inadequate bone dimensions, advanced surgical options are done.

Classification of advanced surgical procedures

Regenerative procedures

a. Bone augmentation procedures
   - Sinus elevation procedures
     - Direct sinus lift
     - Indirect sinus lift
   - Bone grafting/regeneration procedures
     - Vertical grafting
       a. Distraction osteogenesis
     - Horizontal grafting
       a. Onlay grafting
       b. Sandwich grafting
     - Guided bone regeneration procedures

b. Gingiva augmentation procedures
   - Free gingival grafts
   - Connective tissue grafts
   - Pedicle grafts
   - Guided tissue regeneration procedures

Resective procedures

c. Bone resective procedures

d. Soft tissue resective procedures

Sinus elevation procedure

Definition

It is a surgical procedure that increases the amount of bone in posterior maxilla. The bone grafting material is deposited on the inferior wall or floor of sinus to increase the bone dimensions available for implants in maxillary posterior region.

Indications

- Decreased bone height in posterior maxilla
- Implant restoration with deficient bone dimensions (length) in posterior maxilla.

Contraindications

- The presence of sinus infections, inflammation and pathologic growth
- Systemic diseases that have poor prognosis to healing
- Psychological impairment.

Procedure

Based on the surgical approach a direct or indirect technique can be done.

In direct technique the sinus approach is done directly through superior, middle or inferior lateral wall approach.

In indirect technique the sinus approach is through crestal direction of the partially edentulous space.

Superior lateral approach of direct technique and crestal osteotome of indirect technique are the commonly followed technique for sinus elevation.

Superior Lateral wall approach (Caldwell–Luc approach)

- The surgical approach is through the buccal surface of edentulous site to gain access to the floor of sinus raising the Schneiderian membrane
- The space thus created between the sinus floor and the Schneiderian membrane is filled with a suitable bone grafting material to obtain the desired bone dimensions
- Commonest postoperative complication is the tear of sinus membrane which is repaired by stitching the membrane or restored by undisturbed healing for a period of 3–6 months for auto-repair.

Osteotome technique

- With the crestal approach, crestal access till the floor of sinus is obtained by implant drills or by other methods of osteotomy
- With suitable osteotomes bone is compressed in incremental quantities through the osteotomy site towards the sinus floor elevating the Schneiderian membrane till the required amount of bone augmentation is done
- The procedure is completed with the implant insertion on the augmented site.

Important points to note

The healing time associated with sinus grafting is in average of 3–6 months. Complications, such as infection, inflammation, nerve damage, graft failure, oro antral communications and implant loosening or implant failure, can occur.

Evidence-based data[1,2]

The meta-analysis on sinus lift procedures by Stephen S Wallace and Stuart J Froum (2003)[2] concludes the following:

- The survival rate of implants placed in augmented sinuses varied between 61.7% and 100% with the average survival rate of all interventions being 92.6%
- Reports favored better implant survival rates in the non-grafted posterior maxilla

- Rough-surfaced implants have a higher survival rate than machine-surfaced implants when placed in grafted sinuses
- Particulate grafts show a higher survival rate than those placed in sinuses that had been augmented with block grafts
- Better prognosis is obtained when a membrane was used in covering the lateral window technique
- No statistical difference between delayed implant placement, types of rough-surfaced implants, length of follow-up, year of publication, and the evidence level of the study.

Implant site augmentation methods[3-5]

Classified as

- Horizontal augmentation techniques
- Vertical augmentation techniques.

Minor bone deficiency areas are restored with guided bone regeneration materials with suitable alloplastic materials.

Major deficiency regions are restored by vertical or horizontal augmentation techniques in accordance to bone deficiency.

Horizontal Augmentation Techniques

Horizontal bone grafting is done by onlay and sandwich grafting.

Indication

Atrophy of the edentulous ridge with adequate residual height.

Contraindication

- Excessive inclination of the alveolar ridge
- Presence of bony undercuts prone to fracture during the space creation.

Onlay grafting

Block autogenous bone, derived from other intraoral or extraoral sites, is placed in the deficient region, secured with retrievable screws or resorbable materials.

Sandwich grafting

Space created is by splitting the bone between the cortical plates and filled with suitable augmentation materials. This technique is mainly indicated in the maxilla. It is difficult in the mandible due to the rigidity of the bone.

Vertical Augmentation Techniques

- The vertical bone height is achieved by securing the grafts with screws, plates or by any retrievable materials
- The vertical augmentation technique is highly sensitive and success rate is less compared to horizontal augmentation techniques
- The success rate depends on the site vascularity.

Vertical distraction osteogenesis

Increases the vertical height of bone by the process of slow distraction. Mostly done in mandible.

Indication

Insufficient vertical height with satisfactory residual width.

Contraindications

- Severely deficient mandible has high risk of fracture or neural damage
- Close proximity of maxillary sinus
- Rigid palatal mucosa might reduce the distraction forces.

Soft tissue surgeries

- Are done for better esthetics
- Done either by resective surgery or by regenerative surgery
- The resective surgery corrects the irregular bone or the increased thickness keratinized gingiva. It is generally a final option to be adapted after attempting the regenerative procedures in the management of implant failures.

Types of gingival graft surgeries[6]

- Free gingival graft (FGG)
- Connective tissue graft (CTG)
- Pedicle grafts (PD) are the commonly employed.

The FGG requires a gingival tissue from a donor site whereas CTG require a part of tissue from a flap.

The pedicle graft utilizes gingival tissue close to required region.

The CTG is more efficient with encouraging results of root coverage and with lesser patient discomfort and postoperative complaints.

The FGG is conventional and standardized procedure for increasing the thickness of attached gingiva where less than 2 mm of attached tissue is present. The FGG procedure reduces the frenum or muscular tension on the graft or the flap.

References

1. Chen ST, Beagle J, Jensen SS, Chiapasco M, Darby I. Consensus statements and, recommended clinical procedures regarding surgical techniques. Int J Oral Maxillofac Implants. 2009;24 Suppl:272-8.
2. Wallace SS, Froum SJ. Effect of maxillary sinus augmentation on the survival of endosseous dental implants. A systematic review. Ann Periodontol. 2003 Dec;8(1):328-43. Review.
3. Harris D. Advanced surgical procedures: bone augmentation. Dent Update. 1997 Oct;24(8):332-7. Review.
4. Draenert FG, Huetzen D, Neff A, Mueller WE. Vertical bone augmentation procedures: basics and techniques in dental implantology. J Biomed Mater Res A. 2014 May; 102(5):1605-13.
5. Nkenke E, Neukam FW. Autogenous bone harvesting and grafting in advanced jaw resorption: morbidity, resorption and implant survival. Eur J Oral Implantol. 2014 Summer;7 Suppl 2:S203-17.
6. Kao RT, Conte G, Nishimine D, Dault S. Tissue engineering for periodontal regeneration. J Calif Dent Assoc. 2005 Mar;33(3):205-15. Review.

27. Discuss implant failures and precautions that need to be taken.

Implants have become most successful treatment modality in the treatment of partially and completely edentulous patients. Even with the success rates more than 70%, as stated by Brånemark and Misch after detailed clinical study, there exist a failure at various levels of the treatment procedure.

Classification of implant failure

Two main types—Types due to etiology[1] and according to types of failure[2]

1. Etiology
   - Host factors
     - Prevailing medical and dental status
     - Psychology
     - Habits
   - Surgical procedure
     - Pre-surgical
       a. Infected implant sites
       b. Inadequate mineralization of grafts
     - Stage 1 surgery
       a. Inappropriate flap design
       b. Improper implant angulations
       c. Insufficient primary stability
       d. Excess pressure and overheating of bone
       e. Teeth–implant space
       f. Implant contamination
     - Stage 2 surgery
       a. Improper loading protocol
       b. Local and systemic entrusted factors
   - Implant selection
     - Implant dimensions
     - Mismatch of bone and implant type
     - Number of implants
     - Improper implant design and system
   - Prosthodontic factors
     - Increased cantilever
     - Implants–natural teeth connection
     - Prosthesis design
       a. Absence of passive fit of prosthesis
       b. Improper abutment fit interface
       c. Improper prosthesis design
       d. Improper occlusal design.
   - Periodontal factors
     - Peri–implantitis
     - Improper oral health maintenance
2. Type of failure
   - Esthetics failure
     - Gingival esthetics failure
     - Restoration factors
     - Implant factors

- Osseointegration failure
- Functional and psychological problems.

Etiological Factors

The implant failures can be subdivided into factors caused due to host or patient, surgical failure, improper implant selection and prosthetic factors.[3]

Host/Patient Factor

- Prevailing medical and dental status of patient
- Psychology
- Habits.

Contraindications for implants

Pregnancy, granulocytopenia, long-term steroid use, diabetes, hemophilia, Ehler–Danlos syndrome, Marfan's syndrome, osteoradionecrosis, renal failure, organ transplants, anticoagulant therapy, Crohn's disease, fibrous dysplasia, Paget's disease and osteoporosis. Systemic complications delay healing phase or bone repair mechanisms in the implant site.

Patient psychology

The patient has to be educated and motivated to maintain the oral hygiene.

Habits

Such as pan chewing, smoking and other parafunctional habits can cause increased forces on implants and local ischemia.

Surgical failures

Presurgical and surgical failure.

Presurgical

- ***Infected implant sites***—with periodontal infections, endodontic lesions, infected socket and dental pathologic conditions
- ***Inadequate mineralization of graft***—Implants fail to integrate in immature grafts. It is ideal to wait till all the woven bone matures to lamellar bone that can have better implant prognosis.

Factors that can contribute to the failure of implant in stage 1 surgery are:

- Inappropriate flap design— Improper flap design can lead to decrease in nutrients reaching implant site and blood supply, infection and tissue ischemia. Proper flap closure ensures better healing and surgical prognosis
- Improper implant angulations—It is advisable to have straight implant and abutment for favorable prognosis since the implants are designed for axial forces
- Insufficient primary stability—Precision osteotomy reduces the implant mobility and facilitates faster healing
- Excess pressure and overheating of bone—The use of excessive pressure and heat can damage the bone cell by forming a barrier layer between the implant and healthy bone causing osseointegration failure
- Teeth–implant space—Minimum of 1 mm space is required between teeth and implant to maintain ideal bone health

- Implant contamination—Improper sterilization protocol during surgical procedure, broken manufacture seal and oral cavity contamination.

Factors causing failure in Stage 2 surgery

Improper loading protocol

Adequate healing time has to be provided before loading the implant.

Local and systemic factors

The protocol measures for stage 2 surgery as removal of cover screw with adequate tissue relief, infection free zone and adequate keratinized gingiva should be maintained for the success of implant.

Implant selection

Bone support, bone type, number, type and size of the implants play a vital role in implant success. The precautions followed in implant selection to prevent implant failure are:

- The length and width of implant has to be sufficient to support the superstructure
- In possible limits, increased number of implants has to be placed to support the restoration for uniform stress distribution
- Selection of a proper implant system according to available clinical situation for better success of implant
- Mismatch of system can compromise the implant health and success.

Prosthetic factors

Factors influencing the prosthetic design[4] are:

- Reduced number of implants can cause a cantilever design with undue forces on the supporting implant. A minimal of 8 mm cantilever is the permissible limit with increased number of implants
- The preferred design is to avoid implant connection to natural teeth, if connected can cause overload and mismatched resiliency
- A lack of passive fit of prosthesis at the abutment interface.

Periodontal factors

Peri-implantitis

Is the postoperative failure arising due to Gram negative bacteria. Retrograde peri-implantitis can be caused due to micro fracture of bone, infection from adjacent teeth or early loading. Preventive care has to be followed during the various procedures to avoid retrograde peri-implantitis.

Improper oral maintenance

Can lead to wider problems from tissue loss to bone loss which in turn affects esthetic and function.

Types of failure

Esthetic failure can be further subdivided into:

- Gingival esthetics—papilla esthetics, contour and form of gingiva around the restoration
- Restoration esthetics—color, emergence profile, size, form and type of restoration
- Implant esthetics—thread exposure, angulations of implants, bone resorption

Undue care is taken during treatment planning, surgical stage and during fabrication of restoration to avoid esthetic failures.

Lack of osseointegration can be due to:

- Bone grafting issues
- Surgical and prosthetic factors
- Functional and psychological problems.

Treatment options for management of implant failure:

1. Nonsurgical
   - Topical treatments and oral medicaments
   - Removal of occlusal interferences
   - Debridement
   - Repair of prosthesis.
2. Surgical
   - Resective and regenerative surgery
   - Implant removal.

Appropriate procedures have to be selected depending on the clinical situation and type of failure.[5] Careful evaluation procedures are done and suitable management protocol is done to correct the failures.

References

1. Marcelo CG, Filié Haddad M, Gennari Filho H, Marcelo Ribeiro Villa L, Dos Santos DM, Aldiéris AP. Dental implant fractures—aetiology, treatment and case report. J Clin Diagn Res. 2014 Mar; 8(3):300-4.
2. Chrcanovic BR, Albrektsson T, Wennerberg A. Reasons for failures of oral implants. J Oral Rehabil. 2014 Jun;41(6):443-76. Review.
3. Zembic A, Kim S, Zwahlen M, Kelly JR. Systematic review of the survival rate and incidence of biologic, technical, and esthetic complications of single implant abutments supporting fixed prostheses. Int J Oral Maxillofac Implants. 2014;29 Suppl:99-116.
4. Abduo J, Judge RB. Implications of implant framework misfit: a systematic review of biomechanical sequelae. Int J Oral Maxillofac Implants. 2014 May-Jun;29(3):608-21.
5. Hsu YT, Mason SA, Wang HL. Biological implant complications and their management. J Int Acad Periodontol. 2014 Jan;16(1):9-18. Review.

SECTION 2

Short Notes

1. Diagnostic aids in fixed partial denture.
2. Importance of diagnostic casts.
3. Advantages, disadvantages, indications and contraindications of fixed partial dentures.
4. Importance of radiologic examination in crown and bridge prosthesis.
5. Questionable abutments.
6. Mouth preparation in fixed partial denture.
7. Requirements of a crown.
8. Double arch impression technique.
9. Double mix technique.
10. Adhesives in dentistry/dentin bonding agents.
11. Factors in shade matching in all ceramic restorations.
12. Methods to remove crowns and bridges.
13. Ante's law and its significance.
14. Shortened dental arch concept (SDA concept).
15. Rigid connectors.
16. Soldering.
17. Cast core jacket crown.
18. Richmond crown.
19. Davis crown.
20. Axio-proximal grooves.
21. Pier abutment.
22. Causes of abutment failure.
23. Mesial half crown.
24. Cantilever fixed partial denture.
25. Describe cementation of all ceramic restorations.
26. Recent advances in investment materials.

27. Retention in fixed partial denture.
28. Instructions to crown and bridge patients regarding care and maintenance.
29. Articulators.
30. Fixed removable prosthodontics.
31. Dental laboratory form.
32. Dalhs appliance.
33. Management of tooth surface loss (TSL).
34. Flowchart for surgical procedure in implant placement.
35. All ceramic restoration.
36. Material selection and failures in RBFPD.
37. Osseointegration.
38. Alloys used in fixed partial denture.
39. Non-rigid connectors/stress breakers in fixed partial denture.
40. Wax patterns.
41. Functionally generated pathways (Meyer).
42. Interocclusal records.
43. Lug seat.
44. Soft tissue mask for implant models.
45. Recall and maintenance.
46. Treating tilted molars.
47. Telescopic crown.
48. Finishing and polishing.
49. Mention the anatomical concerns for implant placement in posterior maxilla and mandible region.
50. Pickling.
51. Defects in casting.
52. Myofascial pain dysfunction syndrome.
53. Implant-supported fixed partial denture.
54. Full mouth rehabilitation.
55. Contraindication for implant placement.
56. Laboratory procedures in fixed partial denture.
57. Tenso-frictional resistance.

SHORT NOTES

1. Diagnostic aids in fixed partial denture.

Important diagnostic aids are:

- Diagnostic casts
- Radiographs.

Diagnostic casts

Articulated diagnostic casts

- Aid in planning treatment procedures
- Provide information about static and dynamic relationships of the teeth
- Helps to view several aspects of the occlusion not detectable within the confines of the mouth.

Diagnostic cast impression can be made of irreversible hydrocolloid and poured in dental stone.

Advantages of diagnostic cast

- Changing the arch relationship before orthognathic procedures
- Changing the tooth position prior to orthodontic procedures
- Modifying the occlusal scheme before attempting any selective occlusal adjustment
- Trial tooth preparation and waxing can be done before fixed restorative procedures
- Selection of an optimum path of withdrawal of a fixed partial denture can be assessed.

Radiographic examination

- Periapical radiographs
- Bitewing radiographs
- Panoramic films
- In case of temporomandibular joint (TMJ) disorders:
  - Transcranial exposure
  - Serial tomography
  - Arthrography
  - CT scanning
  - Magnetic resonance imaging.

Periapical radiographs

(14 periapical radiographs helps in complete examination).

Importance of periapical radiographs:

- Knowing the extent of bone support, quality of supporting bone
- Detailed root morphology of each abutment tooth
- Width of periodontal ligament space
- Bone resorption (vertical, horizontal)
- Inclination of teeth
- Continuity of lamina dura

- Pulpal morphology and previous endodontic treatment
- Any periapical pathology can be evaluated
- Evaluation of crown–root ratio
- Evaluation of the shape, length and direction of root
- Helps in checking for periodontal situation of the abutment tooth, as widening or thickening of lamina dura, occlusal prematurities or trauma can cause thickening.

Bitewings

Evaluation of caries on proximal surfaces and secondary caries on previous restorations.

Panoramic films aid in

- Evaluation of bone resorption, pattern of bone resorption and quality of bone support
- To check for presence of retained root tips, impacted tooth
- To determine the thickness of soft tissue on the ridge in area of pontic placement
- They do not provide a detailed view for assessing bone support, root morphology, or caries.

2. Importance of diagnostic casts.

- A diagnostic cast should be an accurate reproduction of the teeth and adjacent tissues, poured in dental stone, because of its strength and abrasion resistance
- The impression for the diagnostic cast is made with irreversible hydrocolloid (alginate) in a perforated impression tray
- It is a life-size reproduction of a part or parts of the oral cavity or facial structures for the purpose of study and treatment planning.

Importance of diagnostic casts

- Diagnostic casts permit viewing of the occlusion from the lingual and buccal aspect
- To analyse the existing occlusion in case of needed occlusal adjustment and occlusal reconstruction
- Aids in diagnostic wax up, to determine the occlusion before definitive treatment is begun
- Diagnostic casts helps to survey the dental arch as a whole
- Helps in surveying of the cast to determine existing soft tissue under cuts, parallelism of teeth as for over denture cases
- Aids in mouth preparation decisions, as to the removal of soft tissue undercuts
- Helps to show and discuss the case with patient regarding the treatment plans, needed corrections and problems, if any
- Aids to select and fabricate trays
- If needed, can duplicate diagnostic cast in case a undercut has to be blocked
- Diagnostic casts may be used as a constant reference
- In areas where alterations are required as in soft tissue or hard tissues, a rough alteration can be mocked on the duplicate cast to assess the outcome.

3. Advantages, disadvantages, indications and contraindications of fixed partial dentures.

Advantages

- Movements for a fixed partial denture are less compared to a removable partial denture
- Psychologically better accepted than removable partial denture
- Acts as a splint
- Less lateral forces are transmitted to abutment tooth compared to a partial denture abutment
- Can use weak abutment if other abutments are strong
- Esthetically better with more comfort to the patient
- Better functioning of the prosthesis with good perception
- Less bone resorption compared to removable prosthesis.

Disadvantages

- It can weaken a strong abutment tooth if the other abutment support is weak
- It is an irreversible treatment
- Preparation of sound tooth will make the patient think twice before agreeing to go for fixed prosthesis
- Adequate preparation with good occlusal clearance is required or a fixed prosthesis can fail
- If restoration is overcontoured, it can cause periodontal problems.

Indications for fixed bridges

The selection of prosthesis depends on biomechanical, periodontal, esthetic and financial factors:

- In tooth bounded situations when a single tooth is missing
- In case where the abutment tooth on either side can support the number of tooth missing
- If the abutment tooth is periodontally sound
- To maintain space in orthodontic cases
- If the edentulous span is short and straight
- To restore missing tooth in order to prevent the adjacent tooth from drifting into the space
- To restore the mouth to complete function free of interferences.

Contraindications

- Unfavourable crown–root ratio
- Large edentulous space
- Edentulous space with no distal abutment
- Bilaterally edentulous with no distal abutment
- Grossly tipped teeth (more than 22°)
- Periodontally weak teeth
- Teeth with short clinical crowns

- Severe bone resorption
- Young age with large pulp chamber and lack of total eruption
- Large tongue
- Extensive caries with poor oral hygiene
- Financially poor patients
- If the patient cannot maintain oral hygiene
- In case of parafunctional habits—with excessive force load on abutment tooth.

4. Importance of radiologic examination in crown and bridge prosthesis.

Different types of radiographic examinations are as follows:

- Periapical radiographs
- Bitewing radiographs
- Panoramic films
- In case of temporomandibular joint (TMJ) disorders:
  - Transcranial exposure
  - Serial tomography
  - Arthrography
  - Computed tomography scanning
  - Magnetic resonance imaging.

Periapical radiographs

(14 periapical radiographs helps in complete examination)

Importance

- Knowing the extent of bone support, quality of supporting bone
- Detailed root morphology of each abutment tooth
- Width of periodontal ligament space
- Bone resorption (vertical, horizontal)
- Inclination of teeth
- Continuity of lamina dura
- Pulpal morphology and previous endodontic treatment
- Any periapical pathology can be evaluated
- Evaluation of crown–root ratio
- Evaluation of the shape, length and direction of root
- Helps in checking for periodontal situation of the abutment tooth, as widening or thickening of lamina dura, occlusal prematurities or trauma can cause thickening.

Bitewings

Evaluation of caries on proximal surfaces and secondary caries on previous restorations.

Panoramic films

They aid in

- Evaluation of bone resorption, pattern of bone resorption and quality of bone support
- To check for presence of retained root tips, impacted tooth

- To determine the thickness of soft tissue on the ridge in area of pontic placement
- They do not provide a detailed view for assessing bone support, root morphology, or caries.

Radiographs are important tools in the assessment to determine the success of the prosthesis after evaluating the abutment tooth, the proximity of pulp chamber, the residual ridge support of the pontics, and for good aesthetic replacement of the pontics.

5. Questionable abutments.

Are abutment teeth that can be retained after periodontal and endodontic treatment which otherwise are hopeless teeth.

It is possible to retain a tooth with hopeless prognosis by highly specialized and complex treatment methods.

Selection of questionable abutments

- An abutment tooth that is periodontally weak yet can be used as multiple splinted abutment teeth, along with non-rigid connectors or intermediate abutments
- Tooth with gross caries, which can be used as abutment after endodontic treatment
- Abutment tooth with large restorations
- Abutments that are malaligned, tilted or mesially drifted tooth
- Abutments that cannot withstand forces of a long edentulous span
- Abutments that are grossly attrited due to parafunctional habits
- Abutments with reduced bone support.

Assessment of abutment teeth

Periodontally weak tooth

1. Tooth with slight mobility.
2. Tooth with recession and furcation involvement.
3. Tooth with gingival and periodontal pathology.

Some teeth can be saved and used as abutments by:

- Good oral hygiene measures before and after treatment
- Scaling, polishing and root planing for initial periodontal pathology
- Mobile tooth that can be stabilised by splinting
- Gingival recession can be corrected by flap surgeries
- Osseous defects can be corrected by ridge augmentation methods/guided tissue regeneration techniques.

Abutment tooth requiring endodontic treatment

1. After testing for pulp vitality, if pulpal health is doubtful endodontic treatment should be carried out.
2. An endodontically treated abutment with a post and core foundation for retention and strength can serve as good abutment support.
3. Failures occur with short roots and tooth with less coronal tooth structure.

Abutments with large restorations

For abutments with large restorations extending to cervical areas, the retainer margin should be placed subgingivally.

Abutments that are malaligned, tilted or mesially drifted tooth

Mesially drifted tooth closing the pontic space is not an ideal abutment (mesially tilted second molar).

This can be treated by:

1. Modified preparation designs.
2. Non-rigid connector.
3. By uprighting the tilted abutment orthodontically.
4. Malaligned occlusion as supra-erupted, tilted tooth need to be occlusally corrected.
5. A well-aligned tooth provides better support than a tilted one.

Abutments that cannot withstand forces of a long edentulous span

The more the edentulous span length, greater the flexing of the prosthesis under occlusal loads. This can cause fracture of a porcelain veneer, breakage of a connector, loosening of a retainer or unfavorable soft tissue response.

Treatment method

1. A mock preparation is done on diagnostic cast to check the feasibility.
2. If the abutments cannot withstand the occlusal load or if periodontally weak abutments are present then an implant-supported prosthesis or a fixed and removable prosthesis need to be used.
3. Pontics and connectors should be of adequate thickness and of high strength and rigidity.
4. If the restoration is overcontoured then maintenance of oral hygiene is difficult.

Replacing multiple anterior teeth

- Missing four mandibular incisors can be replaced with canines as abutments
- A single incisor present is best removed, as it cannot withstand the forces
- Multiple edentulous spaces are best restored with a combination of fixed and removable partial denture.

Abutments that are grossly attrited due to parafunctional habits

During application of load the abutment teeth should not drift or become mobile as in a multiple unit restoration. The dislodging forces are in a mesiodistal direction.

These abutment teeth are generally attrited and sometimes with slight mobility and drifting. Only after a treatment appliance is given to reduce parafunctional activity should a restoration be given.

In case the clinical crown height is less then:

1. Crown lengthening procedures or a subgingival finish line should be done.
2. If chances of pulp exposure are present it should be endodontically treated.
3. Favorable crown–root ratio is 1:1.
4. Proximal boxes and additional grooves on the buccal and lingual surfaces are added to the preparations to produce greater resistance and structural durability.

Abutments with reduced bone support

After periodontal disease, root surface area is reduced. There is excessive bone loss, which magnifies the forces on that tooth as length difference between the clinical crown and root exists.

Other factors to be considered

Root shape and angulation

1. When tooth support is borderline, short conical roots give less support.
2. Divergent multiple roots give good support and can be used as abutments even if there is reduced bone support.
3. Single-rooted tooth with an elliptic cross section gives better support than a tooth with circular cross section.
4. In case of vertical and horizontal resorption, potential abutment teeth need to be carefully evaluated as related to root shape angulation and number of roots.

Good oral hygiene measures

Nyjnan and Ericsson used abutment teeth with reduced bone support and reduced root surface area less than half that of the replaced teeth.

They recalled patients and found no loss of attachment after 8–11 years.

With proper and meticulous root planing, plaque control during the observed period, and the occlusal design of the prostheses any questionable abutments can bring success to the long-term prognosis of fixed partial denture.

6. Mouth preparation in fixed partial denture.

Mouth preparation is part of the treatment-planning phase carried out to enhance the success of the fixed partial denture.

Mouth Preparation helps to:

- Relieve symptoms
- Removes the etiologic factors causing the symptoms
- Repairs the damages caused by the etiologic factors
- Maintains dental health.

The order of procedures in mouth preparation

1. Diagnosis and treatment planning.
2. Treatment to relieve the presenting symptoms.
3. Surgical procedures.
4. Endodontic procedures.
5. Periodontal procedures.
6. Orthodontic realignment, if necessary.
7. Definitive occlusal treatment.
8. Prosthetic rehabilitation.
9. Follow-up.

Surgical procedures

- Extractions
  - Abutment tooth detrimental to the design of fixed partial denture
  - Residual roots tips
  - Impacted or unerupted supernumerary teeth
  - Malposed teeth, which is grossly extruded or drifted which cannot be corrected by restorations.

- Cyst and odontogenic tumors
- Hyperplastic tissue
  - Surgical excision by scalpel, curette, or electrosurgery.
- Bony spines and knife-edge ridges
- Dentofacial deformity
  - Surgical correction of a jaw deformity can be made in horizontal, sagittal, or frontal planes.
- Implant-supported fixed prostheses

  These are placed under controlled oral surgical procedures if required for fixed partial denture.

Endodontic procedures

- Endodontically treated tooth are restored with crowns
- Caries tooth are restored by amalgam, composite, glass ionomer, pin-retained restoration or post and core depending on extend of damage.

Periodontal procedures

The periodontal procedures follow surgical procedures.

Objectives of periodontal therapy

- Removal of all etiologic factors causing periodontal disease
- Elimination of all pockets
- Creating physiologic gingival and osseous architecture
- Establishment of functional occlusal relationships
- Plaque control program and definitive maintenance schedule.

Evaluation of abutment tooth for periodontal health

- Evaluating pocket depth especially in the abutment tooth
- Check bleeding on probing, for sulcular health
- The extent and pattern of bone loss
- The degree of mobility present
- Any traumatic occlusion.

Diagnostic aids

Diagnostic aids which are used include:

- Periodontal probe
- Mouth mirror
- Curved explorers
- Furcation probes
- Diagnostic casts
- Roentgenograms.

Evaluating pocket depth

Periodontal probe is used circumferentially around each tooth and depths are recorded in distobuccal, mesial, mesiobuccal, distolingual, lingual and mesiolingual aspects of each tooth.

Crown lengthening procedures

Done when clinical crown height is less and when retention will be compromised.

Orthodontic Treatment

- Minor orthodontic tooth movement can be done to upright a malpositioned abutment tooth
- Can improve axial alignment
- Will create pontic space and will improve embrasure form in the fixed prosthesis
- It can direct occlusal forces along the long axis of the teeth.

Definitive occlusal treatment

Done to make intercuspal position coincident with centric relation and to remove eccentric interferences.

Contraindications

- Bruxers, when too much tooth structure needs to be removed
- Angle Class II and a skeletal Class III
- Excessive wear
- Temporomandibular pain.

Prosthetic rehabilitation and Follow-up

Whether removable, fixed or implant supported, the patient needs to be recalled after prosthetic rehabilitation.

7. Requirements of a crown.

Definition

Artificial crown is a fixed restoration of the major surfaces or the entire coronal part of a natural tooth that restores anatomy, function and esthetics, usually of metal, porcelain, synthetic resin, or combinations.

Requirements of a crown

- An ideal retainer needs to support and connect the body of the bridge with the abutment
- It should restore the form, function and esthetics of the abutment
- Should impart strength to tooth
- Should have harmonious occlusion
- Should have good marginal adaptation and a smooth gingival margin with a supportive relationship to the gingival margin
- An artificial crown should have strength, stability, and retention
- An artificial crown should replicate the exact contours of missing tooth to maintain oral hygiene and periodontal health
- Artificial crown should maintain occlusal plane
- Should be biocompatible with tooth and its adjacent tissues
- Retainer should be constructed without injury to pulp and supporting structures
- Should protect and maintain the pulp against thermal and galvanic shock
- Should provide safety for the tooth during the lifetime of the restoration

- Should provide self-cleaning property
- Should be resistant to corrosion and tarnish
- Should be a conservative preparation with uniformity of reduction of the abutment tooth
- Load should be dispersed to the more receptive areas of the abutment
- There should be large surface contact between the abutment and a retainer
- Complete metal crowns should provide desirable guide planes for RPD
- It should be made of rigid material to withstand the forces
- Should maintain vertical dimension and should have the property of resistance to wear.

8. Double arch impression technique.

Other names

Closed bite double arch method/dual quad tray, double arch, triple tray, accu-bite, closed mouth impression.

Requirements

- The articulator must have an incisal pin or other metal-to-metal contact
- There should be a positive stop in articulator or natural teeth should be present to maintain vertical dimension. Limited to single castings with good interdigitation
- Should have sufficient space distal to the terminal tooth for tray approximation.

Advantages

- Physical deformation of the mandible during opening is minimized
- Shifting of teeth during maximum intercuspation is copied
- Less impression material is required
- Chance of gagging sensation is less.

Disadvantages

- Tray is not rigid
- It is not a functionally generated technique
- Distribution of the impression material is not uniform.

Impression procedure

- After selecting the correct tray, the trays crossbar is positioned distal to last tooth
- The patient is asked to close the mouth to observe complete bilateral closure and patient's comfort.

Loading light-body material

1. Automatic gun dispensing:
   - Activated by placing a replaceable cartridge and mixing tip into the gun and squeezing the trigger, which expresses the material.
2. Manual mixing:
   - 6 by 8 inches of impression material is mixed with a pliable spatula against the pad with circular motion combining the two strands

- A figure of eight motion is used to flatten the mixture onto the mixing pad (mixing time 1 minute)
- The pad is placed near the edge of a table (waist high).

Loading the mixed material

The mixed material is loaded onto the syringe at a slight angle while scraping the pad.

Cord removal

The 2 mm excess of cord is grasped with forceps and teased slowly with a gentle continuous pressure toward the occlusal surface.

Impression method

1. The light body loaded onto the syringe is injected into inaccessible areas first, and then the prepared tooth surface completely.
2. The high-viscosity elastomer is manipulated and "overfilled" bilaterally, tray is seated and the crossbar is positioned distal to the last tooth in that arch.
3. The patient is asked to slowly close mouth and the interdigitation is observed on the opposite arch. The patient is asked to continue interdigitation until the material sets.

Tray removal

1. The patient is asked to open mouth; generally the impression adheres to one arch.
2. A finger is placed on either side of the tray and tray is removed with equal pressure bilaterally.
3. Evaluate the final impression.

Pour die

Excess impression material is removed and die stone is poured, dowel pin is positioned and stone is allowed to set.

Articulation

1. After making working cast, it is attached to a hinge articulator with incisal pin or vertical dimension stop.
2. Sticky wax is placed around tray. Boxing wax in half length-wise is adapted to both upper and lower arches at one time and sealed to prevent the stone from entering the opposite side of the impression.
3. Small openings are made in boxed wax to accommodate the boxed impression within the articulator for correct positioning of the impression.
4. The tray is positioned, in the center of articulator, parallel to the tabletop, and centered from side to side.
5. First the opposing side without dies are poured and articulator arm closed into unset stone. Then the dowel pins are placed without interfering with the closure of the articulator arm on the working side. This side is poured after lubricating the die(s). The articulator arms are closed until incisal pin contacts the lower arm. Unset stone is removed around tip of dowel pin(s) to facilitate removal.
6. After complete setting of gypsum the impression tray is removed from articulator, the cast is separated from the impression tray.
7. Casts and separate die(s) are evaluated.

9. Double mix technique.

(PVS PS CS)

Impression technique

- After a stock tray is selected, tray adhesive is applied; the impression putty is mixed and placed in tray
- A polyethylene sheet is used to cover the putty material and impression is seated in the patient's mouth
- The complete set of the impression is ensured by fingernail testing and the tray is removed.

Relieving the tray

A sharp hand instrument is used to remove uniform amount of impression material from the tissue surface.

After gingival retraction evaluate tissue displacement, check the finish line area(s), and leave cord(s) in place for 8–12 minutes.

Manipulation of light body material

1. After measuring the arch length of tray, one times the length of the tray low-viscosity elastomer is dispensed.
2. A mixing pad, (6 by 8 inches) or an automatic gun dispensing system is used.
3. The low-viscosity impression material is mixed with a circular motion combining the two strands.
4. A figure of eight motion is used to blend and flatten the mixture onto the mixing pad. (mixing time less than I minute).

Loading the impression material

1. The syringe is loaded by holding it at a slight angle while scraping the pad.
2. Screw on the tip and insert the plunger.
3. While the plunger is inserted into the syringe, the cord is removed.
4. After evaluating retraction site for seepage, hemorrhage, or debris, first syringe inaccessible areas as distal lingual finish line and then the entire area of preparation.
5. The syringe is positioned so the elastomer is ahead of the tip's orifice.

Tray Insertion

1. Insert the low-viscosity impression material into the tray slightly less than the depth of the external borders.
2. Seat the tray from posterior to anterior, allowing the excess to extrude anteriorly.
3. Seat the tray firmly in position.
4. The tray should not be moved while the material is setting.

Final impression

After the final set is over, tray is removed parallel to the preparation(s) path of withdrawal and impression is evaluated.

Rinse impression with ambient water, and dry with short, small bursts of compressed air.

Evaluate set impression

1. The area 0.5 mm beyond visible finish line should be visible.
2. There should be no show-through in any areas of the impression, except at tissue stops
3. There should be no shiny smooth areas, no voids present, there should be no thin areas leaving the finish line unsupported.

Making working cast

1. Position the dowel(s) into the impression.
2. Insert one extra dowel pin on either side of the working dies.
3. This ensures die removal despite errors during sectioning
4. Check dowel position in impression for parallelism and retention and add paper clips or orthodontic wire for retaining the second pour to the first.
5. Pour first layer of stone, wait for initial set of stone.
6. Lubricate die areas, bead and box impression.
7. Pour second layer of stone for the base.

10. Adhesives in dentistry/dentin bonding agents.

Indications

- Direct resin composite restorations (caries, fractures, reshaping)/pit and fissure sealants
- Bond all-ceramic restorations (veneers, inlays, onlays, crowns)
- Bond amalgam/core build ups
- Resin-retained fixed partial dentures
- Orthodontic brackets
- Treatment for dentinal hypersensitivity
- Repair fractured porcelain and composite.

Classification of dentin bonding agents

1. First generation—**Hydrophobic monomers,** bond strengths—2–3 MPa, chemical bond to calcium (Cervident - SS White 1965).
2. Second generation—**Phosphorous-ester monomers**—increased surface wetting, 5–6 MPa bond strength and smear layer predominately intact (Scotch bond).
3. Third generation—**Mildly acidic hydrophilic monomer**, preparation by acid etch, modified/altered smear layer, moderate bond strength (Scotch Prep).
4. Fourth generation—**Multi step**, conditions dentin by removing smear layer, primes and then adhesive. High bond strength (3M Multipurpose).
5. Fifth generation—**One step**, combined primer and adhesive high bond strength. (Onestep).
6. Sixth generation—Two types, one with combined primer and conditioner (AdheSe), moderate bond strength and another type with conditioner, primer and adhesive, low bond strength (Prompt-L-Pop).
7. Seventh generation—**All in one adhesives,** combined conditioner, primer and adhesive, one-step, low bond strengths (G Bond).

Another classification based on type of use

Etch and rinse (i.e., total-etch)—three step (conditioner, primer and adhesive) or two step (primer and adhesive) 4th and 5th generation

Self-etch—6th and 7th generation

Resin-modified glass ionomer—two step.

Depending on type of bonding

- ***Wet Bonding***—Acetone- and ethanol-based primers displace remaining water and carry monomers into collagen (One step)
- ***Dry bonding***—Water-based primers can check etching more reliably as self rewetting (Optibond).

Etch and rinse three steps

Conditioner

Acids, such as phosphoric, citric, maleic and nitric are used. They etch the enamel and also remove the dentinal smear layer exposing the collagen fibrils. Rinse after etching time is over and keep moist.

Primer

Are hydrophilic monomers dissolved in acetone, alcohol or water. After application, lightly air dry. Primers are bifunctional monomer that links the hydrophilic collagen to the hydrophobic resin (E.g. HEMA) by displacing water in dentin and promoting infiltration into collagen.

Adhesive resins

Are unfilled or lightly-filled monomers, such as Bis-GMA, UDMA, TEGDMA. They form resin tags linking primer to composite resin.

Etch and rinse two steps

Conditioner followed by an application of a combined primer and adhesive. It is highly technique sensitive and multiple layers need to be applied (E.g. Optibond Solo plus, Prime and Bond NT).

Advantages of etch and rinse

Long-term studies available, good etch pattern, separate etch is confirmative of proper etching.

Disadvantages

Technique sensitive and over etching can happen. If the moistness after conditioning is not present ineffective penetration occurs.

Self etch two steps

Combined conditioner and primer followed by adhesive resin (AdheSE)

Composition

- Acidic monomers—MDP Di-HEMA-Phosphate, MA 154, Phenyl-P, MAC-10 and 4-META
- Cross-linking monomers—Bis-GMA, UDMA,TEGDMA, GDMA and HEMA
- Solvent—Water based.

Self etch one step

Combined conditioner primer and adhesive (Prompt-L-Pop, ibond, etc).

Advantages
Good dentin conditioning with simultaneous infiltration of resin, no post-conditioning rinse and reduced application time.

Disadvantages
Low bond strength, few clinical data.

Resin-modified glassionomer

Polyacrylic acid removes smear layer and exposes collagen. Mechanical bonding occurs by formation of hybrid layer and chemical bonding through carboxyl groups with calcium in tooth (Fuji bond LC).

11. Factors in shade matching in all ceramic restorations.

Shade matching occurs in the dentist's office, in which the information on color and translucency of the adjacent teeth to be matched is recorded through either visual shade matching or color analysis.

Color is purely an impression, formed in a specific portion of the brain, owing to the specialization of rods and cones distributed over the retina.

Munsell color system and CIELAB system are used for descriptive purposes of color. Color is defined based on three parameters,

1. Hue.
2. Value.
3. Chroma.

Hue

It is the quality that distinguishes one color family from another (E.g. red, green and blue). The vita shade guide comprises of 4 hues, A (reddish brown/orange), B (yellow), C (yellow grey) and D (orange grey).

Value

Is the relative lightness or darkness of a color. It is also the brightness of an object.

Chroma

Chroma is the relation to the amount of pigment contained in a hue. It is the intensity of a hue or saturation of hue.

Translucency

It plays a decisive role in light transmission phenomena.

- Standard shade guides only offer one type of translucency which is generally at a lower level than which is seen in natural teeth
- Translucency is often expressed in a scale of 1–5 where 1 represents a low degree of translucency and 5 represents highly transparent enamel.

Metamerism

Objects that appear to be color matched under one type of light appear different under another light source hence, color matching must be done under more than one light source.

Type of lighting for color matching

- Earlier sunlight was considered the best source for shade matching, but was discarded as the color of natural light may vary
- The ideal source of light would be one that is diffuse and comfortable to the eyes
- The ideal color temperature would be 5500ok [d65] and a color rendering index (CRI) greater than 90 is recommended for shade matching
- Normal dental setups would have fluorescent and incandescent hence, color corrected lighting is recommended for shade matching
- It is recommended that light intensity for dental operatory be between 18 and 28 lux. If ambient lighting is not available, auxiliary light sources should be used.

Shade selection systems

There are two methods of matching shade:

- Shade guides
- Shade taking devices.

Shade guides

- Are convenient
- Porcelain shade guides aid in picking the most natural and reproducible color of the shade in the final restoration
- Available shade guides in market are vita lumin vacuum shade guide, vita 3d master shade guide, and ivoclar chromascop, etc
- Shade guides match hue, chroma and value in different steps before the final selection
- In case of all ceramic restoration, specialized die materials are also used for matching the dental shade. Hence, a stump shade is also chosen after tooth preparation for these patients
- The tooth is divided into a cervical, middle and incisal third and each region is matched individually. This gives a better shade for the crown.

Guidelines for shade matching with shade guides

1. Shade matching is done under balanced light.
2. Bright clothing, lipstick should be hidden as it can affect the shade matching.
3. The teeth to be matched should be cleaned.
4. It should be made at the beginning of the visit.
5. Patient to be viewed at eye level.
6. It should be made quickly.
7. The dentist should rest his eyes by focussing on a neutral grey surface.
8. Generally a shade with low chroma and highest value should be selected.

Shade taking devices/color measuring instruments

The three types of commercially available devices are as follows:

1. Colorimeters.
2. Spectrophotometers.
3. Digital color analyzer.

- Machines, such as spectrophotometers and spectroradiometers are used to measure light reflectance at wavelengths over a visible spectrum
- A spectrophotometer has a stable light source and an aperture between detector and sample
- Colorimeters provide direct color coordinate specifications without mathematical manipulation.

12. Methods to remove crowns and bridges.

Crown removal often happens when the fabricated crown fails due to functional, biological or esthetic reasons.

Eye protection is a must for the dentist, assistant and the patient during removal of the prostheses.

Commonest causes of why crown has to be removed[1,2]

- Bad treatment planning
- Endodontic retreatment
- Progressive disease (caries/periodontal) process
- Chipping of ceramic veneer/Fracture
- Gingival recession of the crowned tooth
- For extension of the bridge span
- Trauma.

Classification and Types of Crown Remover

- Crowns can be removed using any of the following techniques:
  - Adhesive resins/Sticky gums
  - Different types of forceps
  - Chisel and spring action crown removers.
- Crown remover techniques in which crown cannot be reused
  - By cutting the retainer.

Techniques in which crown can be reused

Using sticky gums/adhesive resin

Sticky gums can also be used in the removal of broken crowns as the gums stick on and the adhesive forces will aid in the removal. E.g. Richwil crown and bridge remover (adhesive resin tablet).

Using a straight chisel

By applying a sharp force in an occlusal direction using a mallet, with a sharp chisel placed under the retainer margin, the crown can be removed. The tapping should be done parallel to the path of withdrawal of prosthesis.

Using a crown remover

They are commercially available and manufactured with different tips to engage retainers and pontics. There are commonly three types of crown removers

1. Back action: Uses a weight to deliver a force directed backwards with the tip placed such that it transfers the force occlusally (E.g. slide hammer).
2. Spring loaded: Uses a spring mechanism to deliver a sudden force.
3. Pneumatic: Uses compressed air to deliver a controlled force. Ultrasonic vibration with a ultrasonic scaler can loosen the crown and bridge.

Techniques in which crowns cannot be reused

By cutting the retainer

- This is the best method to prevent any damage to the abutment tooth
- A thin groove is placed on the middle of the restoration with a high-speed airotor handpiece exposing the abutment
- Removal is attempted with a crown remover following cutting through one surface or both. Thus, the crown can be removed using a sharp instrument by wedging it
- Once the crowns are cut through spreaders, help to release the metal substructure from the tooth by inserting into the groove and rotating to break the cement seal.

Removal of different types of crowns

Metal crowns

They can be levered at the margins with a heavy duty scaler (Mitchell Trimmer) or a slide hammer type of remover. If it does not work, the retainer should be cut off.

Ceramic crown

If the crown remover fails they are split open. A vertical groove is made with a diamond bur in the labial/buccal surface to visualize the underlying cement. Later the crown is split with a suitable heavy duty instrument.

Metal–ceramic crowns

Same as above and for splitting the crown a tungsten carbide cross cut bur is most efficient.

Removal of Bridges

1. If the abutment is to be extracted, crown and bridge removers can be used.
2. If the abutment should be intact, retainer can be cut followed by the use of crown and bridge removers.
3. If bridge is needed intact, both tooth and bridge should not be damaged. It is easier to remove all metal and minimal preparation bridges intact than conventional metal ceramic bridges. Sharp tapping can break the bonding of the cement.

Recent advances

Lasers, such as Er, Cr: YSGG lasers 2780 nm are used for debonding porcelain laminate veneers. When applied for 1–2 min on each side of the crown it softens the resin luting agent enabling the easy removal of the veneer.[3]

References

1. Smith BGN, Howe LC. Planning and making crowns and bridges, ed 4. Informa Healthcare; 2007.
2. Rosensteil SF, Land MF, Fujimoto J. Contemporary Fixed Prosthodontics, ed 4, Elsevier; 2006.
3. Berk N, Berk G. The new era for porcelain veneers-remove them with your LASERS! Laser Congress. 4 th Congress of the International Society for Oral Laser Applications SOLA, Bruges, Belgium, Oud St. Jan; 2007.

13. Ante's law and its significance.

(Irwin H Ante)

Definition

- Abutment tooth/teeth should have a combined pericemental area equal to or greater in pericemental area than the tooth or teeth to be replaced (Antes law)
- The optimum crown–root ratio is 2:3
- At least a root ratio of 1:1 needs to be present for a prospective abutment.

To calculate according to Antes law, the pericemental areas of maxillary and mandibular teeth need to be known (Table 1):

Table 1: Pericemental areas of maxillary and mandibular teeth

Teeth	Maxillary teeth root surface areas in mm^2	Mandibular teeth root surface areas in mm^2
Central incisor	204	154
Lateral incisor	179	168
Canine	273	268
First premolar	234	180
Second premolar	220	207
First molar	433	431
Second molar	431	426

Factors that results in modifications to Ante's Law

- Root proximities
- Common path of insertion
- Span length
- Root shape/root angulation/root numbers
- Bone support and periodontal involvement
- Occlusal scheme
- Oral hygiene.

Root proximities

There should be adequate clearance between the roots of proposed abutments for development of physiologic embrasures in the completed prosthesis.

Inadequate clearance is present

1. In malpositioned teeth.
2. In mesiobuccal roots of maxillary molars.

Treatment method

Selective extraction or root resection procedures need to be done if adequate clearance is not present between roots.

Common path of insertion

If long axis of the teeth diverge or converge from parallelism more than 25°, tooth preparation is difficult.

Situations where tooth is more angulated

1. Malaligned tooth.
2. Drifted tooth.
3. Tilted tooth (mesially titled molar).

Span length

- "Ante's law" proved that fixed bridges with short pontic spans have a better prognosis than long-span bridges
- The more the edentulous span length greater the flexing of the prosthesis under occlusal loads. This can cause failure of fixed prosthesis due to breakage of a connector, loosening of a retainer or unfavorable soft tissue response. A bridge with a two-tooth pontic span will flex eight times more than a single tooth pontic
- A long-span prosthesis needs to be made of a high strength and rigid material
- Depending on the edentulous span the number of abutments to be prepared needs to be decided on Ante's law by Johnson (1926). The root surface area of the abutment should be more than the root surface area of the teeth being replaced. Crown–root ratio of 1:1 need to be followed. Two abutment teeth can support two pontics
- Failures due to abnormal stress have been attributed to increased length of the span.

Root shape and angulation

- A molar with divergent roots, single-rooted tooth with an elliptic cross section (broader labiolingually than mesiodistally), a long root or multiple roots provide better support than a root surface area with circular cross section
- Larger teeth will have greater surface area and will handle stress better.

Bone support

- Teeth with vertical and horizontal resorption give less support
- Slightly mobile teeth can be splinted and used as successful abutments.

Occlusal scheme

Varying the occlusal scheme by:

- Narrowing the occlusal tables
- Altering occlusal plane
- Programmed canine disocclusion.

These modifications decrease the load on abutment teeth.

Oral hygiene

Teeth with slight mobility can be used as abutments if stabilized and if oral hygiene is maintained.

14. Shortened dental arch concept (SDA Concept).

SDA is a condition where an individual has intact anterior teeth but no teeth posteriorly affecting their mastication.

The World Health Organization suggests that at least 20 teeth must be present in the oral cavity though literature says that a complete set of anterior and posterior teeth must be present for functional wellness.

Impaired masticatory efficiency is seen when a person has less than 20 teeth.[1]

Significance

- Oral functionality is maintained with SDA concept
- Vertical dimension and occlusal contacts are stable
- Hard tissue health, joint health and patient comfort are maintained
- When all the above factors are present the concept states that missing spaces need not be restored
- Presently SDA concept has become a treatment option for the partially dentate patients
- This concept entirely depends on the patient's opinion and oral hygiene maintenance
- Case reports have proved that SDA for a partially dentate patient provides oral functionality, improved oral hygiene and comfort and reduced costs.
- SDA offers the patient with affordable and functional treatment.

Concept

- The SDA treatment protocols show that the occlusal table is terminated at the second premolar region. Therefore, we can stop with the replacement of first molar and leave the posterior space edentulous
- This concept benefits the medically compromised patients, such as immunotherapy patients under chemo- or radiotherapy
- This may be beneficial for patients as posterior implants are not required
- Other treatment options include distal extension RPDs, Cantilever fixed dental prosthesis and implants.

Conclusion

Functional demands and the number of teeth to satisfy them vary with each individual. Hence, dental treatment must be customized to individual's needs and adaptive capability. SDA as a treatment option is an advantage as it does not compromise patient care.

Reference

1. World Health Organization. Recent advances in oral health. WHO Technical Report Series No. 826. Geneva: WHO;1992. pp. 16-7.
2. Armellini D, von Fraunhofer A. The shortened dental arch: A review of literature. J Prosthet dent. 2004; 92:531-5.

15. Rigid connectors.

Connectors

Definition

Connector is that part of a fixed partial denture (FPD) or splint that joins the individual components (retainers and pontics) together.

Connectors are classified as:
1. Rigid connectors.
2. Non-rigid connectors.

Rigid Connectors

Definition

Rigid connector is a non-moving rigid connection that joins the retainers and pontics.

Techniques of fabricating rigid connectors
1. Rigid connection can be made by casting, as part of a multiunit wax pattern.
2. By soldering, using an intermediate metal whose melting temperature is lower than that of the parent metal.
3. By welding, in which two parts are jointed by melting the adjacent surfaces by heat and/or pressure. A filler metal whose melting temperature is about the same as that of the parent metal can be used or two metal areas are plainly joined.

Design of Connector

Size
- The connector must have adequate bulk to prevent distortion or fracture during function
- A large-sized connector interferes with effective plaque control and can lead to periodontal breakdown
- In metal-ceramic fixed partial dentures, a large connector may also display metal.

Shape
- Elliptical cross section connectors have better strength, but because of anatomic contour it cannot be fabricated
- Most connectors have their greatest dimension perpendicular to the direction of applied force and this tends to result in a weaker connector.

Position
- Connectors should occupy the normal anatomic interproximal areas
- If it encroaches on the buccal, gingival, or lingual embrasure plaque control becomes difficult
- Connectors are normally placed towards the lingual aspect for esthetics and good oral hygiene measures.

Variation in design

Loop connectors are designed when an existing diastema is to be maintained in fixed prosthesis. It consists of a loop on the lingual aspect of the prosthesis that connects adjacent retainers and pontics. The loop can be cast as part of wax pattern that is circular in cross section or shaped from a platinum-gold-palladium (Pt-Au-Pd) alloy wire.

Procedure
- The design of rigid connectors is incorporated into the wax pattern after they have been completed but prior to rewaxing of their margins
- Connectors to be soldered are waxed to final shape and sectioned

- Convexity of the gingival aspect of the connectors is important for good oral hygiene measures
- Anterior connectors should be placed toward the lingual for good esthetics.

Rules to Follow

1. If connectors are to be soldered a soldering gap of about 0.25 mm is ideal.
2. The component should be parallel when casted. This ensures accurate soldering with a minimum of distortion.
3. Large or small gap widths lead to incomplete or weak joints.
4. If complex designs are used it is safer to solder the connector than to cast it.
5. Cast connectors are ideal for complete coverage restorations.
6. Soldered connectors are ideal for partial coverage restorations as wax patterns are easily distorted when they are cast.

16. Soldering.

Definition

It is the joining of metals by use of a filler metal, which has low fusion temperature than that of the metal parts being joined.

Types

Group I

Traditional gold-containing solders (JELENCO).

Group II

Special solders

Pre-soldering

Used for joining the components before porcelain application.

Post-soldering

Used for joining the components after porcelain application.

Pre-ceramic solders

- Are high-fusing alloys, with temperature slightly beneath the softening point of the parent alloy to be joined and should flow well above the fusion range of applied porcelain
- Solder flow is increased by the addition of silver and decreased by the presence of copper.

Postceramic solders

Should flow well below the pyroplastic range of the porcelain.

Composition of solders

Gold, silver, copper, zinc and tin.

Requirements of solder

- Should resist tarnish and corrosion
- The fusion temperature of solder should be lower than metal
- Should be free flowing with proper adhesion to metal
- Solder should not cause pitting of soldered joint
- Strength of solder should be equivalent to the parts to be soldered

- Color of solder should match the parts to be soldered
- It should be corrosion resistant
- It should have adequate mechanical properties to withstand the forces
- It must have a low surface tension when molten.

Soldering techniques

- Torch soldering
- Oven soldering
- Electro-soldering
- Microwelder/Laser welding
- Infrared soldering.

Torch soldering

- After preheating the assembly a gas-air torch is used as the heat source to melt the solder. The flame is kept moving to prevent uneven heat distribution
- Oxidization of the joint surfaces is prevented by using the reducing zone of the flame and by applying an appropriate flux.

Advantage

- Solder flow is controlled and solder flows to the hottest point only
- Ideal for badly designed connector in wax, which can be connected well by varying the temperature of solder manually.

Advantages of oven soldering/electro-soldering over torch soldering

- Temperature is uniform through out the procedure
- The temperature is known through out the procedure
- Application of vacuum can control oxidation
- Close monitoring is possible.

Electro-soldering technique

- Easier to use than torch soldering
- Permits the use of very high fusing alloy solders.

Laser welding

- Used for joining cast titanium components in implant superstructures.

Infrared soldering

- Can be used for low-fusing connectors as well as for pre-ceramic soldering
- A pointer is used to direct heat source to the connector after the application of flux
- While activating the infrared heat source, a protective shield to prevent eye injury is used.

Fluxes

Fluxes containing fluoride must be used.

Soldering investment

- Gypsum and phosphate-bonded investments containing fused quartz with low thermal expansion are used as casting investments
- Invested units should expand at the same rate as the castings.

Soldering in fixed partial denture

Pre-ceramic soldering

Advantages
- The connected prosthesis can be tried in the mouth in the unglazed state
- Adjustments can be made before final glazing.

Disadvantages
- Needs support to prevent high-temperature deformation or sag on long span
- Difficult to contour the proximal embrasures.

Postceramic soldering
- Indicated when regular gold and metal–ceramic units are being combined
- Final staining and glazing must be completed before the soldering.

Advantages
- Proximal areas are more esthetic as they are shaped before soldering
- Sag does not occur and hence, support is not required.

Disadvantage
Adjustment cannot be made after soldering, if made they need to be reglazed and resoldered.

Soldering steps in fixed partial denture
1. Preparation of connector.
2. Occlusal soldering index.
3. Investing.
4. Wax removal and preheating.

Preparation of connector
- After removing surface oxides from the connector surfaces with a stone, evaluate the seating of restoration in the mouth or cast
- The soldering gap should be 0.25 mm.

Occlusal index
- Can be made using plaster, resin or zinc oxide eugenol (ZOE) in a small tray or on a sheet of base plate wax
- The index should not cover the margins and the margins should be exposed prior to investing.

Investing
- The cervical aspect of the restorations are placed into a warmed wax sheet and sealed along the axial wall to protect the porcelain from contact with the soldering investment
- After sealing the porcelain, the entire assembly is boxed and filled with soldering investment, forming into a patty on a slab
- The restorations are seated angled forward so the solder can be placed above the joint.

Wax removal

- After the investment has completely set, remove the index by placing it in boiling water (if plaster or ZOE index was used)
- Flow a little flux into the joint space while the soldering block is still warm
- The joint space must be free of investment
- Acrylic resin indexes are removed by heating slowly to 300°C till the resin is burned out and then heat the block to 650°C and then transfer it to the soldering oven for soldering.

Preheating

Preheat the investment in a burnout furnace to 650°C for low-heat soldering and 850°C for pre-ceramic soldering.

17. Cast core jacket crown.

Post crown/Radicular retainers/Endodontically restored tooth/Dowel crowns/Coronal-radicular stabilization.

Classification of radicular retainers/Endodontically restored tooth

- Single-rooted teeth to be restored require dowels: 80% of remaining tooth structure
- Restoration without dowels for multi-rooted teeth only: 75% remaining tooth structure—Pin-retained complete crown
- Cast dowels
  - Single-rooted teeth:
    - Direct technique
    - Indirect technique (multiple dowel and cores and overdenture abutments).
  - Multi-rooted teeth:
    - Single dowel or multiple parallel dowels.
    - Nonparallel dowels:
      Interlocking castings
      Nonparallel dowel(s) fitted through primary dowel and core casting.
- Preformed dowels
  - Smooth sided tapered:
    - Unitek Kerr Endo Post
    - Minimal retention hence, used for 90% remaining tooth structure.
  - Parallel sided with serrations or grooves for retention (Parapost)
  - Tapered threaded post:
    - E.g. Dentatus
      Threads for retention post are not screwed in.
      Core retention in multi-rooted teeth.
- Tapered and threaded posts:
  - E.g. Flexi Post Brasseler
    - Maximum retention
    - Useful with short roots to retain core.
- Core retention with pins.

Advantages of cast post to preformed dowels

- Custom fit to irregularly shaped canals and not cylindrical as preformed dowels
- Cast as one unit rather than two separate units
- Do not require auxiliary retention as in prefabricated systems.

Custom (Cast) Dowel and Core/Custom cast post and cores

For single-rooted teeth

Techniques

A. Direct Technique:
- Commonly used.

B. Indirect technique:

For multiple dowels and cores, overdenture attachments.

Direct Technique

Preparation of tooth

The remaining tooth structure is reduced to the buccal and lingual surface to produce a ferrule effect (360° collar) with the dowel and core.

Preparing the root canal

- Correct sized files, Pesso reamers and Gates Glidden drills are used to prepare the canal to the approximate size of a No 30 file
- The coronal end of the canal is funnelled (Fig. 1).

Placement of anti-rotational groove

- If the canal is elliptical in shape, an anti-rotational notch is not required
- If it is circular an anti-rotational notch is placed with a tapered bur.

Impression of the canal

- Plastic dowels of the canal size, Kerr Endo Post, toothpicks, nails, paper clips can be used to carry acrylic or wax to form the pattern of the canal. The plastic dowel is roughened and canal is lubricated

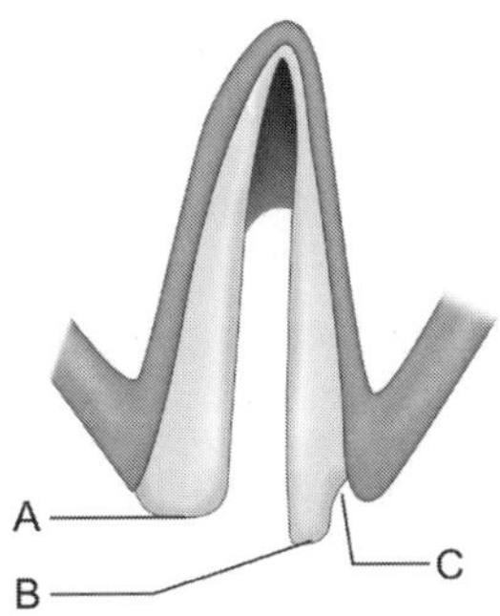

Fig. 1: Preparation of the root canal: A—Horizontal stop; B—Vertical wall to prevent rotation; C—Finish margin for core

- A resin, such as Duralay is applied to the dowel. After the resin reaches the doughy stage, the dowel is inserted into the canal and the dowel is moved up and down to prevent it being locked in an undercut in the canal
- After the resin has set, the pattern is removed and checked for accuracy.

Shaping of coronal aspect

Coronal aspect is next shaped to resemble an ideal tooth preparation.

Investing and casting

The pattern is then invested and cast in a metal of choice.

Indirect Technique

For multiple dowels and cores, overdenture attachments.

Advantages

- Reduced chair time
- Accurate fitting of the coping margin in the gingival crevice
- Can accurately align the overdenture attachment
- Can accurately parallel the coping.

Technique

Impression of the canal

- A loose-fitting plastic or metal dowel with the coronal end bend is used to make the impression
- The dowel is coated with impression material adhesive and the selected elastomeric impression material is injected into the canal with a lentulospiral
- The dowel is also coated with the impression material before placing into the canal. Additional impression material is injected around the tooth and into the gingival crevice and the loaded impression tray is seated.

Removing the impression

- The impression tray is removed along with the dowel carrying the impression of the canal
- The impression is poured in die stone.

Trimming of dies

Dies are trimmed to expose the margins.

Forming pattern of the die

- The dowel pattern is formed by adding molten soft wax on the loose-fitting dowel and inserting it into the canal
- Procedure is repeated until a satisfactory pattern is obtained.

Forming coronal portion

The coronal portion is made with inlay wax to replicate a prepared tooth.

Investing and casting

The pattern is sprued and invested as in the direct technique and cast.

For Multi-rooted teeth

First technique

The larger, longer canal is selected for the primary post, e.g., the palatal canal of maxillary molars or the distal canal of mandibular molars, while the other canal is made parallel to the primary canal for the secondary post, which is not more than 3 or 4 mm in length.

Second technique

Is to make an interlocking post and core for divergent canals so that the length of the secondary canal can be made long.

Third technique

Is to use two or even three canals when they are not parallel with the primary post in the larger, longer canal, while the other canal or canals are used for the secondary dowels.

Procedure (mandibular molar)

- A plastic dowel of last file size used is seated in the distal canal
- A stainless steel dowel is placed in the mesial canal
- The plastic dowel is notched, roughened, and coated with resin which is pumped up and down to prevent locking.

Forming the coronal aspect

After the resin is almost set, the dowel is inserted back into the distal canal and coronal portion is made to resemble an ideal tooth preparation with resin, embedding the lubricated stainless steel post in the pattern (Fig. 2).

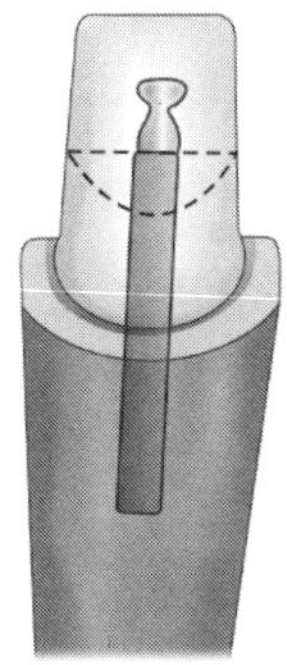

Fig. 2: Cast post completed

Removing stainless steel dowel

- After the resin has set the stainless steel dowel is removed with a plier and is heated until it is oxidized (turning cherry red)
- After it cools, it is reinserted into the pattern to maintain the patency of the hole for the post in the mesial canal during casting.

Investing and casting

- The pattern is invested and cast with a metal of choice
- The oxidation of the stainless steel dowel prevents it from becoming an integral part of the casting.

Removing stainless steel dowel

- The dowel is removed from the casting with a plier
- When fitting the post and core, a new stainless steel dowel of the same size is placed in the hole in the casting.

Seating the casting in the tooth

A cast dowel should be at least the size of a No. 90 endodontic file.

Fitting and cementing custom dowel and cores (Fig. 3)

- Casting is seated passively
- Occlusal clearance and axial contour are examined
- Final corrections are made and the dowel and core are ready for cementation
- The canal is cleaned with a solvent to remove residual lubricant, dried with absorbent points and luted with an appropriate cement (zinc phosphate, resin or glass ionomer)

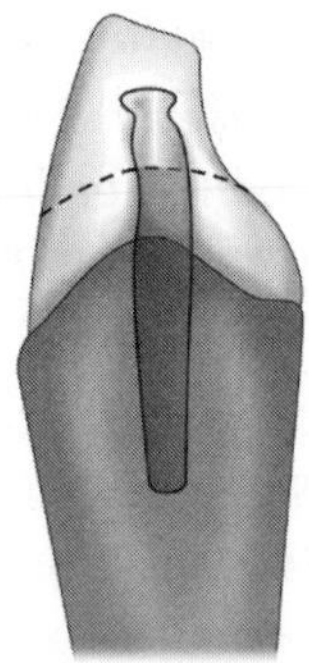

Fig. 3: Crown on cast post

- The cement is mixed and placed into the canal with a lentulo spiral, the dowel and core is also coated with cement and then placed into the tooth under finger pressure until the cement sets
- The crown needs to be made separately after impression procedure to be cemented over the core
- A minimum of 1–2 mm of sound tooth structure apical to the gingival margin of the dowel (post) and core is required.

Note: For question on radicular retainers details of prefabricated dowels also need to be included.

Prefabricated Dowels

Shape

Cylindrical.

Design

- Matched with a specific size endodontic file, Pesso reamer or Gates-Glidden drill
- Have an escape channel for the cement.

Disadvantages

- Cannot resist rotation because of their cylindrical shape, hence threaded or serrated dowels need to be used
- Core material need to be made of amalgam or composite resin.

Available systems

Para-Post

It is a parallel-sided post with a threaded or spiral fluted surface. The amalgam core is retained by the screw-in pins.

Dentatus Screw Post

It is a tapered, threaded rectangular-headed post that retains the core, which can be screwed-in or passively fitted with the threads, providing retention for the cement.

Flexi-post

Prevents root fracture with its split shank that closes during insertion, absorbing stresses.

Brasseler–Vlock Drill and Post System

Is a parallel-sided micro-threaded post with a posthole that can be precisely cut to match the micro-threaded post, reducing stress and improving retention.

Cementing and core fabrication

- Luting is similar to other techniques
- The core is fabricated with composite resin or amalgam in posterior teeth which is pin retained
- The gingival margin should not terminate on the core build up.

18. Richmond crown.

It is an old type of crown with a dowel and a gold crown cast or soldered with a porcelain veneer facing.

Indication

As a bridge retainer on pulpless anterior tooth.

Parts of Richmond crown (Fig. 4)

Facing

Porcelain.

Coping

- Metal cap fitted on root face
- Dowel extending into root canal.

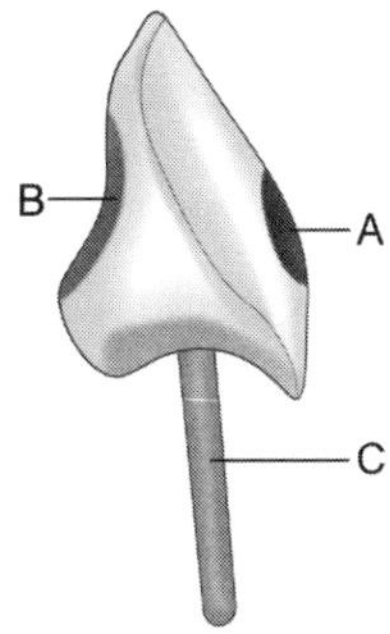

Fig. 4: Richmond crown: Parts: A—Facing; B—Cast gold body; C—Post

Steps in preparation

Preparation of tooth

Diamond stones are used to drill holes labiolingually through the crown 3 mm above the highest level of the crest of gingival tissues.

Root pre-operational

The part of tooth in which a series of holes were placed is broken off and the face of the root is prepared.

Labial plane

Is prepared sloping gingivally terminating 1 mm above labial crest of gingival tissue.

Lingual plane

- Prepared sloping in cervical direction lying in horizontal plane and terminating 3 mm above lingual crest of gingival tissue
- Unsupported enamel margins are removed by files.

Measuring the face of root

A wire is used to measure the circumference of the root cap required.

Construction of cap

- Direct method:
  Prepared tooth by fitting an axial band on which the cap is soldered
- Indirect method:
  Cap swaged from a single piece of metal.

Direct method

1. The measured wire is cut and straightened and the measurement transferred to a gold plate.
2. The height of band is from gingival margin to the highest point on root preparation.
3. The plate is made to a ring form with both ends joined and soldered.
4. The soldered band is placed on root preparation and made to fit the ferrule margin cervically
5. After many adjustments the band is fitted well till it parallels the curvature of gum tissue.

Placement of band at gingival margin

1. The margin of the band should be marked at the labial and lingual aspects and lowered into the crest of gum 0.75–0.5 mm short of the preparation till the marked area on the band.
2. The height of the band is reduced 2 mm above the crest of gingival tissue.

Gold cap soldered

The band is removed from tooth and gold plate is soldered to the incisal end.

Dowel placement

1. After a clasp metal dowel is placed in the root canal, the opening of the canal is countersunk 0.5 mm.
2. Cap is burnished into the countersunk area and the dowel is forced through the cap into root canal.
3. Dowel extends 2–3 mm above the root cap.
4. The dowel and cap are stuck with sticky wax at the countersunk area.
5. After the sticky wax is cooled the dowel cap unit is removed, invested and soldered.
6. The solder fills the countersunk area and the cap is united to the dowel and this is referred to as coping.

Indirect method

1. After wire measurement, copper band matrix is fitted and a modelling compound impression is made.
2. Impression is boxed and an amalgam die is prepared.
3. Heat treated gold plate with its softness is swaged on to the die with finger pressure or wood piece to adapt well.
4. Cap is placed on the prepared tooth, and united to dowel by soldering.

Preparation of models

1. Impressions are made, and a wax wafer bite is taken.
2. Before pouring the cast the inside of copings and sides of dowel are flowed with thin layer of wax.
3. The wax should not be flown to the inside of root cap and gingival margins of root cap.
4. After cast is retrieved, flame is applied to the region of the coping, this removes the thin layer of wax and the coping is also removed from cast.
5. After the entire wax is removed the coping is lubricated and placed back on the model.

Selection of facing

1. A correct shade porcelain facing with the adequate length and height is selected.
2. The facing is ground to fit the gingival margin accurately.
3. The lingual aspect is hollowed out and the facial aspect contacts the root cap in a line.

Incisal bevel

- After grinding to the correct shape and size the incisal edge is bevelled to a 45° angle with lingual surface.

Trial

- The facing is placed into the coping with soft wax to check alignment
- Once the fit is confirmed assembling is done.

Assembling

The entire coping and backing of the face are covered with wax, invested and soldered or cast.

Variation

Steele interchangeable facing: Is a replaceable facing, which can be cast or soldered.

19. Davis crown.

(Wallace Clyde Davis) 1866–1950

- This is a dental restoration supported by a dowel in the root canal over which a porcelain tube teeth is placed directly on the root face of the tooth
- It is one type of dowel crown, which is detachable or called as the detached dowel type
- It is cemented in position uniting the tooth, dowel and crown into one unit (Fig. 5).

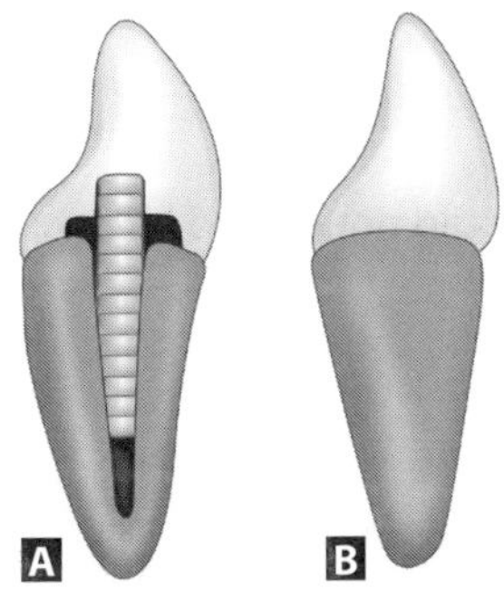

Figs 5A and B: Detached dowel with all-porcelain crown

Methods to adapt the crown

1. When excessive tooth decay has occurred, there will be discrepancy between the fit of the crown and root planes in such cases a cast metal base can be placed between the crown and root planes. The cast base is attached to the dowel.
2. Porcelain is fused and interposed between the crown and root planes.

Preparation method

Steps in preparation:

1. Preparation of labial and lingual planes is done.
2. A complete porcelain crown of proper mould, size and shape is selected.
3. The dowel is fitted in the root canal.
4. A platinum ferrule (0.0005 inch thick) is adapted on the dowel extension.

Porcelain crown is placed over the dowel and ferrule.

The crown position, with adjacent teeth and alignment is verified and the crown is fitted to the dowel with sticky wax and removed.

Laboratory steps

A platinum foil 0.001 inch is burnished onto the root face of die and the crown, ferrule and dowel is seated on platinum foil.

The gap between the porcelain crown and swaged platinum matrix is sealed with melted inlay wax and its removed.

This is invested and burn out done to remove the inlay wax. The temperature of furnace is raised to 1093 degree and medium-fusing porcelain is placed at the area where wax has burned out.

Depending on the morphology, porcelain can be added and fired to form the correct contours. Excess porcelain is ground and glazed to complete the restoration.

20. Axio-proximal grooves.

Axio-proximal grooves are grooves that are placed to provide retention to the preparation.

Preparations requiring axio-proximal grooves

- Anterior and posterior partial veneer crowns
- Three quarter crowns
- Mesial half crowns.

Design

Should be 1 mm wide and should not extend below the cervical line.

Location

In the axial walls proximally.

Instrument used

No. 170 bur or No. 169L.

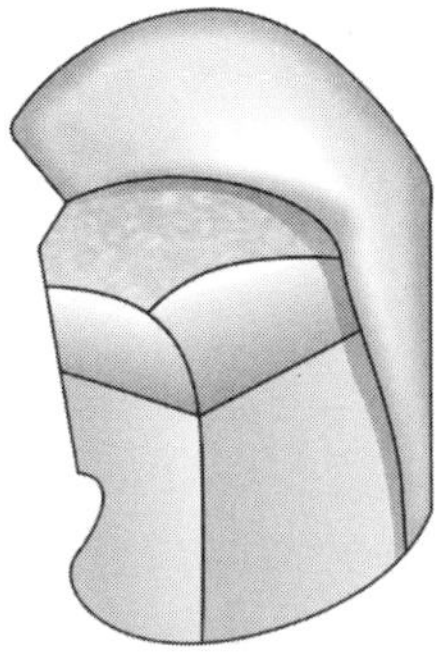

Fig. 6: Outlining the groove

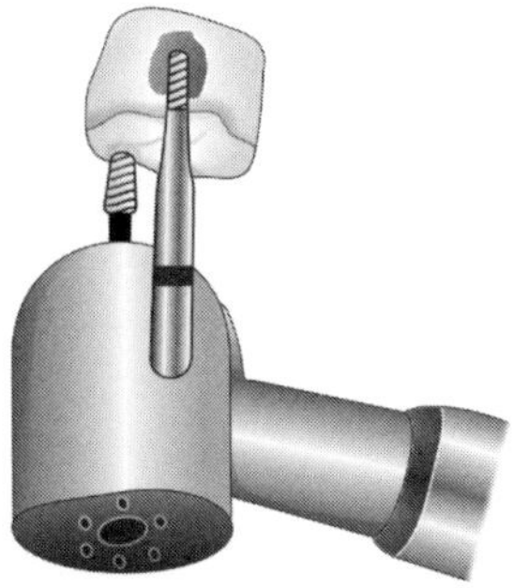

Fig. 7: Alignment of second groove

Steps in preparation

1. Axial reduction is done starting from the lingual surface with a chamfer diamond.
2. Before extending to the interproximal areas proximal access is gained with a short, thin tapered diamond.
3. The final interproximal chamfer margin is completed with a chamfer diamond.
4. The axial wall and finish line are placed with a chamfer carbide finishing bur.

Axio-proximal groove placement

- The outline of the groove is drawn on the occlusal surface of the tooth (Fig. 6)
- Proximal grooves are ideally the size of a No. 170 bur; the groove can be also placed with a No. 169L bur (minor adjustments can be made later).

Placement of second groove

For easy alignment of second groove a bur is held with utility wax in the first groove (Fig. 7).

Making a template

- The outline form of the finished groove is made on the occlusal surface with a pencil and a template is cut which is 1 mm deep
- The template is used as a guide to extend the groove to half its length placing the bur aligned with the path of insertion or the preparation.

Proximal flare placement

- A proximal flare is placed on the walls of the proximal groove for good marginal adaptation of the restoration
- A flame-shaped diamond or enamel hatchet is used to smoothen the proximal flares.

Occlusal offset

- By connecting both the grooves on the occlusal aspect an occlusal offset is formed with No. 170 bur on the lingual incline of the buccal cusp (Fig. 8).
- Offset provides space for more metal that reinforces the margins and the grooves.

Bevel placement

A white polishing stone is used to place a 0.5 mm finishing bevel along the bucco-occlusal finish line, which merges with the proximal flares.

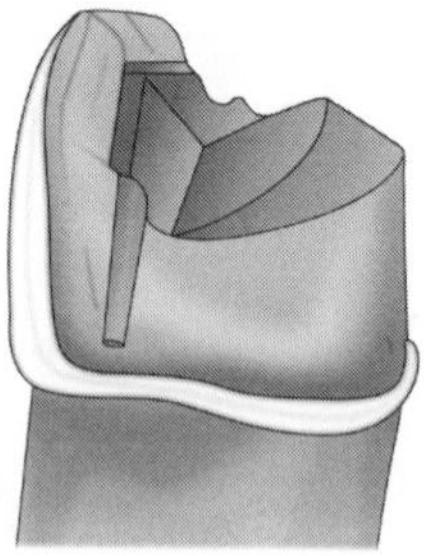

Fig. 8: Completed axioproximal groove with occlusal offset

Rules to follow

1. Place grooves first in inaccessible interproximal surfaces (distal aspect) and then place the second corresponding groove on mesial aspect.
2. Alteration of groove is easy in accessible areas if minor corrections are required.
3. Use a No. 169L bur first so that adjustment can be made if needed.
4. Place the proximal grooves parallel to the incisal two thirds of the facial surface in anterior tooth preparation.
5. In case of adequate thickness of tooth the groove can be expanded.
6. The lingual wall of the proximal grooves should have 2°–5° incisal convergence with the lingual gingival wall.
7. The grooves should resist lingual displacement.
8. The facial wall of the groove should be continuous with the proximal flare to add bulk to the facial margin.
9. The grooves should be at least 3 mm long and terminate within 0.5 mm of the gingival finish line.
10. The facial and lingual walls of the grooves should have a 2°–5° incisal divergence.
11. Place the proximal groove approximately 0.5 mm from the facial and gingival finish lines.
12. Axial walls of each groove should converge occlusally.

21. Pier abutment.

Synonyms

Intermediary abutment/Intermediate abutment (Fig. 9).

Definition

Pier abutment is a natural tooth located between terminal abutments that serve to support a fixed or removable prosthesis.

Disadvantages of placing a rigid connector in pier abutment

Movements in tooth

- A tooth moves buccolingually, faciolingually and intrudes to a minor extent (buccolingual movement from 56μ to 108μ and intrusion is 28μ)

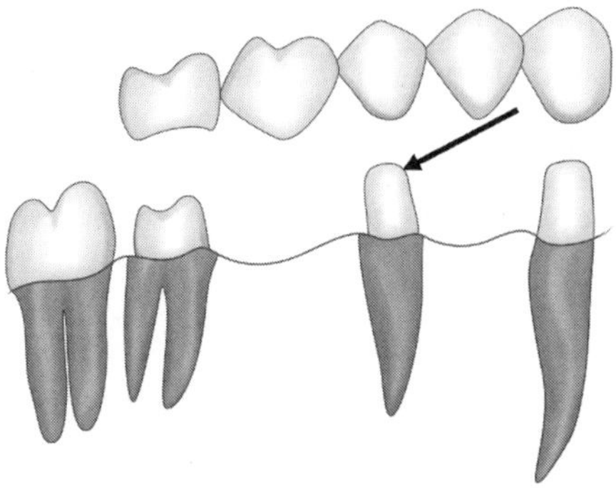

Fig. 9: Pier abutment

- Anterior tooth moves more in a faciolingual direction and posterior tooth moves more in buccolingual direction
- These movements increase stresses transmitted onto the abutments.

Fulcrum-like effect

In pier abutments with rigid connectors, the independent direction and magnitude of movements of the abutment teeth cause a fulcrum-like effect on pier abutment.

Weakening of terminal retainers

The forces transmitted to the terminal retainers due to the pier abutment's fulcrum-like effect can cause failure to the weaker retainer.

Microleakage and caries

The loose retainer will have leakage about the margin and can cause extensive caries leading to failure of abutment tooth.

This commonly occurs with the small anterior retainer than the posterior retainer.

Ideal design for pier abutment

To protect pier abutment, non-rigid connectors are designed.

Indications

- In short span bridges
- In single tooth replacements.

Contraindications of non-rigid connector

- When pier abutment is mobile (then rigid connector is to be used)
- When posterior abutment opposes an edentulous space (supraeruption of abutment tooth and displacement of key can occur).

Advantages of non-rigid connector

- The movement in the connector prevents the middle abutment from acting as a fulcrum in buccolingual or occlusocervical direction

- Less stress to the terminal abutments
- Long life of prosthesis as chances of abutment failure is less.

Design of non-rigid connector

The non-rigid connector is a broken-stress mechanical union of retainer and pontic instead of the usual rigid solder joint.

Components

- Non-rigid connector consists of a key and keyway
- A T-shaped key that is attached to the pontic
- A dovetail key-way placed within a retainer
- Male component or the key is attached to mesial surface of the mesial pontic of distal edentulous spaces.

Location of non-rigid connector

- It must be placed on the middle abutment
- The keyway of the connector is placed in the distal side of the middle abutment and the key is placed on the mesial side of the first molar pontic.

Keyway

- When occlusal forces are applied to posterior tooth it leans mesially as the long axis of posterior tooth slants mesially hence, placement of the keyway in the distal side of the pier abutment seats the key into the keyway during mesial movement
- If keyway is placed on mesial aspect it gets unseated during mesial movements leading to mobility in abutments in the long run.

Examples of pier abutment design

Using non-rigid connector

Missing
Maxillary central incisor and opposite side lateral incisor.

Abutments
Lateral incisor, central incisor (pier) and canine.

Retainers
- Pin-retained partial veneer crown on lateral incisor
- Three-quarter crowns on the central incisor and canine.

Pontics
Porcelain fused to metal.

Design
A keyway is placed in the distal of the central incisor retainer to accommodate a key on the mesial of the lateral incisor pontic.

Using rigid connector

Missing
Mandibular central incisor and opposite side lateral incisor.

Abutments
Lateral incisor, central incisor (pier), and canine.

Retainers
- Pin-retained partial veneer crown on lateral incisor
- Three-quarter crowns on central incisor and canine.

Pontics
Porcelain fused to metal.

Design
- A completely rigid bridge is used in this situation because of short span length and small teeth
- If bone support is poor, the central incisor is extracted and rigid connector bridge placed from canine to canine.

22. Causes of abutment failure.

Failures in abutment can occur at different stages, from case selection to postinsertion problems.

Failures at different stages

- Case selection
- Mouth preparation
- Tooth preparation
- Inaccurate impression
- Temporary restorations
- Errors in wax pattern and laboratory procedures
- During insertion
- Postinsertion failures.

Case selection
1. Failures occur when the patient has unrealistic expectations of the esthetics, function and life expectancy of prosthesis.
2. Inadequate medical and dental history.
3. Inadequate radiographic and intraoral examinations.
4. Wrong selection of abutment tooth, for example selection of malaligned, mobile tooth as abutment.
5. Patients with temporomandibular joint problems.
6. Improper ridge contours—Bulbous ridge, healing ridge or excessively resorbed ridge can hamper esthetic outcome of prosthesis.
7. Patients with poor oral hygiene.

Mouth preparation

Soft tissue preparation

1. Inadequate periodontal procedures.
2. Failure to correct high and attached frenums.
3. Failure to restore the health of the prospective abutment tooth by adequate mouth preparations.

Hard tissue preparation

1. If present, overhanging restorations, supraerupted tooth, mesially drifted tooth occupying pontic space, un-restored caries tooth, all need to be corrected before tooth preparation for fixed partial denture.
2. Extensively damaged tooth need to be endodontically treated.

Tooth preparation

1. Excessive tooth reduction.
2. Improper path of removal and placement (lack of parallelism).
3. Over reduction leading to decreased height of abutment tooth decreases resistance form.
4. Inaccurate, irregular finish lines—Poor marginal adaptation.
5. Reduced labial reduction—Lack of bulk for porcelain material leads to failure of porcelain or an overcontoured restoration leads to periodontal problems.
6. Inadequate cooling of tooth during preparation leads to loss of vitality of tooth.
7. If anatomical morphology of tooth preparation is not followed during occlusal preparation, inaccurate finish lines, over reduction with more taper leads to decreased retention and resistance of the prosthesis leading to failure.

Inaccurate impression

Inaccurate, distorted final impressions can lead to distorted dies that form inaccurate wax patterns leading to failure of prosthesis.

Temporary restorations

1. Over extension of temporary restoration below gingival margin can cause recession of gingiva.
2. Lack of occlusion in temporary restoration can lead to supraeruption of opposing tooth.

Errors in wax pattern and laboratory procedures

1. Materials used for dies and wax patterns should be dimensionally stable.
2. Technique for wax pattern fabrication and marginal adaptation should be correct.
3. Improper spruing, weak investment materials, incomplete wax burn out with wax residues, reused alloys, alloys that have not flown completely into the mould due to faulty machine setting all lead to failure of prosthesis.

During insertion

1. Restoration with poor marginal adaptation.
2. Lack of proximal contact can lead to food impaction.
3. Lack of proper occlusion.

Postinsertion failures

1. Recurrent caries or secondary caries under the retainers.
2. Failure of luting agent—consistency of luting agent while luting is significant.
3. Over reduced tooth can fracture leading to failure.
4. Fracture of facings.
5. Soldered connector joints that fracture.
6. Poor pontic design can cause soft tissue response, such as inflammation.
7. Periodontal involvement of tooth due to bad oral hygiene measures.

23. Mesial half crown.

Synonym

One half crown (Fig. 10).

Definition

Mesial half crown restores the occlusal and mesial surfaces as well as portions of the facial and lingual surfaces.

Indication

In mesially tilted molars (second mandibular tilted into the space of first mandibular).

Contraindications

- In caries or decalcified tooth extending distally
- In caries prone mouth
- In poor oral hygiene maintenance
- If there is severe marginal ridge height difference between the distal of the second molar and the mesial of the third molar
- The molar tooth should not converge more than 25°–30°.

Preparation

- A mesial half crown is a three-quarter crown rotated 90° with the distal surface uncovered
- As the second molar is generally over-tapered it needs additional grooves on buccal and lingual aspect.

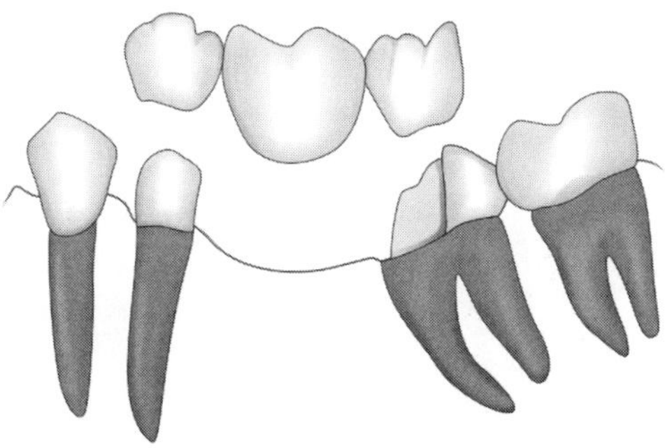

Fig. 10: Mesial half crown

Steps in preparation

1. The path of insertion is established and many lines are scribed on base of cast parallel to the established path.
2. Occlusal or incisal reduction is done first parallel to the planned occlusal plane.
3. Depth guides are placed on the buccal and lingual surfaces of abutment teeth and are prepared parallel to the scribe lines on the base of the diagnostic cast.
4. A chamfer diamond with a 2°–3° taper is used to prepare the inaccessible areas first, such as the distal and lingual aspect, then the facial and mesial aspects.
5. After the reduction parallelism is checked with intraoral mirrors, a trial cast is made of the preparation and evaluated for parallelism on dental surveyor.
6. All sharp margins are rounded, and finish lines are evaluated for smoothness.

24. Cantilever fixed partial denture.

Synonym

Cantilever bridge (Fig. 11).

Definition

This is a fixed partial denture in which the pontic is retained and supported only on one end by one or more abutments.

Selection of cantilever abutments

- Good bone support should be present more than the average
- Adequate clinical crown height should be present
- Should be able to develop an harmonious occlusion
- Extensively damaged teeth, maligned teeth, endodontically treated teeth and mobile teeth are contraindicated from being used as cantilever abutments.

Ideal cantilever situations

1. Replacement of lateral incisor using canine as cantilever.
2. Replacement of first premolar using second premolar as cantilever.
3. A cantilever bridge should ideally have lengthy roots with a favorable configuration, good clinical crown height, good crown–root ratios and healthy periodontium.

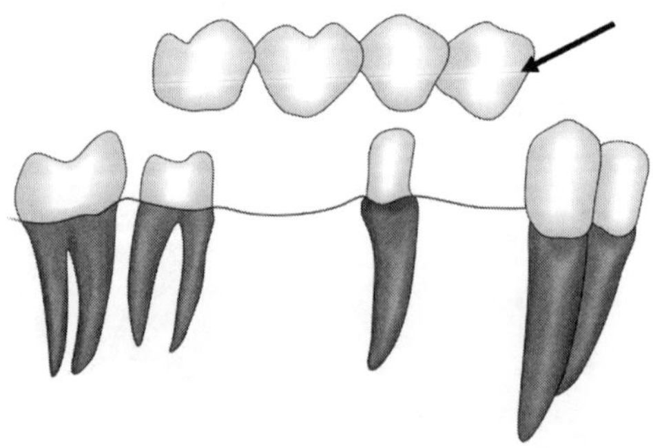

Fig. 11: Cantilever bridge

Advantages

- Conservative design with preservation of tooth structure
- Secondary abutments used can be prepared easily with parallelism.

Disadvantages

- Produces torquing and lateral forces
- Cannot restore long-span edentulous space
- Lateral forces can tip rotate or drift the abutment tooth.

Modifications

Spring cantilever

- For replacing maxillary incisors
- Support is from splinted premolars or molars; a long resilient bar connects both.

Advantages

- In diastema cases
- Preservation of tooth structure as only all-metal restoration is required for molar.

Disadvantages

- Interference in speech
- Distortion of connector can displace pontic
- Food entrapment is common.

Design examples

- Can replace maxillary lateral incisor with canine as abutment
- Can replace mandibular first premolar with second premolar and first molar as abutments
- In some instances can replace molars with no distal abutments to prevent super-eruption of opposing teeth. The replaced pontic should be premolar sized, good occlusogingival height and minimal occlusal contact.

25. Describe cementation of all ceramic restorations.

With the introduction of all ceramics and CAD–CAM restorations, the types of cementation have evolved into adhesive cementation.

Adhesive cementation is the bonding of the restoration (crown/veneer) to the tooth. The tooth is being sealed as well.

Classification of dental cements

Based on chemistry and application, they are of three types:

- Water-based cements
- Resin-based cements
- Oil-based cements.

Water-based cements

- Undergo acid–base setting reaction and are acidic during cementation
- Are non-adhesive or have low bond strength with tooth [E.g. glass ionomer (Fuji I, Ketac Cem), resin-modified glass ionomer (RelyX luting, FujiCEM), zinc phosphate (Harvard, D-Tech) and zinc polyacrylate (Poly F)].

Resin-based cements

- Can be light cure or dual cure type
- If the crown is >3 mm thick autopolymerizing resin cement is used as light cannot penetrate to the depths; otherwise a dual cure resin cement is used
- Are chemically similar to composites
- They have higher bond strengths with tooth structure
- The tooth needs to be etched and rinsed
- Some of these cements are self-adhesive to dentin
- The restoration should be surface treated and primer is applied before cementation
- These cements have stronger physical properties but are technique sensitive. [E.g. Resin luting agents, etch and rinse composites (RelyX ARC, C & B cement) and self-etch and self-adhesive composites (Multilink, RelyX Unicem), compomers (Principle)] .

Oil-based cements

- Used for provisional cementation
- Eugenol containing or eugenol free [E.g. are zinc oxide-eugenol and non–eugenol zinc oxide (Provicol)].

Commonly used luting agents for all ceramic restorations

- Zinc phosphate (for zirconia restorations)
- Glass ionomer cement (for zirconia restorations)
- Resin luting agents, mostly dual cure (for any all-ceramic restoration).

Resin-modified glass ionomer is not used for cementing all ceramic restorations as they undergo expansion due to water absorption following cementation. The most popular cements are resin cements and glass ionomers (Table 2).

Table 2: Differences between conventional (luting) cement and adhesive (bonding) cement

Conventional cement	Adhesive cement
• Relies on mechanical retention – Long axial walls – 6 degree taper – Conventional cements fill the gap between tooth and restoration • Based on water and reactive alkaline fillers	• Bonds to tooth and restoration – Adhesive surfaces – Moisture-free environment – Adhesive cement fills the gap and creates a monobloc • Anhydrous and silanized nonreactive fillers

Step-by-step procedure

1. Isolate the tooth and clean it.
2. Place plastic strips interproximally.
3. Etch the enamel with phosphoric acid, clean and dry the tooth.

4. Seal any open dentinal tubules using a bonding agent.
5. The fitting surface of the ceramic restoration is etched using hydrofluoric acid gel.
6. Apply silane coupling agent to the ceramic restoration.
7. Select the shade of the resin luting agent and mix the components using a plastic spatula
8. Load the crown and carefully seat over the prepared tooth.
9. Do not give any excessive seating force.
10. Remove any excess cement after tack curing.
11. Final curing using light is done after removal of the excess luting agent.
12. Adjust the premature contacts.
13. Finish the cement margins with carbide finishing burs, fine paper discs or rubber cups.

Conclusion

- For good esthetics of the final ceramic restoration, the color of the underlying luting agent must be faintly colored and translucent enough to bring out the natural color of the dentin and enamel
- If the cement is opaque, the esthetic quality declines and the margins begin to be visible. Color can be controlled by varying the proportions of opaque and translucent catalyst.

26. Recent advances in Investment materials.

Types

- Gypsum bonded
- Phosphate bonded
- Silicate bonded.

Types of investment materials commonly used

Extensive use of metal ceramics and heat-pressed ceramics has resulted in the increased use of phosphate-bonded or silicate-bonded investments.

Disadvantages: They are difficult to remove from the castings than gypsum-bonded investments.

Modifications in composition

Carbon is added to produce clean castings as they facilitate divesting casting from the mold if the casting alloy is gold.

In case of casting palladium silver alloys or base metal alloys a carbon free investment material is used because palladium reacts with carbon at temperatures above 1504°C. A carbon crucible should not be used for melting the alloy.

The detailed reproduction and surface smoothness of metal ceramic gold alloy restoration cast in phosphate-bonded investment was considered inferior to a gold alloy cast in gypsum-bonded investment. Now, phosphate-bonded investments approach surface quality or fineness of gypsum-bonded investments.

Recent advances in investments

- Investments used for all ceramic restorations
- Investments used for soldering/brazing

- Die/Investment combinations
- Investments used for ringless casting system.

Investments for all-ceramic restorations

Types
- For cast glass technique (phosphate-bonded refractories)
- Refractory die material (Used with all-ceramic veneers, inlays and crowns).

Refractory die materials
- Refractory dies are made by pouring investment into the impressions
- When the investment is set, die is removed and heated to remove gasses
- They accurately reproduce the impression, remain undamaged during porcelain firing and have a thermal expansion compatible with that of ceramic
- They are phosphate bonded and contain fine-grained refractory fillers to reproduce details
- The investment materials have quartz only and no cristobalite, unlike the conventional phosphate-bonded investments which contain both quartz and cristobalite.

Investments for brazing investments

Types
- Type I—Gypsum-bonded dental brazing investments
- Type II—Phosphate-bonded dental brazing investments.

Procedure
- The parts to be soldered must be embedded in an investment material before heating
- The assembled parts are temporarily held together with sticky wax
- The portion to be soldered is left exposed and free from investment to permit wax removal and effective heating before it is joined with a solder
- Soldering investments have lower setting and thermal expansions than casting investments, so that the assembled parts do not shift in position during setting and heating of investments
- Their particle size is larger as smoothness of the investment is less important.

Die Stone/Investment Combination
- This is a technique wherein a die material and investing medium with a comparable composition is used. E.g.: Divestment
- They are gypsum-bonded materials mixed with colloidal silica liquid
- Die is made from this mix and wax pattern is fabricated on this. The die with the wax pattern is invested in a mixture of the investment and water. This is recommended for conventional gold alloys
- A phosphate-bonded investment is used in the same manner as gypsum-based materials and is suitable for high-fusing alloys.

Investments for ringless casting system[1]
- A ringless system that provides maximum expansion of investment material is available commercially as power cast ringless system

- It consists of three sizes of rings and formers, preformed wax sprues, investment powder and special investment liquid
- It is suitable for alloys that require greater mold expansion.

Reference

1. Touati B, Miara P, Nathanson D. Esthetic dentistry and Ceramic restorations. Informa Healthcare. 1999.

27. Retention in fixed partial denture.

Definition

Retention

Retention prevents removal of the restoration along the path of insertion or along the path of the tooth preparation.

It is the quality of a preparation that prevents the restoration from becoming dislodged by such forces parallel to the path of withdrawal.

Resistance

Prevents dislodgement of the restoration, by forces directed in an apical or oblique direction and prevents any movement of restoration under occlusal forces.

Factors affecting retention

- Magnitude of the dislodging forces
- Geometry of the tooth preparation
- Roughness of the fitting surface of the restoration
- Type of restorative materials being cemented
- Type of luting agent/film thickness of the luting agent.

Magnitude of the dislodging forces

Factors influencing dislodging forces:

- Stickiness of the food
- Surface area of the restoration
- Texture of the restoration being pulled.

Of all the type of forces, sticky food exhibits large dislodging forces a floss placed beneath the connectors present the same type of effect as sticky food.

Geometry of the tooth preparation

Factors influencing geometry of tooth preparation:

- Taper
- Surface area
- Stress concentration
- Type of preparation.

Taper

- Maximum retention is obtained if a tooth preparation has parallel walls
- Smaller degrees of taper have more retention
- Two opposing surfaces each with a 3° taper provide a 6° taper for the preparation
- Ideal convergence between opposing walls is 6°
- This amount of convergence is required to restrain the cemented restoration.

Factors decreasing retention with regard to taper

- Less amount of taper will form an undercut in an occlusocervical direction
- An increased amount of taper increases free movement of the restoration and retention will be reduced (experimented by Jorgensen in 1955).

Preparation rule

- A rotary instrument of the desired taper held at a constant angulation produces the amount of taper required
- The rotary instrument of ideal taper when moved through a cylindrical path during tooth preparation will produce the desired axial wall taper on the completed preparation.

Surface area

- The greater the length of the clinical crown, the more is the retention
- Short clinical crowns require the help of grooves and box preparation for increased retention
- The greater the width of the clinical crown, the better the retention
- A restoration with a limited path of withdrawal is more retentive depending on the length of the surface area in sliding contact.

Stress concentration

- Round margins reduce stress concentrations, and increase the retention of the restoration
- Stresses are generally concentrated around the junction of the axial and occlusal surfaces.

Type of preparation

- Additional grooves and boxes to a preparation with a limited path of withdrawal increase the retention
- Retention is double for complete crowns than for a partial crown
- Luting agent is only effective if the restoration has a single path of withdrawal
- The occlusoaxial line angle of the tooth preparation should be a replica of the gingival margin geometry
- Fixed prostheses depend on the geometric form than on adhesion of the luting agents for retention.

Roughness of the surfaces

- Retention is increased if the restoration is roughened or grooved by air-abrading the fitting surface with alumina
- If the internal surface of a restoration is very smooth, retentive failure can occur.

Materials being cemented

- The more reactive base-metal alloys have more adhesion with certain luting agents than less reactive high-gold content metals
- Cement adheres better to amalgam than to composite resin or cast gold.

Type of luting agent

Adhesive resin cements are the most retentive.

28. Instructions to crown and bridge patients regarding care and maintenance.

Significance

After placement and cementation of fixed dental prosthesis improper maintenance program is the major cause for failures in fixed partial dentures.

Hence, maintenance program is aimed at reinforcing meticulous plaque control habits, identifying incipient caries/gingivitis and to introduce corrective treatment wherever required.

Postcementation instructions

- Patient is advised to chew food only one hour after cementation
- Is instructed to avoid biting on hard foods for at least 24 hours to achieve maximum strength
- Patient is warned to expect mild to moderate sensitivity to hot and cold food/drink for a few days after cementations over vital teeth
- Patient is advised against flossing for a couple of days but brushing can commence almost immediately
- If the bite does not feel normal the patient is asked to report to the dentist
- Patient is instructed in special plaque control measures to use floss and floss threaders
- Patient is instructed on the importance of attending recall visits every six months.

29. Articulators.

Fully-adjustable articulators

Initially the term fully adjustable was used, suggesting that articulators in this category would be able to duplicate all mandibular movements.

As studies proved that they could not duplicate all mandibular movements, fully adjustable and semi adjustable articulators were re-classified as adjustable articulators.

- All articulators in this class are arcon instruments with adjustable intercondylar distances
- The condylar housings can be adjusted in the horizontal, sagittal, frontal planes
- Each has a Bennett guide adjustment
- They all accept arbitrary or hinge axis face-bow transfers
- They are often referred to as gnathologic instruments, because of their full adjustability.

Semi-adjustable articulators

- Accept three-dimensional dynamic registrations and utilize a face-bow transfer
- The condylar pathways, or cams, are formed by registrations engraved by the patient
- The immediate Bennet movement and progressive Bennet movement can be determined
- They have curvilinear condylar guidances.

Classification

Mechanical adjustments

Examples:

- Hanau 166-1 Radial shift

- Whip Mix 8340
- Whip Mix DB 2200.

Preformed Fossae

Examples:
- Denar Anamark
- Panadent SL
- TMJ Delux.

Custom created

Examples:
- Denar D5A
- Stuart Gnathologic Computer
- TMJ Stereographic.

Hanau 166-1 radial shift

- Horizontal guidances have ¾ inch curvature adjustable in inclination from 0° to 60°
- Lateral condylar guidance has a radial curve (immediate side shift) adjustable from 0 to 3 mm
- Progressive side shift adjustable from 0°–30°
- Condylar elements are fixed at 110.

Panadent

- By Lee and Lundeen
- In this there are five analog fossa features with a precurrent side shift of 0.5, 1.0, 1.5, 2.0, 2.5 mm
- A hinged centric latch mechanism holds two members together and permits 180° range of opening
- Fixed intercondylar distance of 110 mm
- Dynalinks are elastic elements preventing separation of two frames during lateral excursive movements and also aids in returning to centric relation afterwards.

TMJ stereographic

- By Kenneth Swanson in 1965 (Class 4)
- An intraoral registration generated by studs in autopolymerizing resin similar to chew-in technique. This is called a "stereographic" recording
- The stereographic recording is then placed on the articulator and used to mould fossae in autopolymerizing resin, which is supposed to produce an accurate analog of the patient's temporomandibular joint function.

Stuart Gnathologic Computer

- By Charles Stuart in 1955
- Gnathology refers to the study of occlusion and occlusal rehabilitation through the use of pantographs and fully-adjustable articulators
- The Bennett guides are situated in the middle of the posterior aspect of the instrument similar to the Gysi Trubyte articulator

- The Bennett guides can be angulated and customized
- Numerous plastic condylar inserts are available and they can be customized by grinding, if necessary.

Denar D5A modification of D4A

- By Niles Guichet, 1968
- Condylar guidances are adjustable in three planes
- Intercondylar element adjustments from 90 to 150 mm
- Is similar to the D4A except for refinements in machining and in the centric latch mechanism located at the rear of the articulator
- Plastic condylar inserts are available that can be custom ground
- The Bennett adjustment is located in the medial wall of the condylar housing and has provisions for both immediate side shift (straight) and progressive side shift (angular) adjustments
- Instruments in this class will accept three-dimensional dynamic registrations and utilize a face-bow transfer. The condylar pathways can be selectively angled and customized
- The three-dimensional dynamic registration procedure utilized in this class is the pantographic tracing procedure. The tracings produced by the pantograph are called pantograms
- The pantronic is an electronic pantograph, which provides a computer printout of numerical condylar measurements. In addition, several electronic tracings can be made consecutively and the condylar measurements compared immediately via the computer printout.

30. Fixed removable prosthodontics.

Fixed removable partial dentures:

- This term denotes the concept of removable pontic sections supported by abutment teeth
- The first removable partial denture was a round bar attached to abutment crowns that supported a suprastructure designed by Fossume.

Types

- Bar and clip with extended tissue coverage by Dolder, Baker and Hader and Andrews
- Bar and sleeve devised by Bennett is called Bennett blade.

Parts

- Milled substructure bar
- Suprastructure
- Spring wire pins.

Indications

- Osseous deformities
- Trauma
- Natural resorption.

Steps in locating the placement of each component

- Initially, path of placement is determined
- Teeth are selected and tried to the edentulous area of the diagnostic cast
- This provides a guide to the placement of substructure bar
- The bar is placed lingual to these teeth.

Positioning of retentive pins

1. After orienting replacement teeth, they are stabilised with a removable plaster core.
2. The ideal pin location is opposite the interproximal spaces of adjacent replacement tooth.
3. After pin positioning, 0.7 mm size drills are used and drilled into respective ridge areas of the working cast to a 2 mm depth.

Fabrication of the substructure bar

1. Substructure bar is developed in wax around the pre-positioned stainless steel pins.
2. The bar is carved to its correct dimensions and its sides are made parallel to each other.
3. The wax bar is removed and cast in Type IV gold alloy with the pins in place.
4. After casting, the bar is reoriented into the path of placement and joined to abutment by soldering.
5. After assembling bar to abutment the parallel pins are removed and replaced by carbon rods.
6. The assembled substructure is placed back on cast, which is placed on the milling machine for refining lateral surfaces.

Fabrication of suprastructure

1. The stainless steel pins are placed back in substructure.
2. The plaster core is repositioned and pattern resin is placed on the lubricated substructure.
3. The pattern resin or wax is added till the desired contour is obtained.
4. Retentive elements, such as loops or bars, are placed on the facial aspect of the suprastructure pattern to provide retention for artificial tooth.
5. The suprastructure pattern is removed and cast in Type IV gold alloy.
6. The retentive pins are replaced with metal pins and these are soldered to the suprastructure.

Advantages

- Flexibility of design
- Can maintain good oral hygiene as the prosthesis can be removed
- Minimal tissue coverage
- Esthetic
- Ease of adjustment.

Disadvantages

- Abutment requirements as for fixed partial denture
- Abutment tooth have to be splinted together for common path of insertion
- Require more occlusogingival clearance (e.g. 3–4 mm)

- Can have gingival irritation if oral hygiene is not maintained
- Precise technical procedure is required.

31. Dental laboratory form.

Synonym

Work authorization form.

Definition

The written instructions submitted to a dental laboratory by a dentist along with the work.

Items to be sent to the laboratory

1. Properly prepared and articulated master cast with interocclusal records or mountings.
2. Diagnostic cast with specific design and requirements drawn on it.
3. Shade guide for the replacement prosthesis.
4. Impressions with poured casts.
5. Dissected dies.
6. Work authorization order.
7. Appropriate laboratory infection control protocol needs to be followed.

Work authorization order should include

1. Signature of the dentist.
2. Date of the authorization.
3. Name and address of the patient.
4. Date of case returned for try-in or completion.
5. Telephone number of dentist and dental technician.
6. General description of the restoration to be made.
7. Designs of gingival margins, pontic designs, anterior and posterior.
8. Exact location of metal and porcelain joining on occlusal surface.
9. For fixed-removable, rests and guide planes designs need to be drawn.
10. The desired occlusal scheme.
11. Connector design for fixed partial dentures.
12. Pontic design, including the material specification for tissue contact.
13. Substructure design for metal–ceramic restorations.
14. Materials specification.
15. Instructions on articulation and shade selection with type of tooth replacement.

Objectives

- Acts as a good line of communication between the dentist and the laboratory
- The technician can carry out the work according to the dentist's clinical requiremen
- Instructions written can be clarified
- The quality of the work done by the dentist and by the laboratory can be improved
- Also serves as a legal protection form for the dentist and laboratory technician
- Protects the public from the illegal practice of dentistry
- Establishes the separate responsibility of the dentist and the laboratory technician.

Preparation margins

Should be outlined on the die or ensure that the impressions can give the accurate margin demarcation.

Articulation

Cast with interocclusal record helps to accurately articulate the casts.

Occlusion

Should designate the location of the occlusal contacts.

Desirable occlusal schemes

- Cusp-fossa
- Cusp-marginal ridge (If positive stops are not present).

Connectors

To specify the connectors to be cast, preceramic soldered and postceramic soldered.

Pontic and substructure design

- Type of pontic replacement need to be drawn (ridge lap, modified ridge lap)
- To instruct specifically if wax pattern is to be evaluated.

Shade selection

- A diagram of the tooth with multiple shades, (as cervical shade, an incisal shade and individual characterization), needs to be charted for easy identification and accuracy
- Also a shade guide matching the tooth to be replaced is placed.

Evaluation for accuracy

- A wax pattern try in to review the contours of retainers and pontics
- A metal substructure try in for metal–ceramic restorations
- A final try in to evaluate the contours, texture and staining of a metal–ceramic restoration.

32. Dahls appliance.

This concept was proposed by Dahl in 1975 for localized anterior tooth wear cases. The first design included a cobalt chromium partial denture with anterior bite plane which caused a posterior disocclusion.

Principle

There was a reestablishment of posterior occlusion due to a combination of intrusion of anterior teeth (40%) and extrusion of posterior teeth (60%) in a period of 4–6 months. The degree of space created ranged between 1.8 mm and 4.7 mm.[1]

Advantage

- The vertical dimension of occlusion can be increased within the physiologic limits
- The steep incisal guidance angle is reduced
- Favorable biomechanical situation is reached

- Once the posterior occlusion is reestablished there is enough space to restore the anterior teeth with definitive restorations
- This is specifically used for localized anterior tooth wear
- A conservative method for good esthetics.

Disadvantages

Time consuming, increased treatment time and extra laboratory procedures.[2]

- Material is placed on the palatal aspect of anterior teeth for re-establishment of inter-occlusal space
- The thickness of the material placed is equal to the amount of space required
- No mucosal-borne component is present
- The bite plane in anterior ensures that occlusal forces are directed along the long axis of the teeth
- Stable inter-occlusal contacts
- No interference to the movement of the posterior discluded teeth.

Modification in Dahls appliance

- Presently fixed appliances or materials are used
- The palatal surfaces of anterior teeth can be build up using cemented cast metal appliance or resin materials.

Recent advancement

- This technique includes a single stage procedure instead of the original two step procedure
- Here restorative space is gained by cementing the restoration in supraocclusion
- Direct bonded composites are employed commonly as they are less expensive, reversible and easy to adjust and favorable wear properties.

Advantages

- Restore esthetics and function
- Less treatment time, cost and final control over esthetics
- Easy to retreat, repolish, repair and is a reversible process.

Limitations

The higher wear rate than porcelain and prone to staining.

Contraindications of direct bonding

- In cases of periodontal disease or short root length direct bonding can cause tooth displacement in a nonaxial direction leading to drifting
- If less than two thirds of root length.

Techniques for composite build up

The techniques apply to cases where dentoalveolar compensation has occurred, and there is insufficient space for restorations.

- Free-hand technique
- Matrix-guided technique.[3]

Procedure

- Clinical evaluation of space required either by intraoral examination or by articulated study casts mounted
- Shade selection is done
- A diagnostic wax-up is done on the articulated cast.

Clinical procedure

- Old restorations are removed in order to improve bond strength
- Tooth surfaces are cleaned with pumice and a polishing brush
- Retraction cord is placed
- A long bevel at the enamel margins improves the transition between tooth and composite, decrease internal stresses and increases the bonding surface area
- Good moisture control is ensured by use of rubber dam, cotton wool rolls and saliva ejectors.

Free-hand technique

Advantages

The free-hand technique may avoid a visit for impression taking and can be carried out in a single treatment session.

Limitation

Good clinical skill and moisture control.

Procedure

- First step: Both canine cingulum region build up—Composite is added to the cingulum region of both upper canines and the mandible manipulated into the retruded axis and closed into the uncured resin until the desired anterior space is achieved[4]
- Recheck OVD and bilateral cingulum contact
- Second step: Individual incisor build up—Each individual incisor is build up in the cingulum area and finally the entire contacts are finished with the aid of a matrix strip. After each incisor build up the midline is checked
- The occlusion is checked with thin articulating paper to ensure even contact and protective guidance in protrusive and lateral excursions
- The posterior teeth will be out of occlusion and should be monitored over subsequent months until contact is re-established.

Matrix technique

Advantage

Palatal anatomy and the position of the incisal edges are guided by the matrix.

Limitation

Depends on the clinical skill of the diagnostic wax up.

Procedure

- Models are mounted on a semiadjustable articulator in retruded axis by face bow transfer

- A diagnostic wax up which is 1–2 mm clear from gingival margin palatally is made in the desired vertical dimension
- A transparent silicone matrix (Memosil Heraeus-Kulzer, Hanau, Germany) is adapted just beyond the incisal edges of the diagnostic wax up
- This matrix aids as a template for composite build up on the palatal cingulum area but clear of the proximal contact areas
- The composite is cured and the matrix removed
- Proximal areas are built up with the help of a matrix strip
- The occlusion is checked to create even contact on the restorations at the new vertical dimension, with canine guidance in excursive movements.

References

1. Dahl BL, Krogstado"The effect of a partial bite raising splint on the occlusal face height. An X-ray cephalometric study in human adults. Acta Odantol Scand. 1982;40:17-24.
2. Clinical design for an ideal Dahl appliance: (Poyser NJ, et al. The Dahl Concept: past, present and future. Br Dent J. 2005;198: 669-76)
3. Mizrahi B. A technique for simple and aesthetic treatment of anterior toothwear. Dent Update. 2004;31:109–14.
4. Felippe LA, Monteiro S, Jr, De Andrada CA, et al. Clinical strategies for success in proximo incisal composite restorations. Part II: Composite application technique. J Esthet Restor Dent. 2005;17:11–21.

33. Management of tooth surface loss (TSL)

Classification of tooth surface loss (Grippo)[1]

Erosion

Erosion is the loss of tooth substance by acid dissolution by either intrinsic or extrinsic origin. Extrinsic sources are carbonated drinks and alcoholic beverages. Intrinsic sources include gastrooesophageal reflux, bulimia, etc.

Abrasion

The pathological wear of tooth substance through biomechanical frictional process. (e.g. tooth brushing and abrasive food).

Attrition

The loss of tooth substance as a result of tooth to tooth contact during normal function or parafunction (e.g. bruxism—is the grinding of teeth during nonfunctional movements of the masticatory system).

Abfractions (stress lesions)

Is the pathologic loss of tooth substance caused by biomechanical loading forces. Causes stress at the cervical area resulting in a lesion which is typically wedge shaped with sharp line angles.

Types: Hairline cracks, striations, saucer shaped and semi-lunar shaped.

Flowchart 1: Treatment options for tooth wear

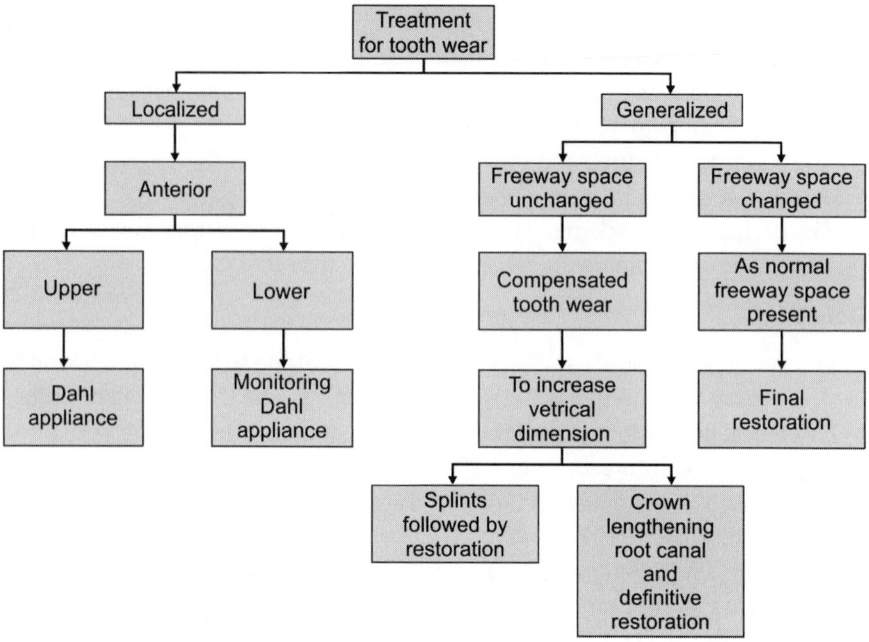

Features of different types of tooth surface loss

- Flattening of cusps or incisal edges and wear facets on occlusal or palatal surfaces—Attrition
- Cervical lesions with defined margins and smooth surface—Abrasion
- More rounded and shallow lesions and have a cupping effect—Erosion
- Measured by tooth wear indices. Commonest is Smith and Knight.[2]

The effects of tooth surface loss[3]

- Reduction in vertical tooth height and horizontal tooth width leading to loss of vertical dimension of occlusion (increased free way space)
- Forward posturing of the mandible
- Dentoalveolar compensation seen in some cases maintaining the vertical dimension.
- Unesthetic.

Treatment plan (Flowchart 1)

- To evaluate if to confirm to the existing centric occlusion or to reorganize in centric relation
- To evaluate if centric occlusion is in centric relation.

The conformative approach

- Criteria for conformative approach[4]
- The patient with centric occlusion occurring in centric relation
- The patient does not have any deflecting contacts and will not need other restorations for tooth loss
- When there is no temporomandibular disorder.

The reorganised approach

If the above criteria is not present and there is lack of freeway space then a reorganised approach is considered.

References

1. Grippo JA. A new classification of hard tissue lesions. J Aesthetic Dent. 1988;3:14-9.
2. Smith BG, Knight JK. An index for measuring wear of teeth. Br Dent J. 1984;156:435-8.
3. Kelleher M, Bishop K. Tooth surface loss: an overview. Br Dent J. 1999;186:61–6.
4. Gray R M J, Davies S J, Quayle A. A clinical approach to temporomandibular disorders: Splint therapy. Br Dent J. 1994;177:135-42.

34. Flowchart for surgical procedure in implant placement.

Flowchart 2, 3 and 4 gives the surgical procedure in implant placement.

Flowchart 2: Steps in surgical procedure in implant placement

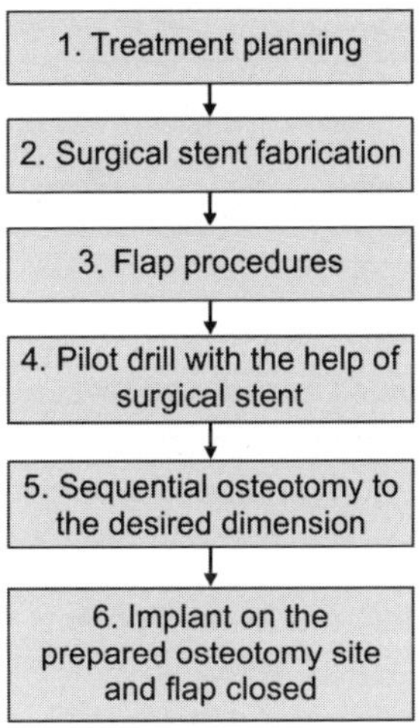

Second stage surgery

Flowchart 3: Steps in second stage surgical procedure in implant placement

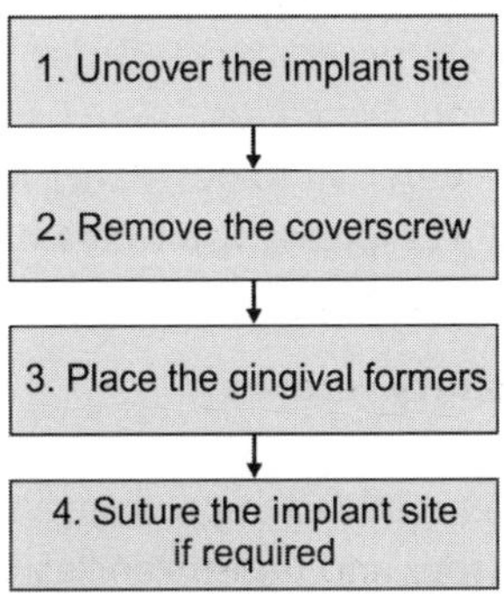

After 4–6 weeks post second stage surgery

Flowchart 4: Steps in final restoration of implant-retained prosthesis

1. Unscrew the gingival former
2. Position the suitable impression posts and make impression by direct or indirect technique
3. Attach the laboratory analogue, inject gingival mask and make the cast
4. Fabricate the wax patterns and casting is done
5. Retrieval of cating, tried for passive fit on the cast and then on patient. If its multiple unit, soldering might be requied to obtain the desired fit of the casting
6. Ceramic layering is done and try-in done on patients
7. Cementation of glazed restoration
8. Periodic review and maintenance

35. All-ceramic restoration.

- The first all-ceramic crowns introduced by Land in 1903
- In 1965, McLean and Hughes formulated aluminous porcelain in which 50% aluminum oxide increases the strength and baking temperature.

Definition

Ceramics are defined as man made solid objects formed by baking raw materials at high temperatures.

From Greek word 'keramos' meaning burnt stuff.

Composition of all ceramics

Feldspathic dental porcelain with high amounts of alminum oxide.

Classification of all-ceramic systems

- Conventional powder–slurry ceramics—Optec HSP, Duceram LFC
- Castable ceramics—Picon, Dicor Plus
- Machinable ceramics—Cerec vitablocs Mark I, Mark II, Dicor MGC, Celay
- Pressable ceramics—IPS Empress, Optec Pressable Ceramic
- Infiltrated ceramics—In-Ceram.

Conventional powder–slurry ceramics

Available as

- Powders to which water is added to produce a slurry
- Available in various shades and translucencies, with characterizing stains and glazes.

Manufacturing

1. Leucite crystals are dispersed in a glassy matrix by controlling their nucleation and crystal growth.
2. The leucite and glassy matrix fuse together during the baking process.
3. The build-up and contouring of the crown can be done by using the powder–slurry technique on semipermeable die material.

Advantages

- Greater strength than conventional feldspathic porcelain due to its leucite content
- Does not require a core as with aluminous porcelain jacket crowns
- The body and incisal porcelains can be pigmented to provide desired shade and translucency
- Does not require special processing equipment
- These restorations fit accurately.

Disadvantages

- Their high leucite contents can cause increased wear to opposing teeth.

Other types

Duceram LFC

- Hydrothermal low-fusing ceramic
- Composed of an amorphous glass containing hydroxyl ions.

Advantages

- Greater density, higher flexural strength, greater fracture resistance and lower hardness than feldspathic porcelain
- No special laboratory techniques or equipment required.

Uses

- For fabrication of ceramic inlays, veneers and full-contour crowns.

Procedure

Base layer

Duceram Metal Ceramic–(a leucite-containing porcelain)—is placed on a refractory die using powder–slurry techniques and baked at 930°C.

Over base layer

Duceram LFC is applied using the powder–slurry technique and baked at a relatively low temperature (660°C).

Castable ceramic systems

Available as

- Solid ceramic ingots, which are cast using lost-wax and centrifugal-casting technique
- Only one shade is available
- Staining is done to obtain proper shading of the final restoration.

Picon

This is a polycrystalline glass-ceramic material, in which glass is heat-treated under controlled crystallization.

Procedure

1. When solid ceramic ingots are cast at 1350°C, a transparent glass crown is obtained.
2. This crown is then heat-treated at 1075°C for 10 hours.
3. "Ceramming" causes partial crystallization (55%) of tetra-silicic-mica-like crystals.
4. For final restoration colorant stains are baked on the surface of the glass–ceramic material.

Advantages

- Easier as it is a lost wax technique
- The transparent crown after heat treatment at 1075°C for 10 hours forms an opaque crown, which increases fracture resistance and strength
- Less abrasive to opposing tooth structure.

Dicor Plus

This is a shaded feldspathic porcelain veneer applied to the Dicor substrate.

Disadvantages

- Abrasive to opposing teeth
- Requires a special high-temperature, electric-heated casting unit
- Fracture of the restorations is common.

Machinable ceramics

Available as:

- Ceramic ingots in various shades
- Used in computer-aided design and computer-aided manufacturing (CAD–CAM) procedures
- The machined restoration are stained and glazed to the desired characterization.

Cerec vitablocs Mark I

This is a feldspathic porcelain, used with the Cerec system

Composition and properties are the same as feldspathic porcelain used for porcelain-fused-to-metal restorations.

Cerec vitablocs Mark II

This is a feldspathic porcelain of increased strength with less abrasive wear of the opposing tooth structure.

Dicor MGC

- Contains fluorosilicic mica crystals in a glass matrix
- It has greater flexural strength than the castable Dicor and Cerec
- Less abrasive wear of the opposing tooth structure than Cerec Mark I.

Celay

- Can be used for CAD-CAM-and copy-milling technique
- Identical in physical properties to Cerec Vitablocs Mark II.

Disadvantage

Marginal fit is not good.

Pressable ceramics

Available as:

- Ceramic ingots, which are melted at high temperatures and pressed into a mould created by lost-wax technique
- Can be made to full contour, or can be built up using feldspathic porcelain.

IPS Empress

- This is a feldspathic porcelain supplied in ingot form
- The ingots are heated and moulded under pressure to produce the restorations.

Procedure:

1. The ceramic ingot is placed under the plunger and heated to 1150°C
2. The plunger presses the molten ceramic into the mould
3. The final shade of the crown is done by staining or veneering. (Cut back technique of wax pattern).

Optec Pressable Ceramic

This is a type of feldspathic porcelain with increased leucite content, processed by moulding under pressure and heat.

Advantages of IPS and OPC

- Produce strong, translucent, dense and etchable ceramic restorations
- Useful in fabricating ceramic veneers.

Disadvantages

Require special equipment to fabricate the restorations.

Infiltrated ceramics

Available as:

- Powder (aluminum oxide or spinel), which is fabricated into a porous substrate, and a glass, which is infiltrated at high temperature into the porous substrate
- The infiltrated ceramic is then veneered using conventional feldspathic porcelain technique.

In-Ceram

- The spinel cores are more translucent than the aluminum oxide cores
- The core is made from fine-grained particles that are mixed with water to form a suspension referred to as a 'slip'.

Procedure

1. The slip is placed on a gypsum die and baked at 1120°C for 10 hours to produce the opaque, porous core.
2. An appropriate shade of glass powder is applied to the core, which is baked again at 1100°C for four hours.
3. During this process, the molten glass infiltrates the porous alumina core by capillary action.

Advantages

- Extremely high flexure strength
- The aluminum oxide or spinel crystals limit crack propagation and the glass infiltration reduces porosity
- Provides an accurate fit.

Disadvantages

- Cannot etch internal surface; hence a resin cement, such as Panavia 21TC is recommended
- Not as esthetic as other systems
- Requires specialized equipment to fabricate a restoration.

36. Material selection and failures in RBFPD.

The original Rochette's bridge used gold alloy. Further studies proved that base-metal alloys had better bonding with resin cements than gold alloys since then nickel-chromium alloy was the choice for resin-bonded fixed partial denture (RBFPDs).

Materials Used

Gold alloy
Ni–Cr alloy
Co–Cr alloy
Metal ceramic
Fiber-reinforced composites
Zirconia.

Types of Retainers in RBFPD

- Fixed–Fixed
- Fixed–movable
- Single abutment single pontic cantilever
- Double abutment single pontic cantilever.

Base-metal alloys

Advantages of base-metal alloys

- Greater bond strengths with resin and tooth
- Can be made in thin section hence, bulky crown contour can be avoided (ideally should be a minimum of 0.5 mm thick).

Disadvantages

- At high temperatures base metals are difficult to cast and pre-solder
- Nickel sensitivity is possible in allergic patients.

All ceramic RBFPDs

- Were introduced in the early 1990s
- Better esthetics.

Fiber-reinforced composite (FRC)

Advantages

- Better adhesion of the composite resin luting agent to the retainer
- Superior esthetics
- Ease of repair.

Disadvantages

- Delamination and framework fracture are the most common failures
- They will also discolor over time
- Greater occlusal clearance is required (1–2 mm).

Zirconia

Advantages

- Superior strength and fracture resistance and toughness
- Can be milled
- Good esthetics.

Disadvantages

- Fracture of the veneered porcelain
- Bonding needs to be increased by selective infiltration etching.

Bonding/cementation

- The original RBFPD frameworks were perforated for mechanical retention of the cement to the framework
- Perforations weakened the framework strength and exposed the resin to abrasion and thereby caused microleakage
- Presently adhesive bonding is commonly used in which there is enamel to resin bond, cohesive bond of the composite resin and resin to framework bond.

Commonly used Luting agent

- Panavia EX introduced in 1984 is capable of bonding cobalt chromium to enamel. It is based on bis-GMA resin and contains MDP (10-methacryloxydecyl dihydrogen phosphate)
- Panavia has a compressive strength of 200–300MPa and tensile strength of 20–40MPa.
- Basemetal bonded better than noble alloys due to oxidation of metal

- Air abrasion with 50μ alumina prior to bonding roughens the surface and provides a molecular coating of alumina which helps oxide bonding of phosphate-based adhesive systems, such as Panavia
- Moisture control is essential to optimal bonding hence, rubber dam or cotton wool isolation is required.

Failures

- Debonding is the commonest problem and if occlusal discrepancies/parafunctional habits are present there are increased chances of debonding
- Hence recall appointments are important before caries or debonding occurs
- Creugers et al. found a survival rate of 75% for anterior and 44% for posterior bridges at 7.5-year follow-up
- Other failures observed were loss of retention and fractures of the veneering porcelain
- Hence, care need to be taken in case selection, abutment preparation, moisture control during bonding and final occlusal contacts.

Reference

1. O'Sullivan M. Resin-bonded restorations. In: Fixed prosthodontics in dental practice. London: Quintessence Publishing Co. Ltd; 2005
2. Creugers NH, Kayser AF, Van't Hof MA, A seven-and-a-half-year survival study of resin-bonded bridges. J Dent Res. 1992;71:1822–5.

37. Osseointegration.

Definition

Osseointegration is "the structural and functional connection between ordered living bone and the surface of a load carrying implant".

Theories of osseointegration

Classification based on stimulus of regeneration.

Cell-to-cell contact

The injured cells close to the osteotomy region send chemical signals to the adjacent undifferentiated cells to form new cells.

Matrix involvement

The matrix component of injured bone releases protein signals to undifferentiated cells to form the new cell.

Piezoelectric stimulation

The piezoelectric signals elicited by the movements of the fracture ends can act as a stimulus for repair and that stimulates the progenitor cells to form the cell lines.

Mechanism/sequelae of osseointegration[1,2]

The red cells, platelets and inflammatory cells of blood shift from the capillaries to the tissue surrounding the implant.

The blood cells get entrapped at the implant interface and releases cytokines and other soluble, growth and differentiation factors.

Fibrin, the reaction product of thrombin and fibrinogen released into the healing site can adhere to all surfaces and is critical in determining the integration.

The implant surfaces provide sufficient anchorage to the fibrin to withstand detachment during cell migration. The cells that reach the implant surface differentiate to synthesize bone matrix.

Differentiating osteogenic cells are also derived from bone remodeling sites and perivascular connective tissue cells around the implant site.

Migration of the connective tissue cells occurs through fibrin that forms during clot resolution and connective tissue cells replace the fibrin to act as a source of osteogenic cells.

The osteogenic cells secrete the bone matrix leading to bone growth.

Theories of Osteogenesis

Distance osteogenesis

Formation of new bone arising from the bone adjacent to implant site. The bone formation occurs from bone towards the implant. The implant is surrounded by new bone rather bone forming on implant surface.

Contact osteogenesis

Formation of new bone starting from the implant surface. The implant surface gets colonized by osteogenic cells and the new bone formation arises to join the adjoining bone interface.

Stages of osseointegration are

Stage-I—Woven bone formation

Occurs within the first 4–6 weeks after surgery. It starts growing from the adjacent bone towards the implant and fills the space between the implant and adjacent bone.

Stage-II—Adaptation phase

Starts from second month, the microscopic structure of newly formed bone changes towards the well-known lamellar bone (most highly structured type of bone tissue).

Stage-III—Remodeling

This is the last stage of osseointegration which improves bone quality by replacing the necrotic and primitive woven bone with lamellar bone. It starts around the third month.

Factors affecting Osseointegration[1,3,4]

Implant surface and design

Increased roughness and threads increases the bone contact area to 30% comparing to that of smooth, non-threaded implants (20%).

Biocompatibility of the material

The oxide layer that is present on the surface of titanium (Ti) makes it more biocompatible (cpTi and Ti-6Al-4V Titanium 6 Aluminum 4 Vanadium).

Host variables

Osseointegration of the implant is dependent on the quality and density of the bone.

Surgical procedure

Minimal trauma to the bone during placement of implant is required for good osseointegration.

Infection control

A strict sterilization protocol to be followed during the implant placement procedure.

Implant site

The osteotomy site should be free from any barriers, or increased space between bone implant interfaces.

Primary stability

Good stability will prevent movement of the implant during healing period.

Occlusion

The delayed loading protocol is reported to be more ideal for osseointegration. Criteria for successful osseointegration given by Albrektsson et al. 1986.[5]

- The individual must have an immobile implant
- No evidence of peri-implant radiolucency in radiograph
- The vertical bone loss must be less than 0.2 mm
- A success rate of 80% after 10 years posttreatment.

References

1. Feller L, Chandran R, Khammissa RA, Meyerov R, Jadwat Y, Bouckaert M, Schechter I, Lemmer J. Osseointegration: biological events in relation to characteristics of the implant surface. SADJ. 2014 Apr; 69(3):112,114-7. Review.
2. Mavrogenis AF, Dimitriou R, Parvizi J, Babis GC. Biology of implant osseointegration. J Musculoskelet Neuronal Interact. 2009 Apr-Jun;9(2):61-71. Review
3. Thalji G, Cooper LF. Molecular assessment of osseointegration in vitro: a review of current literature. Int J Oral Maxillofac Implants. 2014 Mar-Apr;29(2):e171-99.
4. Trindade R, Albrektsson T, Tengvall P, Wennerberg A. Foreign Body Reaction to Biomaterials: On Mechanisms for Buildup and Breakdown of Osseointegration. Clin Implant Dent Relat Res. 2014 Sep 25.
5. Albrektsson T, Zarb G, Worthington P, Eriksson AR. The long-term efficacy of currently used dental implants: A review and proposed criteria of success. Int J Oral Maxillofac Implants 1986;1:11–25.

38. Alloys used in fixed partial denture.

A. Precious metal alloys

1. Gold-based alloys.
2. Palladium-based alloys.

B. Base-metal alloys

1. Nickel–chromium–beryllium (Ni–Cr–Be).
2. Cobalt–Chromium alloys (Co–Cr).

Precious metal alloys

Gold-based alloys

Gold alloys

Used since 1907.

Composition

Main composition is gold. It has platinum content of 8%, palladium—4.6%, silver—1.3% and tin, indium and iron to promote oxide bonding, harden the alloy and refine the grain structure.

Advantages

- Excellent bonding to porcelain
- Good castability
- Resistance to tarnish and corrosion
- Freedom from toxicity
- No discoloration.

Disadvantages

- Expensive
- Low elastic modulus and poor sag resistance.

Gold–palladium–silver alloys

Composition

Gold 42–50%, palladium 25–32%, silver 6–16% and indium and tin contribute 8%.

Advantages

- Substituting palladium for gold raises the melting range and lowers the coefficient of expansion
- Less susceptibility to dimensional changes with good corrosion resistance and clinical working.

Disadvantage

Greening effect due to the silver content.

Gold–palladium alloys

Composition

Gold 42–55%, palladium 36–40% with minor quantities of tin, indium and gallium.

Advantages

- Greening effect not present
- Lower coefficient of thermal expansion of gold and hence, more compatible with porcelain
- Strength is improved
- Corrosion resistance is good with better sag resistance.

Disadvantage

Thermal expansion incompatible with higher expansion porcelain.

Palladium-based alloys

Used since 1970s.

Palladium in alloys:

- Increases strength
- Reduces the cost
- Produces white color.

Palladium–silver alloys

Composition

Palladium content of 50–60%, silver 30–40% and traces of tin and indium.

Advantages

- Good tarnish and corrosion resistance
- Good bond strength
- Lower sag tendency.

Disadvantage

Porcelain discoloration.

Palladium–copper alloys

Used since 1982.

Composition

Palladium—70–80% and 15% copper.

Disadvantage

Copper discolors porcelain.

Palladium–Cobalt alloys

Available as silver-free, nickel-free, gold- and beryllium-free commercial alloys.

Composition

78–88% palladium and 4–10% cobalt.

Disadvantage

Difficult to melt and has high thermal expansion.

Palladium–Tin Alloys

- The silver is substituted with tin and gallium
- Recent clinical use, hence clinical data is not available.

Non-precious alloys

- Base-metal Alloys
- Due to the high cost of gold and palladium, base-metal alloys were developed.

Nickel–chromium alloys

Composition

Nickel 70–80%, chromium 13–20% with or without small quantities of beryllium (0.5–2%).

Advantages

- Good strength hence, can be used in thin sections permitting excellent crown contour
- Physical properties as hardness, yield strength and modulus of elasticity is superior to all noble metals with regard to sag resistance.

Disadvantages

- High casting shrinkage of 2.4%
- Questionable biocompatibility
- Requires modified casting techniques.

Cobalt–chromium alloys

These base metals may contain 55–68% cobalt and up to 25–27% chromium but no beryllium.

Cobalt–chromium–nickel alloys

Advantages

- Base-metal alloys are cheaper than noble alloys
- They have good strength
- Can be used along with metal ceramics.

Disadvantages

- Fusion temperature is high
- Marginal fit is poor compared to gold alloys
- Cannot be burnished
- Nickel-containing alloy can cause allergy to some.

39. Non-rigid connectors/stress breakers in fixed partial denture.

- Intracoronal retainers are non-rigid connectors that confines within proximal axial contours or within crown of tooth
- It consists of a matrix component part housed within the coronal portion of abutment tooth.

Types of intracoronal systems

- Key and keyway system
- Locking mechanism
- Frictional mechanism
- Spring retained types.

Principle of non-rigid connector

- This connector employs a stress breaking principle, which consists of a keyway (female part) and a key (male part)

- This connector when placed between pontic and retainer permits some amount of movement.

Indications

- Resilient intracoronal used for removable bounded prosthesis
- Non-resilient intracoronal used for fixed movable design.

Advantages

- Easy alignment
- Allows individual movement of tooth
- Force distribution can be controlled
- Torsional forces are not transmitted to the teeth
- Contour of tooth is not altered as in extracoronal types
- Can overcome problem of non-parallel abutments.

Disadvantages

- Used only for posterior fixed prosthesis
- Cannot be used when opposing teeth are missing because the key tends to displace
- Cannot be used in long-span bridges
- The size of intracoronal retainers can encroach upon pulp chamber
- Requires extensive tooth preparation.

Different types of intracoronal attachments

1. McCollum attachment (Fig. 12).
2. Chayes attachment (Fig. 13).
3. Stern precision attachment.
4. Crismani attachment.
5. Schatzmann attachment (Fig. 14)
6. ASE attachment.

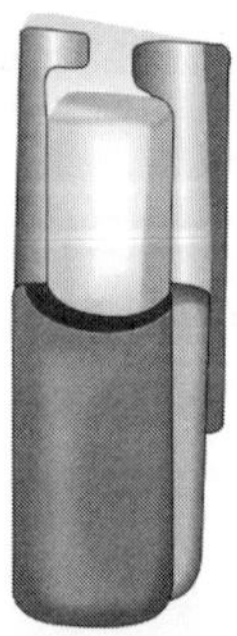

Fig. 12: McCollum attachment

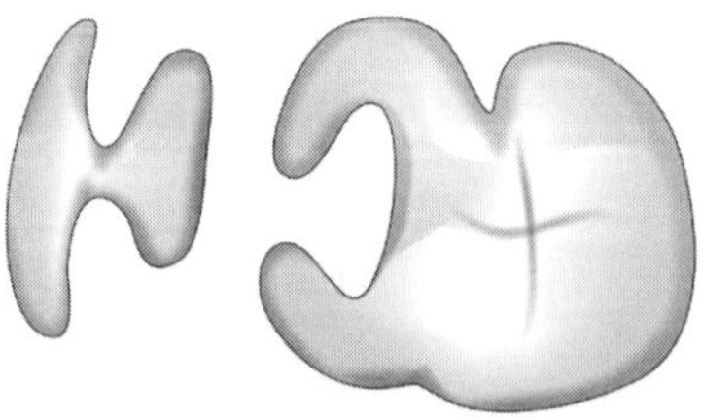

Fig. 13: Chayes attachment

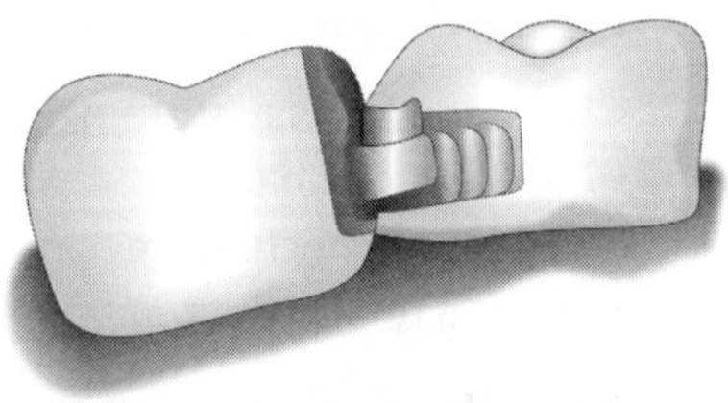

Fig. 14: Schatzmann attachment

Method

1. A wax pattern for retainer is fabricated on working cast.
2. If a plastic pattern is used for the keyway, a deep box form is carved into the distal surface of die wax pattern to create space for placement of plastic keyway.
3. Path of insertion should be accurate while preparing distal box.
4. The working cast with wax pattern is surveyed to locate the ideal path of insertion by locking the extension of key into the surveying arm of surveyor.
5. The surveying table is adjusted till the assembly seats well into distal box.
6. This key and keyway assembly is luted in place, invested, burned out and cast.

40. Wax patterns.

- Wax pattern is the duplicate replica of the finished cast restoration, which will be placed on the prepared tooth
- Wax pattern is invested and cast to form the final restoration.

Methods of fabricating wax pattern

Direct technique
Pattern waxed in mouth on prepared tooth.

Indirect technique
Pattern is waxed on die from an accurate impression of prepared tooth.

Types of wax used

Type I
Used for intraoral patterns.

Type II
Used for extraoral patterns.

Steps in wax pattern fabrication
1. Coping fabrication.
2. Forming axial contours.
3. Occlusal morphology.

Coping fabrication
A die lubricant is coated on the die before fabrication of a coping.

Method
1. The lubricated die is dipped in melted wax, placed in a metal cup, to form a uniform thimble of wax on the die.
2. The wax is added on to the die with quick strokes of a hot No. 7 wax spatula.
3. The margins are re-flowed and perfect adaptation is ensured.
4. The coping should be easily removed and placed back on die.
5. The coping is transferred to the articulated working cast for further build up.

Axial contours

The proximal contact of wax pattern should be slightly oversized mesiodistally so that there is allowance for the casting to be finished and polished without causing an open contact in the finished restoration.

Proximal contacts

- The proximal contacts for posterior teeth are located in the occlusal third of the crowns
- Proximal contacts between maxillary first and second molars are located in the middle third
- The contact must be more than just a point occlusocervically
- The axial surface of the crown cervical to the proximal contact should be flat or slightly concave to prevent encroachment of the interdental papilla.

Facial and lingual contours

The height of contour on the facial surface of all posterior teeth and lingual surface of maxillary premolars and molars occurs in the cervical third.

Facial contour

Facial contour on maxillary and mandibular posterior tooth extends 0.5 mm beyond the contour of the cementoenamel junction.

Lingual contour

0.5 mm beyond the contour of the cementoenamel junction for maxillary teeth and mandibular first premolars, 0.75 mm on mandibular second premolars and 1.0 mm on mandibular molars.

Occlusal morphology

Types

1. Cusp fossa.
2. Cusp marginal ridge.

Cusp Fossa

- The functional cusp contact is only with occlusal fossae
- The occlusion with opposing tooth is tooth to tooth
- Each centric cusp should make three-point contact with the occlusal fossa of the opposing tooth
- The contact points are on the mesial, distal and the inner facing incline of the cusp.

Advantages

Parallel to long axis of tooth and force direction is through center of teeth.

Disadvantages

Not found in natural teeth, used only in restoration of tooth (full mouth reconstruction).

Cusp-fossa waxing up procedure:

Developed by P K Thomas.

Placement of functional cusp for mandibular teeth

- The mandibular buccal cusps will contact the fossae of the opposing maxillary teeth

- Cones of mandibular buccal cusps are placed with a PKT No 1 located approximately one-third the distance from the buccal to lingual surface and positioned mesiodistally.

Cones for the maxillary lingual cusps

- Positioned buccolingually
- The mesiolingual cusp cones should be located as far distally as possible
- The distolingual cones should have no contacts with opposing teeth.

Placement of nonfunctional cusps

- The maxillary buccal cusp cones and the mandibular lingual cusp cones should be formed slightly shorter than the functional cusp cones
- The mandibular lingual cusps are placed as far to the lingual and as far from each other and the lingual cusps are shorter than the buccal cusps
- The highest points on the occlusal surfaces are the tips of the cusp cones.

Placement of marginal ridges

- Should never be higher than the cusps
- The buccolingual dimension of each occlusal table formed by the ridges should be approximately 55% of the overall buccolingual dimension of the respective tooth.

Thomas notch

- When evaluating the waxed upper and lower teeth in both working and nonworking lateral excursions, interferences should be removed
- During the working movement, the buccal cusp of each maxillary premolar passes distal to the buccal cusp of its counterpart in the mandibular arch
- A small depression is placed in the distal incline of the buccal cusp of the mandibular premolar to allow the buccal cusp of the maxillary tooth to pass through without interference. This depression is called Thomas notch
- The maxillary and mandibular lingual and buccal ridges are waxed using PKT No 1
- The final contours are smoothened by PKT No 4
- The rest of the procedure remains same as for cusp marginal ridge wax up.

After final finishing

The nonworking movement of the mesiolingual cusp of a maxillary molar should pass through the area distal to the distobuccal cusp of the mandibular molar.

Stuart's groove

This groove begins in the central fossa and is directed mesiolingually to provide an escape way for the mandibular distobuccal cusp in a nonworking movement. To prevent, such an interference, a groove is placed on the mesiolingual cusp of the maxillary molar.

Margin finishing

After the pattern is completed remove the pattern from the working cast and place it back on the lubricated die.

- Re-melt the entire marginal periphery with a hot PKT No 1 making sure that the wax is melted through to the die
- Add wax with a hot beavertail burnisher
- Carve the excess wax almost to the margin with a PKT No 4
- Finish "carving" the margin with a warm beavertail burnisher
- The margin should be closely adapted to die margin and smoothed with no irregularities.

Final finishing
- A small cotton pellet dipped in die lubricant and held with cotton pliers is run carefully through the grooves
- Axial walls are finished with cotton rolls dipped in die lubricant
- A dry end of the roll is buffed across the wet wax to obtain a smooth surface
- All traces of lubricant should be removed.

Cusp marginal ridge
- Functional cusp contact with marginal ridges and occlusal fossae
- Opposing occlusion is a single tooth opposing two teeth.

Advantages

This is the most natural type of occlusion and is found in 95% of all adults. It can be used for single restorations placing very little lateral stress on the tooth.

Disadvantages

Food impaction and the displacement of teeth may arise if the functional cusps wedge into a lingual embrasure opposing them.

Uses

Most cast restorations done in daily practice.

Cusp-marginal ridge arrangements for molars

Cusp-marginal ridge arrangement for maxillary molars (E V Payne):
1. Cones for buccal cusp (Fig. 15)
   - Wax pattern cones are placed on the buccal cusps, after determining the position of buccal cusp, by protrusive and a working lateral excursion, as on articulator as far buccally as possible, with a PKT No. 1 instrument.
   - The cone placed should be evaluated with the opposing cusp.
2. Placement of buccal ridge of buccal cusp (Fig. 16)
   Wax is added to the buccal aspect of buccal cones giving the buccal surface its contour.
3. Adding triangular ridges
   - Triangular ridges extend from the central groove of the tooth to the cusp tip (wider at base than cusp tip)
   - Added with PKT no 1 instrument
   - They should be convex to allow point occlusal contacts, which are evaluated on articulator and modified.
4. Adding mesial and distal cusp ridges (Fig. 17)
   - Mesial and distal ridges are formed as inclines away from the cusp tip with PKT No 1
   - After placement they are evaluated in lateral and protrusive excursions
   - The inclines of mesial and distal ridges should coincide with inclines of the mesial and distal cusp ridges of the opposing teeth without contact.
5. Adding cones for lingual cusp (functional cusps) (Fig. 18)
   - The cones are located mesiodistally in line with the opposing fossa or marginal ridge
   - The mesiolingual cones are centered between the two buccal cusps
   - Contacts should occur on the sides of the cone but not on the tip.

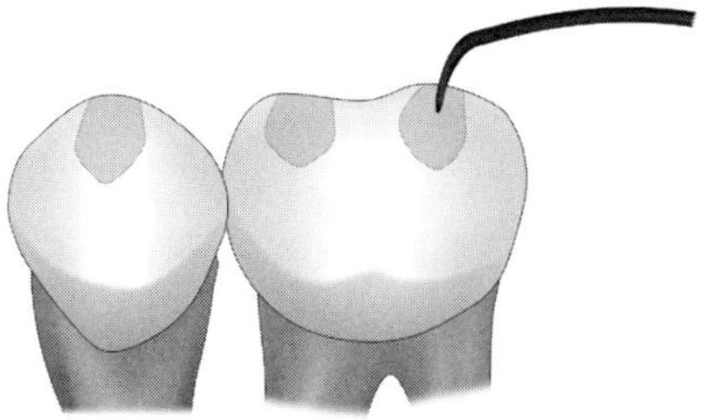

Fig. 15: Cones for buccal cusp

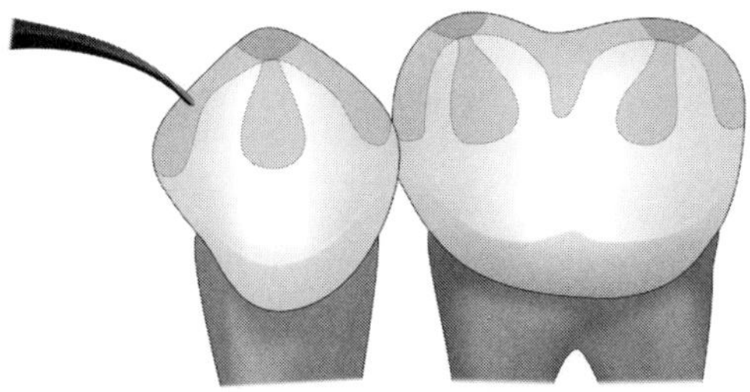

Fig. 17: Mesial and distal cusp ridges

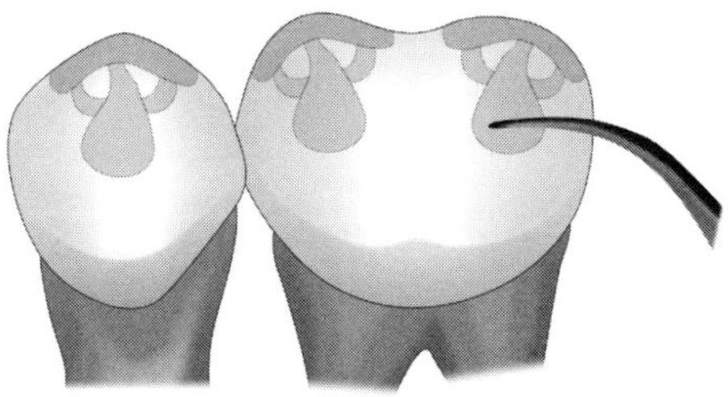

Fig. 16: Buccal ridges and triangular ridges

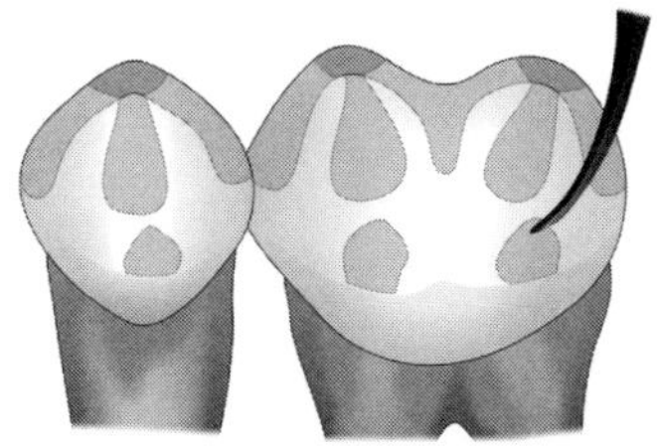

Fig. 18: Cones for lingual cusp

6. Adding mesial and distal ridges to lingual cusp (PKT No 1)
   - The added cusp ridges should decrease in height from cusp tip to marginal ridges
   - The pattern is dusted with zinc stearate and occlusion is checked to complete the lingual axial contour
   - They are smoothed with a PKT No 4.
7. Addition of triangular ridges to lingual cusp (Fig. 19)
   The triangular ridges should be convex to form point contacts with opposing cusps.
8. Forming marginal ridges
   - Marginal ridges are formed by uniting mesial and distal ridges of the buccal cusps with the mesial and distal ridges of the lingual cusps
   - Their height is determined by the height of the cusp tips of the opposing teeth.
9. Final finishing (Fig. 20)
   - The junctions between triangular ridges and adjacent cusp or marginal ridges are joined with PKT No 5
   - The ridges and the grooves are smoothed with a PKT No 3.

Cusp-marginal ridge for mandibular teeth

1. Placement of buccal cusp (functional cusp) (Fig. 21)
   - Placed at the junction of the buccal one third and the lingual two thirds of the mandibular tooth mesiodistally
   - They will occlude with the opposing fossa or marginal ridge, which is evaluated by dusting with zinc stearate and closing the articulator.

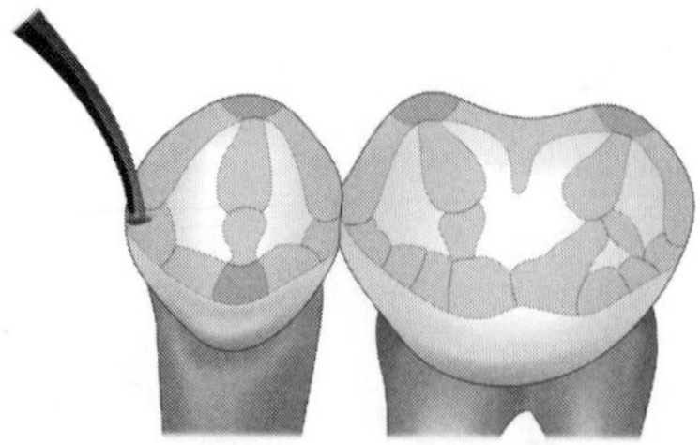

Fig. 19: Lingual ridges and triangular ridges

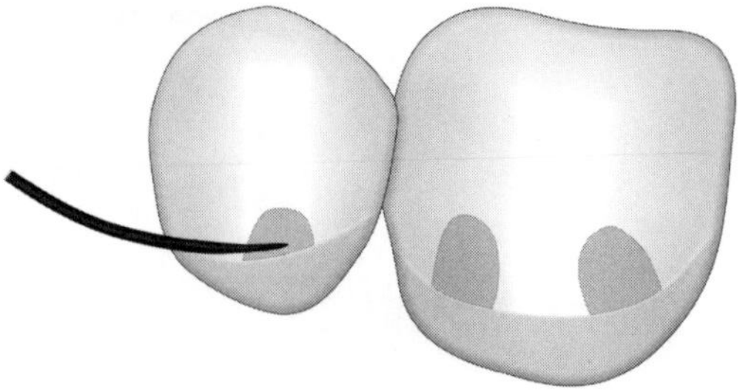

Fig. 21: Placement of cones for buccal cusp

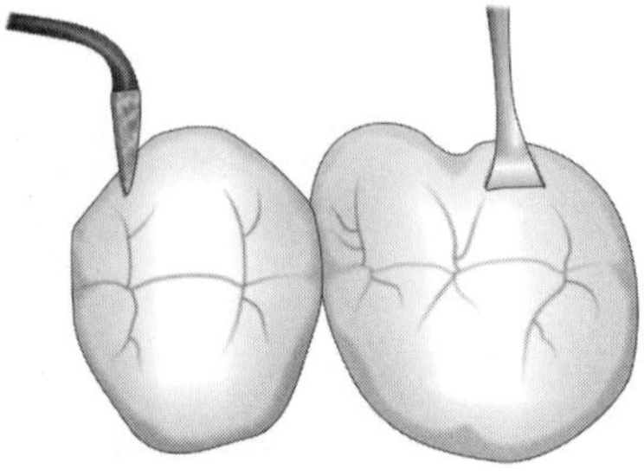

Fig. 20: Final finishing

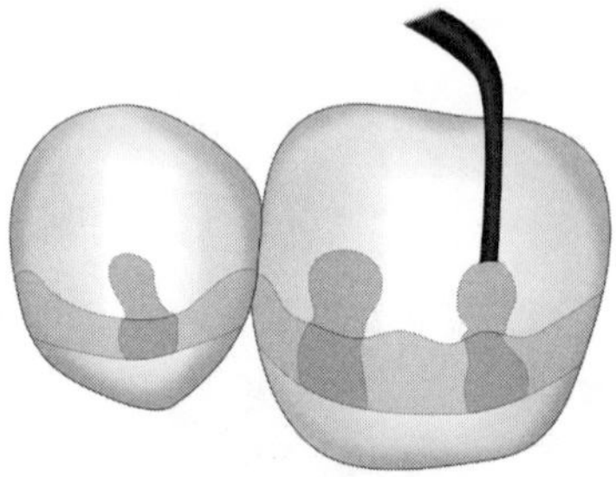

Fig. 22: Placement of mesial, distal and triangular ridges

2. Placement of buccal ridges on buccal cusps:
   - Wax is applied from the tip of the cone to its base with a PKT No 1 producing the outline of the buccal surface
   - Check the buccal ridges on articulator in centric and lateral excursions.
3. Adding mesial and distal ridges to the buccal cusps (Fig. 22)
   The inclines of these ridges added should be evaluated by moving the articulator through excursions.
4. Placement of triangular ridges
   - They are added to the buccal cusps with a PKT No 1
   - The base of these ridges should form the central groove of the occlusal surface
   - The convex ridges should have point contacts with opposing teeth.
5. Placement of lingual cusp
   - Placed as far to the lingual and as far apart mesiodistally to prevent working interferences
   - The lingual cusps should be shorter than the buccal cusps.
6. Placement of lingual ridges
   Lingual ridges added to the lingual cusps form the outline of the lingual contour.
7. Adding triangular ridges to the lingual cusp (Fig. 23)
   - Added with a No. 1 PKT and placed to converge slightly towards the central fossa
   - The contacts formed by opposing cusps should have a tripod form.
8. Forming marginal ridges (Fig. 24)
   Are formed by joining the buccal and lingual cusp ridges.

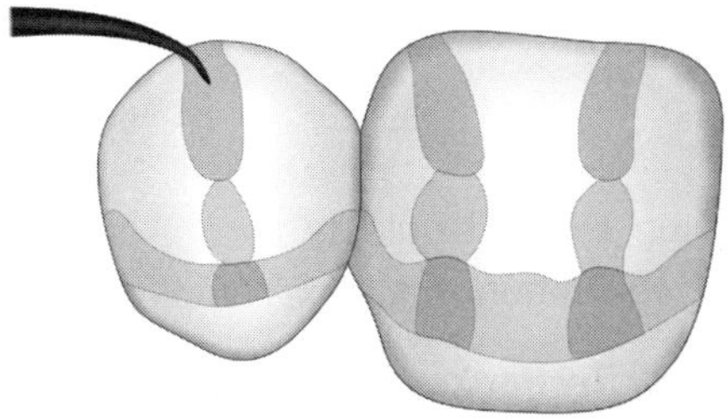

Fig. 23: Adding triangular ridges to lingual cusp

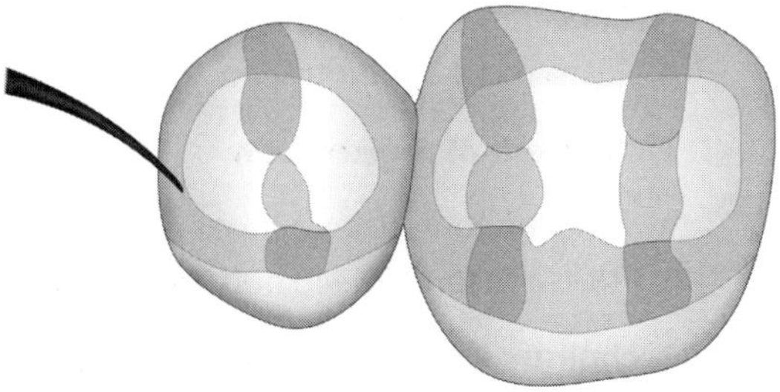

Fig. 24: Placement of marginal ridges

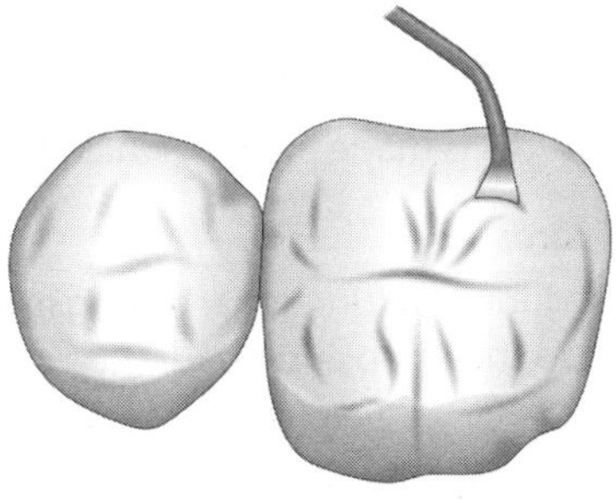

Fig. 25: Final finishing

9. Final finishing (Fig. 25)
   - All grooves and fossae are smoothed with the PKT No 3
   - Ridges are rounded and finished with the PKT No 5.

41. Functionally generated pathways (Meyer).

Functionally generated pathway is a technique in which a tracing is made in the mouth to capture the pathways travelled by the opposing cusps in mandibular function.

Advantages

- Teeth are modified to accept every possible eccentric jaw movement
- Eliminates the need to use extraoral tracing devices
- Accurate
- Occlusion thus established will have complete harmony with the opposing natural or artificial teeth
- Articulator is not required.

Disadvantages

- Opposing teeth need to be cleaned as wax particles accumulate on it
- The patient needs to understand the mandibular movements
- Procedure takes long as wax need to be added to deficient areas as patients start the mandibular movements
- Need to correct occlusal plane irregularities before this technique is done

- Registration of occlusal pathways requires a completely intact opposing arch
- Takes more appointments to complete the procedures.

Final result of registration

- After 24 hours, the occlusal surface of the wax rim should be glossy
- After a second 24–48 hour period of wear, the registration should be complete.

Technique using functionally generated pathway (by Pankey and Mann)

- Based on the spherical theory of occlusion the mandibular teeth are reduced
- To bring the occlusal surfaces into harmony with the surface of the theoretical sphere
- Buccal and lingual preparation guides plane are used as a guide to reduce the mandibular tooth
- The reduced tooth is restored to an ideal plane and a functionally generated recording of the mandibular cusp paths is made against which the maxillary tooth is restored.

Fabrication of functional core:

1. The occlusal reduction is done and functional tracing is made before the axial reduction. Apply lubricating agent to the opposing quadrant
2. A wax adherent like Copalite is applied to the adjacent tooth before a layer of tacky wax is placed on the occlusally prepared tooth
3. Ensure the stability of tacky wax and ask the patient to do all mandibular movements
4. Paint the wax with a die lubricant to ensure a smooth complete functional core.

Pouring the functional core

1. Dental stone is brushed and poured onto the wax record in the mouth to produce a functional core
2. The functional index tray poured in stone should record the adjacent tooth to the prepared tooth
3. This stone replica of the movements of the cusp tips is called the functional core/ functional index, or the counter die.

Continuing preparation of tooth

After recording the functional core the rest of tooth preparation is continued.

Impression making

- An impression is made of the quadrant containing the prepared tooth, using a custom acrylic tray made previously
- A bite registration at the intercuspal position using bite registration paste is done in a bite registration frame using zinc oxide and eugenol paste.

Making of die

- Die is prepared using Di-Lok tray technique
- After the die is retrieved, wax pattern is fabricated against the functional core on an articulator.

42. Interocclusal records.

Type of relationships in partial denture

1. Centric registrations (interocclusal records)
   - Centric occlusion records
   - Centric relation records.
2. Eccentric registrations (interocclusal records)
   - Lateral excursive records (lateral "check-bites")
   - Protrusive records (protrusive "check-bite").

Centric Occlusion

- It is the simultaneous bilateral contact of several pairs of opposing posterior teeth
- At least two posterior and one anterior point contact should be present.

Direct intercuspation is indicated when:

- The indicated fixed restorations do not interfere with the stable tripodization
- When vertical dimension is normal and when patient's centric relation is coincident with the centric occlusion.

Methods

- Hand articulation of the patients casts
- When the distal most tooth is prepared interocclusal relationship is made in maximum inter cuspation with an interocclusal record or occlusal stop.

Interocclusal stop technique:

1. An interocclusal record (polyether silicone or acrylic resin) is placed over the prepared tooth.
2. Patient is asked to close to the normal interocclusal position.
3. After the recording material sets, the record is trimmed and articulation is done.

Centric Relation

This is a contact relationship in which the mandible is located 1–1.5 mm distal to the intercuspal position.

Techniques for guiding mandible

Active technique
Interocclusal registration is made directed by the patient's neuromuscular effort.

Passive technique
In which the dentist guides the mandible into centric relation.

Techniques for record making

Bite wafer technique

1. A thermoplastic bite wafer made from baseplate wax (such as a warm wax wafer) is used to support the registration medium.

2. After evaluation of the record the indentations in the wax are brushed with zinc oxide eugenol/elastomer and the recording is repeated.
3. The resulting interocclusal record represents a stable laminate consisting of the thermoplastic wafer and a wash of paste or elastomer.

Anterior stop technique

1. This technique utilizes an anterior deprogramming appliance (anterior acrylic jig).
2. This jig deprograms the influence of the posterior dentition by the contact of incisal edge of the mandibular central incisor on a platform.
3. This contact provides posterior space for the interocclusal material and the carrier.

Fabrication of the anterior jig (discluder)

1. A foil is burnished over the lingual surfaces and incisal edge of the maxillary centrals on the cast. Acrylic material is manipulated (in doughy stage); it is placed on the foil and moulded into sloping ramp.
2. After the acrylic sets, it is trimmed.
3. It is then seated in the patient's mouth.
4. The patient is asked to close in interdigitation and the space obtained between the posterior teeth should be within 1 mm of interocclusal distance.

Wax wafer bite

1. A warm wax wafer is pressed to the occlusals of the maxillary teeth with the jig in place. The wax wafer is refined and shaped to the patient's arch form.
2. After reheating the wax wafer outside the patient's mouth, the patient's mandible is guided and patient is asked to close on his or her back teeth until the lower anterior teeth touch the anterior jig.

Wash registration record

1. After confirming the record the record is trimmed and a thin layer of ZOE bite registration paste is applied to the lower cusp indentations of the wafer.
2. Centric relation record is repeated with the wash registration material.

Eccentric registrations—Lateral relation

Canine-guided occlusion

In lateral movement canine causes separation of all the other teeth.

Group function

In lateral movement contact is maintained between a group of teeth.

Lateral Check-bites

Adjustment of articulator

1. Before the lateral interocclusal record is made, the patient's casts are mounted on an arcon articulator with facebow and centric relation record.
2. Superior walls of the fossae are arbitrarily set to an angle of 30 degrees and the medial walls to 15 degrees.

3. The mandibular member of the articulator is manipulated so that left mandibular canine is edge to edge with the left maxillary canine.
4. The incisal pin is opened to create a 2 mm space between the incisal edges of the canines and the corresponding point is marked on the incisal table.

Recording of wax record on articulator

1. A warm wax wafer is placed on lower cast, and the articulator is adjusted till it coincides with the pencil mark on the incisal guide table.
2. Close the articulator until the incisal guide pin touches the surface of the incisal table.

Evaluating the record in patient's mouth

After chilling the wax wafer record, the record is checked in patient's mouth with the canine edge to edge in left lateral excursion until the lower teeth locate the indentations in the wax made by the mandibular cast.

Wash record

If the record is accurate it is followed by wax registration record (ZNOE).

Setting the articulator readings to new record

1. After the paste sets, trim the lateral check-bite, seat it on the mandibular cast and place the maxillary cast over it.
2. Loosen the horizontal and medial condylar housing walls of the right condylar housing and allow the horizontal and medial walls to just contact the condyle.
3. Tighten the walls and remove the record.
4. The same procedure is repeated with right lateral excursion to set the left condylar housings.

Protrusive relation

Incisal edges of the lower anterior teeth move against the palatal aspect of the upper incisors to an edge-to-edge incisal contact known as incisal guidance.

Adjusting the articulator

1. The horizontal condylar inclinations are set at 30 degrees.
2. The upper cast is brought with the incisors in an end-to-end relation.
3. The incisal guide pin is raised and marked on incisal table till a 2 mm inter-incisal space is made.

Wax record

A warm wax is placed on the cast till coinciding the incisal table marking in incisal edge-to-edge position.

Reevaluating record in patient

The wax record is evaluated in the patient's mouth with the incisors in edge-to-edge position until the lower teeth find the indentations.

Wash record

Reline the pre-registered protrusive record with registration paste and refine the record in the mouth.

Articulator setting

1. The trimmed protrusive check bite is placed on mandibular cast and the maxillary cast is placed over it.
2. The horizontal condylar inclination screw is loosened and manipulated till the maxillary casts seat into the refined indentations of the check-bite.
3. Once seating is complete tighten the condylar inclination locking nuts.

43. Lug seat

- In non-rigid connectors a keyway and key is present
- The key of the non-rigid connector is referred to as "LUG"
- Lug is a tapering piece of metal usually cast, which fits the key way exactly and made part of pontic
- The key way is referred to as dovetail/lug seat and is a depression cut in one of the retainers (anterior retainer)
- It is widest at its occlusal opening and gradually tapers gingivally ending in a flat gingival seat.

Lug seat preparation is used in:

- Stress breakers
- Non-precision stress breakers.

Shapes of lug seat

- Dove tail
- Semicircular
- Triangular
- Round
- T-shaped
- Oval.

Design of lug seat (Fig. 26)

- Usually prepared on anterior retainer with walls that diverge from the gingival to occlusal
- Buccal, lingual and gingival walls are dove tailed
- Twice as deep as it is wide buccolingually and at least 1 mm wide at the gingival wall.

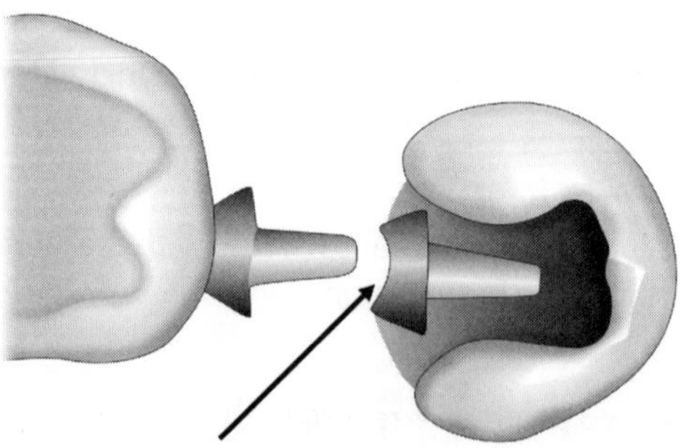

Fig. 26: Lug seat

Modification

1. In molar pontic replacement, an occlusal extension is made mesially and terminates in the center of tooth.
2. Proximal subocclusal rest: A slightly tapered opening is made in proximal surface of anterior retainer below the marginal ridge at the region of contact point.

Advantage

After the restoration is cemented amount of movement is prevented and also prevents occlusal displacement.

Procedure of preparation

The lug seat can be prepared on wax pattern—if consisting of inlay, or on tooth.

Lug seat on wax pattern

- A groove extending occlusogingivally is prepared on axial surface with No 700 crosscut fissure bur till the depth of diameter of bur
- With a inverted cone bur, the groove is extended in buccal and lingual direction
- An inverted cone bur is used to create a gingival undercut in gingival wall
- After completing the preparation, it is invested, cast and tried in the mouth.

Lug seat on tooth

A cross cut fissuring bur can be used to create a groove occlusally and proximally with undercuts in proximal area. The extended groove on occlusal surface is rounded and is wider toward key way than its mesial side.

Other types

Subocclusal spherical keyway (Starr):
In which peripheral outline is an undercut created with round bur.

Sullivan type

Combination of dove tail and subocclusal.

44. Soft tissue mask for implant models.

Composition

- Traditionally soft denture lining material has been used for soft tissue casts but the vaporization of the alcohols used in plasticizer deteriorated the material property rapidly
- Currently materials specifically marketed for soft tissue casts are now available that are chemically similar to elastomeric impression materials.

Significance

- Soft tissue masks allow increased biologic and esthetic harmony of the prosthesis
- The use of soft tissue masks on the casts significantly aids in maintaining the tissue contour and form throughout the laboratory phase of restoration fabrication
- Aids in the selection of abutments that can be clearly visualized because the position of the implant can be observed in relation to soft tissue height and width

- It also enables access to the implant analogue without damaging the gypsum cast during removal.

Requirement of soft mask material

- It should have adequate dimensional stability for the period of time necessary to fabricate and finish the prosthesis
- It should not adhere to the matrix impression material
- It should have adequate flow, tensile tear strength and resilience to allow ease of fabrication and durability during use
- It should be compatible with the matrix impression material.

45. Recall and maintenance.

Recall and maintenance is done to monitor the patient's dental health, identify any incipient disease and initiate corrective treatment before irreversible damage occurs.

Appointment scheme

1. A week after cementation of prosthesis.
2. Periodic recall every six months.
3. Emergency recall.
4. Retreatment.

Evaluations to be made

Review history and general examination

1. Oral hygiene and diet.
2. Recheck for any residual cement in gingival sulcus.
3. Secondary dental caries: It is better to redo the entire restoration again.
4. Root caries.
5. Periodontal disease.
6. Occlusal dysfunction.
7. Pulp and periapical health.

Root caries

Causative factors

1. Plaque containing *Actinomyces viscosus* proliferating on tongue.
2. Xerostomia.
3. Radiation treatment.

Treatment

Tongue cleaning can reduce root caries.

Periodontal disease

Causes

1. Subgingival placement.
2. Overcontouring of restoration.

Evaluate for

1. Sulcular hemorrhage.
2. Furcation involvement.
3. Overcontoured restoration.
4. Poor overall oral hygiene.

Care of fixed partial dentures

- Special plaque control measures
- Use of floss around pontics and connectors.

Method of flossing

Floss is looped through embrasure spaces on each side and pulled tightly against the convex pontic tissue surface and floss is gently slided out to remove dental plaque.

Occlusal dysfunction

Evaluate for

1. Parafunctional habits.
2. Abnormal occlusal wear patterns.
3. Abnormal tooth mobility.
4. Muscle and joint pain.
5. Canine wear can cause excursive interfering contacts on the posterior teeth.

Pulp and periapical health

- Pain in abutment tooth could have lead to loss of vitality of an abutment tooth
- Radiographs need to be taken to evaluate for presence of periapical pathology.

Emergency Appointment

1. Pain.
2. Loose abutment retainer.
3. Fractured connector.
4. Fractured porcelain veneer.

Pain

The location, character, severity, timing, and onset are to be noted.

Causes

1. Periapical pathology.
2. Root fracture in endodontically treated tooth.

Loose abutment retainer

Symptoms, such as bad taste or smell.

Causes

1. Inadequate tooth preparation.
2. Poor cementation technique.
3. Caries.

Fractured connector

Symptoms, such as pain due to extra force transmitted to the abutment teeth.

Fractured porcelain veneer

Causes

1. Faults in framework design.
2. Improper laboratory procedures.
3. Excessive occlusal function or trauma.

Retreatment

In case the problems are related to inadequate tooth preparation or faulty design or lab work, remaking the prosthesis is ideal.

Good plaque removal, patient motivation, a well designed and fabricated restoration can give good service for a long time.

46. Treating tilted molars.

A. Uprighting first molars by a fixed appliance.
B. Using telescopic crowns.
C. Non-rigid connector.
D. Mesial half crowns.

Uprighting first molars by a fixed appliance

1. Both premolars and the canine are banded and tied to a passive stabilizing wire.
2. A helical uprighting spring is placed inside the molar band and activated by hooking it over the wire on the anterior segment.
3. An open coil spring is used to complete the uprighting.
4. After uprighting the molars the tooth preparation is done immediately and prosthesis is given.

Telescopic Crown

A telescope crown and coping can also be used as a retainer on the distal abutment.

Design

- A full crown preparation with heavy reduction is made to follow the long axis of the tilted molar
- An inner metal coping is initially made which is luted to the prepared abutment tooth. Then a crown is made that is luted to the coping.

Advantages

- Allows for total coverage of the clinical crown
- Compensates for the discrepancy between the paths of insertion of the abutments.

Disadvantage

Require radical tooth preparation.

Non-rigid connector

A full crown preparation is done with path of insertion parallel with the long axis of the tilted molar.

Design
A box is prepared on the distal surface of the premolar to place a keyway.

Indication
When the molar exhibits a marked lingual and mesial inclination.

Contraindication
In long-span pontics.

Mesial half crown

Mesial half crown restores the occlusal and mesial surfaces as well as portions of the facial and lingual surfaces.

Preparation of mesial half crown
A mesial half crown is a three-quarter crown rotated 90° with the distal surface uncovered. As the second molar is generally over-tapered it needs additional grooves on buccal and lingual aspect.

47. Telescopic crown.

Definition

It refers to the use of a primary full coverage casting luted to the prepared teeth with the secondary casting placed over the primary casting.

Objectives

- To achieve parallelism in multiple crown preparations for fixed partial denture
- Creates a common path of insertion
- Enables malposed teeth to be used without orthodontic treatment
- Avoids pulpal damage during preparation.

Disadvantages

- Additional lab procedures
- Difficulty in achieving esthetics
- Expensive.

Advantages

- Allows for total coverage of the clinical crown
- Compensates for the discrepancy between the paths of insertion of the abutments.

Design

- A full crown preparation with heavy reduction is made to follow the long axis of the tilted molar

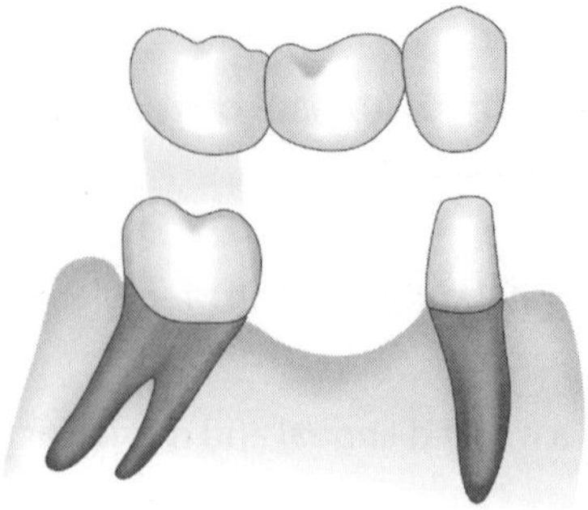

Fig. 27: Telescopic crown with coping

- An inner coping is made to fit the tooth preparation and the crown, which will serve as the retainer for the bridge is fitted over the coping (Fig. 27).

48. Finishing and polishing.

Definition

- Finishing is the removal of excess restoration material from the margins and contours of a restoration and polishing of the restoration
- Polishing is the process of making a prosthesis smooth and glossy.

Advantage of polishing and finishing

- Will limit the accumulation and retention of plaque
- Maintain the health of the supporting periodontal tissues
- A polished surface consists of a microcrystalline or Beilby layer
- This layer helps to keep the surface clean and has high corrosion resistance.

Objectives

Zone 1—internal margin

- A I mm wide band of metal is ideal at the finish lines to prevent luting agent from dissolution and secondary caries
- A perfect marginal fit is attained by re-flowing the margins of the wax pattern.

Defects

- Small nodules can be removed under a binocular microscope with no. 1/4 round bur
- If extensive damage has occurred, remaking the prosthesis is ideal.

Zone 2—internal surface

A uniform space of 25–35 micron is required for the even spread of luting agent.

Defects

- Contact between internal surface and die needs to be relieved with a small round carbide bur

- Small nodules prevent proper seating of prosthesis and this needs to be removed in one step
- Seating interferences can be located by the use of water-soluble dies (Liqua-Mark), solvent-based dies (Accufilm) and powdered sprays (Occludet).

Zone 3—the sprue

The sprue is sectioned with a carborundum separating disk and the casting is refined in the area of its attachment with stones and sandpaper disks.

Zone 4—proximal contacts

- Proximal contact areas are corrected to maintain contact with the adjacent tooth when tried in the mouth
- Overcontoured areas can be relieved by careful scraping with a scalpel and the casting is adjusted till it seats
- Before adjustments a thin Mylar articulating film is to be placed between casting and the adjacent tooth.

Connectors

- Connector should be parabolic shaped
- Finishing can be done with rubber wheels as to access the cervical aspect of the connector
- Final polishing can be achieved by a piece of twine.

Zone 5—occlusal surface

The occlusal contacts are checked with thin Mylar articulating film to ensure that same contacts as during tryin are present.

Finishing

- If occlusal adjustment is required, they are done with flame-shaped finishing burs or diamonds
- Before adjustments are done the thickness of the metal need to be assessed.

Polishing

- Done with rouge on a soft brush wheel
- Matt finish can be achieved by air-abrasion with 25- to 50- micron alumina particles for one second.

Zone 6—axial walls

After finishing the axial walls, they should be smoothly contoured and highly polished, for good oral hygiene maintenance.

Finishing

Is done by grinding with abrasive particles bound on rubber wheel, paper disk, or by an abrasive paste with light pressure.

Polishing

A high polish is achieved by polishing using jeweller's rouge on wheel or brush with heavier pressures and higher rotational speeds than for finishing procedures.

Zone 7—external margins

- A highly polished metal surface without ledges or steps is to be obtained
- Those parts of the margin that cannot be finished on the tooth are finished on the die.

Finishing

Margins should be finished with out distortion with a stone gently brushed over the surface.

Polishing

- A soft rubber wheel is used followed by rouge on a brush, with the margin supported with a finger
- After polishing, the residues left by polishing agents needs to be removed with a soft toothbrush, by ultrasonic cleaning or by steam cleaning.

Abrasives used for Polishing and Finishing

- Diamond
- Emery—mixture of aluminum oxide and iron oxide bound to paper discs with glue or resins (used on gold or porcelain)
- Aluminum oxide
- Garnet—For metal and porcelain
- Sandpaper discs are made from a dense crystalline form of quartz, called flint
- Tripoli — A fine siliceous polishing powder combined with a wax binder to form light brown cakes used with a cloth buff wheel or a soft bristle brush
- Rouge—Composed of iron oxide (cake form). Used for gold restorations applied with a soft bristle brush or muslin buff wheel
- Electrochemical finishing — Aqua regia (one part nitric acid and three parts hydrochloric acid)
- Electrochemical milling (stripping): The casting is placed in cyanide solution which etches the casting by removing a layer of 40 micron from Type III alloy in one minute.

Equipment for gold finishing and polishing

Small nodules

Tip of a No 330 bur in a high-speed handpiece.

Smoothening of sprue area

No 2 Craytex disc followed by Burlew wheel.

Base-metal finishing and polishing

High-speed handpiece, straight handpiece, disc on mandrel, No 2 round bur, No 8 coral stone on mandrel, aluminum oxide tapered stone, aluminum oxide inverted cone and No 330 bur.

Internal aspects nodule'

No 330 bur.

Surfaces around the sprue

No 8 aluminum oxide coral wheel on a mandrel.

Occlusal grooves smoothening

No 2 carbide bur.

Rough finishing of all accessible areas

No 8 aluminum oxide coral wheel.

Occlusal morphology finishing

Aluminum oxide tapered stone and inverted cone.

Margin finishing

A Spratley knife or white polishing stone and petrolatum followed by a cuttle disc increases marginal adaptation.

Final finishing

Tripoli on a soft Robinson bristle brush with the handpiece running in reverse followed by another soft bristle brush used with rouge.

49. Mention the anatomical concerns for implant placement in posterior maxilla and mandible region.

For success of implant in posterior maxilla:

- They should be placed within the bone entirely
- Should be placed away from anatomic structures like maxillary sinus and inferior alveolar canal (Fig. 28)
- Ideally, 10 mm of vertical bone and 6 mm of horizontal bone should be available for implant.

Implant placement in posterior maxilla and specific concerns

1. The bone in this region is less dense. It has a thinner cortex and larger marrow spaces than posterior mandible.
2. A minimum of 6 months is required for adequate osseointegration.
3. The maxillary sinus is usually close to the edentulous ridge due to resorption of bone and pneumatization of the sinus.
4. A 1 mm gap of bone must be left between the implant and the sinus floor.

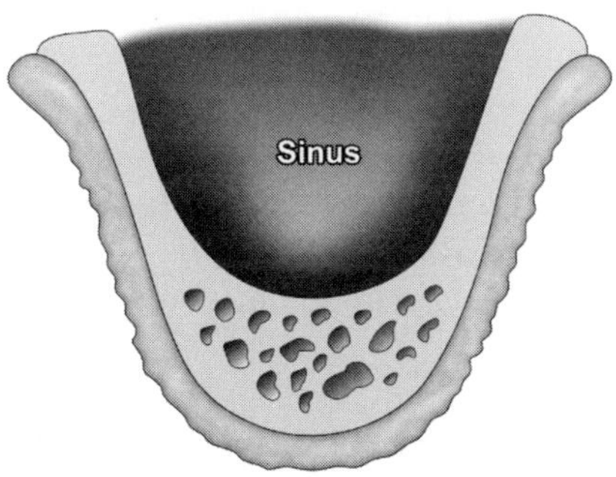

Fig. 28: Anatomical limits of posterior maxilla for implant placement

Adequate bone height is generally present between the nasal cavity and the maxillary sinus. If the bone height is inadequate augmentation like sinus lift should be considered.

Limitations in Implant placement in posterior mandible

- The inferior alveolar nerve traverses the mandibular body in this region and treatment planning must allow for a 2.0 mm margin from the apex of the implant to the superior aspect of the canal
- If adequate length is not present generally an implant is not done here. If overlooked, numbness of the lower lip and nerve damage are potential complications
- The width of the residual ridge must be carefully evaluated in the posterior mandible
- Attachment of the mylohyoid muscle and a deep depression present on the lingual aspect must be noted; if this is overlooked, lingual perforation would result.

50. Pickling.

Pickling is a process that removes a surface film from the casting, which has dark surface oxides and tarnish.

Cause of oxide formation on casting

When the cast gold alloys are quenched to retain their superior physical properties, the water that contacts the hot investment causes reaction that makes the investment soft and granular. This causes a darkening of the casting.

Advantages of pickling

- Removes any clinging investment
- Removes the oxide coating and tarnish.

Disadvantage of using Hydrochloric acid

Fumes from the acid corrode office and laboratory metals.

Other agents that can be used are

- Solution of sulphuric acid with traces of potassium dichromate
- Ultrasonic cleaners.

Pickling Procedure

The discolored casting is heated in an acid such as 50% hydrochloric acid for gypsum-bonded investments.

Method

The casting is placed in a test tube or dish and heated acid is poured over the casting.
The acid is poured off and the casting is removed.
Pickling solution should be renewed frequently.

Rules to follow

1. Casting if gripped with steel tongs will get contaminated because the pickling solution contains small amounts of copper dissolved from previous castings which when contacted by the tongs deposits copper on the casting.

2. The casting if heated can melt the delicate margin or when plunged into the acid, the casting can get distorted by sudden temperature variation.
3. After pickling, the casting should be washed thoroughly to remove traces of the acid.

51. Defects in casting.

Grouped under:

A. Distortion.
B. Surface roughness and irregularities.
C. Porosity.
D. Incomplete casting.

Distortion

Factors causing distortion

- Due to distortion of the wax pattern
- Uneven setting and hygroscopic expansions of the investment
- Configuration of the pattern, type of wax, and thickness influence the amount of distortion caused by expansion of investment
- Distortion during the carving, pooling and removal of wax.

Surface Roughness and Irregularities

Surface roughness is defined as finely spaced surface irregularities whose height, width and direction establish predominant surface pattern.
Surface irregularities are isolated, generally caused by improper mixing technique.

Causes

Air bubbles

- Air bubbles on margin of casting prevents proper seating
- This can be prevented by proper vacuum mixing, application of wetting agent and applying an initial layer of investment on pattern.

Water films

- Appears as ridge or veins
- This occurs due to high water–powder ratio of investment material
- Application of wetting agent to wax pattern before investment can reduce water films.

Rapid heating

- Seen as fins or spines
- When the invested material develops tensile stresses inside and compressive stresses outside, the investment cracks and forms fins.

Under heating

It is due to incomplete wax elimination.

Water–powder ratio

Increased water powder ratio causes rough casting and decreased ratio causes voids.

Prolonged heating

This causes sulphur compounds that contaminate the surface of the casting.

High temperature

Above 700°C causes breakdown of the investment and results in rough casting.

High casting pressure

Ideal casting pressure is 0.10–0.14 MPa (3–4 turns in the centrifugal casting machine.)

Composition of investment

If coarse silica is present it can cause rough casting.

Foreign bodies

Incorporated from rough crucible, sprue former, investment pieces, bits of carbon from flux.

Impact of molten alloy

Due to improper spruing.

Wrong pattern placement in the casting ring

Too many patterns placed together and patterns placed too close in the same ring should be avoided.

Porosities

Internal

- Solidification defects
- Microporosities
- Pin hole porosities
- Subsurface porosities
- Residual air in the mould.

External

Surface roughnesses.

Solidification defects

Solidification shrinkage

Mainly occurs near sprue-cast junction.

Causes

- Incomplete feeding of molten metal
- Premature solidification of the sprue.

Suck back porosities

Near area of sprue.

This occurs when a hot metal, impinging from sprue channel on to a point on the mould wall, causes a hot spot. This hot spot causes local region to freeze last resulting in shrinkage of that area leading to a suck back porosity.

Can be prevented by

- Flaring of the area of sprue attachment
- Lowering casting temperature by 30 degree.

Microporosities

Occurs when solidification occurs too rapidly before the micro voids can reorganise. Can prevent by lowering the mould temperature.

Pinhole porosity

Is spherical in shape whereas gas inclusion porosity is larger. During solidification absorbed gases are expelled leading to pinhole porosity.

Subsurface porosities

Cause

Simultaneous nucleation of solid grains and gas bubbles as the metal freezes at the mould walls.
Can be decreased by controlling the rate of molten metal entry.

Residual air in the mould

- Causes back pressure porosity.
- It occurs as a large concave depression due to the inability of air in the mold to escape.

Causes

- Dense investments
- Low mold temperature.

Can be prevented by:

1. Proper burn out
2. Adequate mold temperature.
3. Ideal casting pressure.

Incomplete casting

Causes

- Insufficient venting
- Increased viscosity of fused metal
- Decreased casting pressure
- Incomplete wax elimination.

52. Myofascial pain dysfunction syndrome.

Myofascial pain dysfunction syndrome, commonly known as a form of temporomandibular joint (TMJ) syndrome, is a vicious cycle between pain and dysfunctional use of the jaw and neck muscles.

Synonyms

- Costes syndrome
- Impostor disease

- Pain-dysfunction syndrome
- Temporomandibular joint syndrome.

Causes

- Bruxism
- Chewing gum for long duration constantly
- An habitual chewing pattern with force on one side of jaw
- Occlusal problems
- Ear infections
- Trauma
- Stress.

Symptoms

- Mainly presents as a unilateral diffuse pain in periauricular region with muscle tenderness, limitation of jaw function, clicking sound in contralateral TMJ
- Tinnitus, dizziness, hearing loss and ear pain
- The pain is sharp and searing, or dull and constant occurring during swallowing, yawning or chewing with the focus over the TMJ joint, immediately in front of the ear
- The pain can be associated with muscle spasm (muscles attachment of skull, face and jaws)
- Crepitation, clicking and cracking of joint
- Luxation and subluxation
- Difficulty in mouth opening
- Mandibular deviation on jaw movements
- Pain can be felt radiating to the side of the head, cheek, lower jaw, and the teeth.

Theories related to cause of MPD

- Psychophysiologic theory—Bruxing and other parafunctional habits leading to muscle fatigue
- Muscle theory—Constant muscle activity leads to pain
- Mechanical displacement theory—Malrelation of teeth alters occlusion thereby leading to pain.

Evaluation of type of pain by (Bell)

Intensity, cause of onset, quality, time, local or diffuse, sensations felt and description of the pain should be noted.

Function of temporomandibular joint

- When excess forces, as bruxism is loaded onto the TMJ the sliding joint uniformly distributes the load
- When the forces applied are constant and intensive the protective cartilage lining of the joint wears.

The pain can be relieved by:
- Observing a dietary regimen consisting of soft diet
- Applying dry or moist heat to the affected side three or more times for 20 minutes at a time
- An analgesic tablet needs to be taken on regular basis if pain is continuous
- Stretching exercises of the jaw and neck muscles can decrease spasm associated with those muscles.

Thorough dental evaluation is required

- Evaluate malrelation
- Faulty restoration
- High points
- Change in vertical dimension
- Change in occlusal contact points
- Abnormal wear of teeth
- Fracture and malalignment of teeth
- Any tooth that was not replaced, causing a change in occlusion.

Correction

- As splints for bruxers
- Restoring the occlusal plane by restoration
- Replacing missing tooth by prosthesis
- Correction of malaligned tooth by uprighting orthodontically
- To eliminate occlusal contact on inclined planes to enhance positional stability.

Differential diagnosis

Trigeminal neuralgia.

Aids used for diagnosis

Myotronics
With microcomputer can help to assess the resting and functional states of muscles.

Pantograph
Can detect muscle dysfunction.

CAT scan
Can locate degenerative joint diseases.

Arthrography and MRI
Can detect internal derangements.

53. Implant-supported fixed partial denture.

Definition

An implant is a substance that is placed into the jaw to support a crown or fixed or removable denture.

Indications in fixed partial denture

- For single tooth replacement where fixed denture is not possible
- In distally missing abutments implants are placed and a crown is given
- In long-span edentulous areas where fixed partial denture do not fulfil Ante's law
- In patients who are unwilling to reduce sound tooth, yet want replacement for missing tooth.

Advantages

- Preservation of bone
- Better retention and stability
- Better function
- Good esthetics and comfort
- Reduction of sound tooth can be avoided.

Classification of implants

1. Depending on tissue placement:
- Subperiosteal (epiosteal)
- Endosteal—Root form and plate form
- Transosteal—Passes the entire alveolar bone height.

2. Depending on materials used:
- Bio-inert—Titanium and its alloys, cobalt chromium and alloys.
- Bioactive —Ceramics, hydroxyapatite, carbon.

3. Depending on edentulous spaces:
Misch and Judy classified spaces with different bone volumes (similar to Kennedy's classification).

Implant options

- The first three classification were fixed prostheses and the other two were removable prostheses
- Classified as FP-I, FP-2, FP-3, RP-4 and RP-5
- In fixed prosthodontics, the endosteal root form implants are commonly used.

Root form implants

Types
- Cylinder type, which is tapped in (Fig. 29)
- Screw type which is threaded or non-threaded, coated or non-coated (Fig. 30).

Mechanism of Integration

Osseointegration

(Ingvar Branemark)

Fibro-osseous attachment

(Weiss)
- In which a fibro-osseous ligament is formed between bone and implant interface.

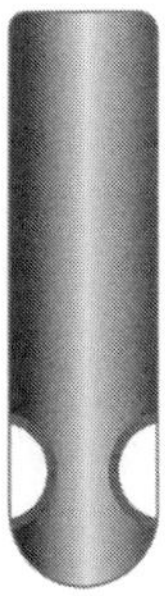

Fig. 29: Cylinder-type implant

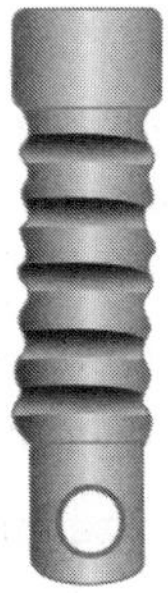

Fig. 30: Screw-type implant

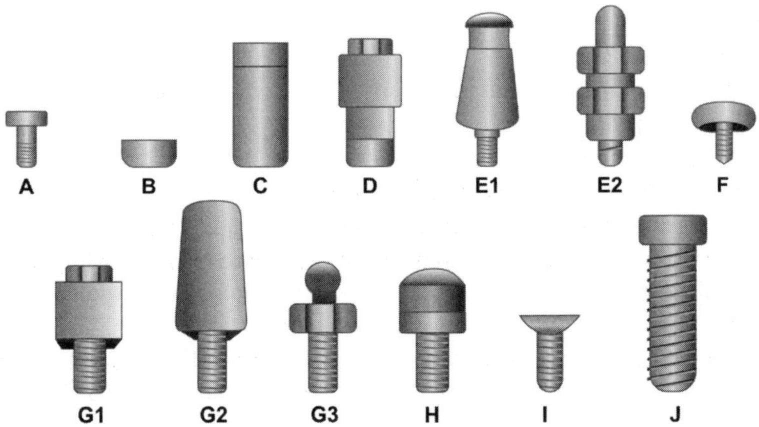

Fig. 31: Parts of an implant: A—Prosthesis screw; B—Coping; C1—Implant body; D—Analog abutment; E1 and E2—Transfer coping; F—Hygiene screws; G1–G3—Types of abutment; H—Permucosal extension; I— First stage cover screws; J—Implant body or fixture

Biointegration

Occurs when the material is coated with hydroxyapatite, which forms a physiochemical bond with bone.

Periosteal integration

The ideal attachment is osseointegration, which is an apparent direct attachment of osseous tissue to an inert alloplastic material without intervening connective tissue.

Parts of an implant (Fig. 31)

1. Implant body.
2. Healing screw.
3. Healing caps.
4. Abutments.
5. Impression posts.
6. Laboratory analogs.
7. Waxing sleeves.
8. A superstructure connected through an attachment.

Types of connections

1. Split external hex

- Fixed by abutment screw
- For two stage.

2. Internal hex/Internal octagon: (Corevent)

For single stage and two stage.

3. Morse taper

Surgical procedure

Procedures are done only after thorough radiographic evaluation and patient examination.

1. Incision:
   For two stage implant:
   Crestal incision on buccal side and flap elevation on lingual side.
   For single stage:
   A trap door incision.
2. A round drill is used to stabilize implant drill.
3. Twist drills of increasing diameter are used after depth is assessed.
4. A final drill, one size smaller than the implant, is used to prepare implant site. Sizes for twist drills are 3.5, 3.8 and 4.2. Depth markings are present on the twist drills.
5. Counter sink is used only for two-stage implants.
6. After the implant site is prepared, the implant is screwed in or tapped in with cover screw and the incision is approximated 3–5 mm from incision line and 3–5 mm apart.

Second stage surgery

1. Once osseointegration is complete, a full thickness flap is raised.
2. Cover screws are removed and the abutment extension is threaded into the body.
3. Impression is made and the final suprastructure is attached after laboratory fabrication of crown.

Single stage systems are placed in one stage surgery with temporary crowns attached.

Implant systems

A few of the implant systems available:

- Sterioss
- Frialitt
- Branemark
- IMTEC
- Centerpulse
- Endopore
- Oraltronics.

54. Full-mouth rehabilitation.

Treatment program

1. Initially pain and infection are eliminated.
2. Restorations like fillings are done.

3. Oral hygiene prophylaxis is done.
4. Reshaping, repositioning and restoring the dentition are done.

Treatment objectives

1. To create occlusal contact by:
   - Recontouring
   - Reshaping
   - Repositioning
   - Surgery
   - Combinations of any of the above.
2. To substitute an occlusal contact:
   An occlusal splint needs to be substituted to achieve a holding contact.
3. To splint unopposed teeth:
   By splinting unopposed teeth to teeth that are opposed.

Factors to be analysed in full-mouth rehabilitation

Anterior teeth

To determine the anterior guidance in harmony with envelope of function.

Occlusal plane

During anterior guidance, if posterior tooth interference is present, the occlusal plane should be evaluated and corrected.

Posterior teeth

Posterior teeth should not cause interference with disclusive function of anterior guidance.

Pankey–Mann–Schuyler technique for full mouth rehabilitation

Principles by Schuyler

1. Maximum teeth in static, coordinated, occlusal contact in centric relation.
2. Anterior guidance should be in harmony with lateral excursive movements on working side.
3. Disclusion by anterior guidance of all posterior teeth in protrusion.
4. Disclusion of all non-working side inclines in lateral excursions.
5. Group function of working side inclines in lateral excursion.

Advantages of Schuyler's technique

- More than eight teeth are not prepared or rebuilt
- No loss in vertical dimension
- Less time
- No complicated equipments
- Laboratory procedure is controlled by dentist.

Procedure

Order of rehabilitation:

1. Lower anteriors.
2. Upper anteriors.

3. Lower posteriors.
4. Upper posteriors.

Establishing anterior guidance:

1. Coordinated centric relation stops should be present on all anterior teeth.
2. Centric slide should not be present.
3. An anterior guide table is customised to minimise stresses in lateral excursions.

Corrections are required for:

1. Steep labioincisal angle.
2. Wear of teeth.
3. Unesthetic appearance as crowding and spacing.

Customised anterior guide table:

1. Centric relation, at the correct vertical dimension, is made and facebow transfer is done.
2. Cast is mounted and articulated after full mouth preparation.
3. A plastic guide table is placed and incisal pin is raised 1 mm.
4. After applying monomer on table, the manipulated acrylic resin is placed on table.
5. The pin is lowered and upper cast is brought in edge-to-edge relationship.
6. The guide pin records the movement of the path followed by cast from centric to edge-to-edge relationship.
7. Lateral excursive movements are also carried out before the acrylic sets.

Evaluation of Upper Anteriors

1. Tooth position in the arch.
2. Lip support.
3. Lip closure.
4. Phonetics.
5. Neutral zone.
6. Smile line.

Evaluation of occlusal plane:

1. Correction can be done by selective grinding.
2. By restoration to alter occlusal plane in malaligned tooth.
3. By occlusal plane analysis (Broadicks).

Evaluation of Lower Posterior Teeth

Restored with cusp tip to fossa contact.

Evaluation of occlusal plane:

1. Each lower buccal cusp tip position and contouring of lower fossa.
2. Distance between the lower buccal and lower lingual cusp should not be greater than half the total buccolingual width of tooth at its widest part.

Evaluation of Upper Posterior Teeth

The last to be restored.

Evaluate type of upper occlusal incline:

1. Group function.
2. Partial group function.
3. Canine guided (total disclusion).

55. Contraindications for implant placement

Implants are contraindicated in patients with abnormal bone metabolism, poor oral hygiene and previous irradiation of the implant site.

They can be classified as follows:

- Medical/Systemic
- Dental/Local.

Medical Contraindications

Medical contraindications given by the National Institutes of Health Consensus Conference, is as follows:[1]

- Acute illness
- Terminal illness
- Pregnancy
- Uncontrolled metabolic disease (e.g.: diabetes)
- Tumoricidal irradiation of implant site
- Low-dose irradiated patients
- Patients with psychiatric problems
- Haematological systemic disorders.

Dental contraindications

Some of the relative contraindication in the oral cavity includes:

- Disease affecting the mucosa of the mouth
- Periodontal conditions
- Severe bruxism
- Heavy masticatory force application
- Occlusal disharmony
- Infections in the neighbouring teeth, such as pockets, granuloma
- Underlying cysts or pathology in the implant site
- Impacted teeth at the implant site
- Root dilacerations of adjacent teeth to implant site
- Anatomic limitations in a specific region.

Reference

1. Dental Implants. NIH Consens Statement Online. 1988 Jun 13-15 [cited year month day];7(3):1-22.

56. Laboratory procedures in fixed partial denture.

Steps in lab procedures

Working cast and dies

Pindex System

Preparing the master cast

- The final impression is poured in stone
- After the stone sets, the retrieved cast is trimmed to a horseshoe-shaped form
- The buccolingual width of the base of the horseshoe is 13–18 mm, and thickness 15 mm between the gingival margins of the preparations and the inferior border.

Pin Placement

- After the under surface of the cast is trimmed perfectly flat, drill two holes for each removable section as far apart to provide space for the pins and sleeves
- The pins are cemented into holes using low viscosity cyanoacrylate cement
- The short index pins are cemented in the lingual holes
- Long pins cemented into the buccal holes
- The white sleeves are placed over the long pins and the gray sleeves over the short pins.

The Secondary Base

- A strip of carding wax is placed over the extensions of the long pins and the gray sleeves
- The master cast is boxed or placed in a rubber base former and a secondary base is poured with cast stone.

Removable Dies

- After the secondary base sets, remove the master cast and trim the secondary base on the model trimmer
- Dies are sectioned with a die saw and trimmed carefully to expose the finish line
- Clean the stone grindings from the dies, pins, base and pin holes
- Reseat the dies
- The master cast is mounted.

Fabrication of wax patterns

- Wax pattern is the duplicate replica of the finished cast restoration, which will be placed on the prepared tooth
- Wax pattern is invested and cast to form the final restoration.

Indirect technique

Pattern is waxed on die from an accurate impression of prepared tooth.

Cusp Marginal Ridge

- Functional cusp contact with marginal ridges and occlusal fossae
- Opposing occlusion is a single tooth opposing two teeth.

Advantages

This is the most natural type of occlusion and is found in 95% of all adults. It can be used for single restorations placing very little lateral stress on the tooth.

Disadvantages

Food impaction and the displacement of teeth may arise if the functional cusps wedge into a lingual embrasure opposing them.

Uses

Most cast restorations done in daily practice.

Pontic placement

After the wax pattern on abutment tooth is complete, a pontic pattern is made and connected to the retainer wax patterns.

Spruing

A sprue former is a wax, plastic or metal pattern used to form the channel allowing the molten metal to flow into the mould to make a casting.

Sprue placement

- Should be attached at 45° angulation to the thickest portion of the pattern. This prevents porosities and air entrapments
- The area of sprue attachment is flared for smooth flow of metal.

Sprue attachment

1. One end of the sprue is attached to the wax pattern with a reservoir.
2. The other end is attached to the crucible formers cone shaped structure.
3. The wax pattern should have 6 mm space between the tip of pattern and casting ring. The space allows for the air to escape out of the pores in investment.
4. The wax pattern should have uniform space within the casting ring (it should be placed in the center of the casting ring).

Investing

1. After the wax pattern is attached to the crucible former, a surface tension reducing agent is applied on the wax pattern.
2. The vacuum mixed invested material is brushed on to the pattern before filling the entire ring.
3. The filled ring is placed away for one hour.

Burn out

- The furnace temperature is brought to 200°C and held at the same temperature for 30 minutes
- The final burn out temperature is raised to 650°C and held for 45 minutes
- The pattern is placed for burn out procedure.

Casting

- Casting machine is given three or four clockwise turns depending on the alloy
- The cradle and counterbalance weights are made to approximate with casting ring used
- Alloys can be melted with gas air torch or electricity
- Only after the alloy is melted the mould is removed from burn out furnace and the lever is released to complete the casting.

Recovery of casting

- After the red glow is disappeared, the casting ring is plunged in running water
- A knife is used to remove the investment material and the rest of investment material is tapped out with blunt instrument.

Finishing of metal

- The recovered casting is trimmed and finished
- Some times a metal try in is done for ceramic restoration.

Other procedures

Soldering

If it is a long-span FPD or a complex design FPD, soldering of certain parts might be required.

Veneer application (acrylic or porcelain)

- In acrylic veneer application, wax is built up to the correct contour, dewaxed and packed in the matched tooth colored heat-cure acrylic resin and cured
- Porcelain application can be achieved by platinum foil technique or direct lift technique
- The condensed porcelain mass is placed in a preheated furnace [approximately 650°C (1200°F) for 5 minutes]
- Initially the opaquer is placed, and then the body porcelain is built and finally the incisal porcelain
- When the final contour is satisfactory, characterization is completed and the porcelain is glazed.

57. Tensofrictional resistance.

Definition

Frictional resistance is the resistance to penetration developed by the friction sleeve, equal to the vertical force applied to the sleeve divided by its surface area.
The resistance is the sum of friction and adhesion.

Application of tensofrictional resistance

In cement retained crown with vital tooth only.

Principle of tensofrictional resistance

Retention is provided by two parallel walls and the friction that is generated between the tooth and crown surface.
Friction becomes relevant when the tooth and crown surfaces are in close proximity.

Function

During the initial phases of the evolution of fixed prosthodontic treatment, retention without the use of a luting agent was routine, hence space for the luting was not provided with die spacers.

As there was no space provided for the luting cement during the process of cementation, hydraulic pressure built up in the crown causing vital dentin to undergo an elastic change creating a resultant tension.

It was believed that the elastic dentin tried to regain its shape by releasing the forces, thereby creating additional retention for the crown.

A few relevant dentin values

- Elastic modulus of dentin—18,600 MN/m^2
- Yield strength of dentin—165 MN/m^2.

Relevance of tensofrictional resistance

Presently this theory has no relevance because of superior quality luting agents and the space provided for luting by die spacer (Fig. 32).

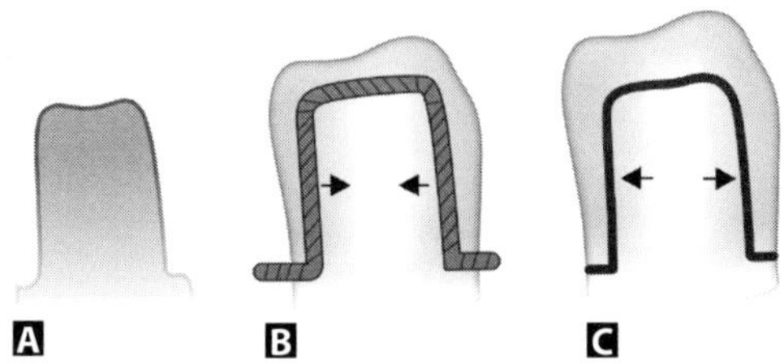

Fig. 32: Tensofrictional resistance: A—Prepared tooth; B—Contraction of dentin due to elastic change creating tension; C—Regain in shape of dentin by release of tension

Suggested Readings

1. Anusavice KJ, Shen C, Rawls HR. Phillips' Science of Dental Materials, ed 12. Elsevier.
2. Freedman. Contemporary Esthetic Dentistry. Elsevier; 2012.
3. Misch CE. Dental Implant Prosthetics. Mosby; 2005.
4. Rosensteil SF, Land MF, Fujimoto J. Contemporary Fixed Prosthodontics, ed 4. Elsevier; 2006.
5. Shalu Bathla. Periodontics Revisited. Jaypee brothers Medical publishers;2011
6. Shillingburg HT, Hobo S, Whitsett LD, et al. Fundamentals of fixed prosthodontics, ed 3. Quintessence; 1997.
7. Touati B. Esthetic dentistry and Ceramic restorations. Thieme; 1998.

SECTION 3

MCQ, Extended Matching Questions, Short Answer Questions, Laminate Veneers and Recent Advances in Fixed Partial Denture

INTRODUCTION TO FPD

MULTIPLE CHOICE QUESTIONS

1. **The width of attached gingiva of an abutment teeth is evaluated with help of:**
   A. Periapical radiograph.
   B. Bitewing radiograph.
   C. Intraoral examination.
   D. Diagnostic casts.
   E. Extraoral examination.

2. **Which of the following are assessed during the intraoral examination for fixed dental prosthesis?**
   A. Attached gingiva.
   B. Gingival architecture and stippling.
   C. Amount of plaque retention.
   D. Occlusal prematurities.
   E. All of the above.
   NOTE—apart from the above the other factors assessed during intraoral examination are non-working interferences, tooth mobility and location, depth of pocket.

3. **Choose the items which can be assessed using a diagnostic cast.**
   A. Inclination of the tooth.
   B. Length of the abutment tooth.
   C. Length of the edentulous space.
   D. All of the above.

4. **Which one of the following can be assessed using a bitewing radiograph?**
   A. Amount of plaque retention.
   B. Location and extent of proximal caries.
   C. Bone level.
   D. A and B.
   E. B and C.

5. **Which one of the following can be assessed using a periapical radiograph?**
   A. Amount of plaque retention.
   B. Chronic apical periodontitis.
   C. Tooth mobility.
   D. Length and configuration of roots.
   E. B and D.

6. **Which one of the following investigations is not necessary for routine assessment of a patient for fixed prosthodontic treatment?**
   A. Full periodontal charting.
   B. TMJ evaluation.
   C. Extraoral examination.
   D. Diagnostic casts.
   E. Radiographs.
7. **Habits like clenching may result in fatigue, muscle pain and hypertrophy of the:**
   A. Buccinator.
   B. Masseter.
   C. Sternocleidomastoid.
   D. Lateral pterygoid.
   E. Trapezius.

ANS: 1C 2E 3D 4E 5E 6A 7B

EXTENDED MATCHING QUESTIONS

1. Theme: Diagnosis.

A. Attached gingiva.
B. Diagnostic wax up.
C. Proximal caries.
D. Dietary habit.
E. Regurgitation.
F. Root configuration.
G. Temporomandibular joint.

Using a letter from A to G, choose the most appropriate response from the list above that best matches each of the following descriptions numbered 1 to 5 below. You may use each response A to G, once only or not at all.

1. Checked using the periapical radiograph.
2. Assessed using the intraoral examination.
3. Revealed during patients history.
4. Evaluated during the extraoral examination.
5. Viewed with the help of horizontal bitewing radiograph.

Description	Response
1	F
2	A
3	E
4	G
5	C

2. Theme : Components of a fixed prosthesis.

A. Abutment.
B. Connector.
C. Pontic.
D. Retainer.
E. Non-rigid connector.
F. Edentulous ridge.
G. Crown.

Using a letter from A to G, choose the most appropriate response from the list above that best matches each of the following descriptions numbered 1 to 5 below. You may use each response A to G, once only or not at all.

1. A component of a bridge that permits limited movement.
2. An artificial tooth on a bridge that replaces a missing natural tooth and restores its form and function.

3. A component of a bridge which is cemented to the abutment(s).
4. The term used to describe the tooth or teeth to which a bridge is cemented.
5. A component of a bridge which joins the retainer to the pontic.

Description	Response
1	E
2	C
3	D
4	A
5	B

SHORT ANSWER QUESTIONS

1. **a. List four possible signs and symptoms of a TMJ disorder. (2 marks)**
    - Clicking
    - Crepitation
    - Pain and limitation on opening, closing and moving laterally
    - Pain of palpation of the joints and masticatory muscles as the patient opens and closes
    - Deviation of mandible when open and close
    - Headache.

   b. Which are the six muscles that should be examined when a TMJ disorder is suspected? (3 marks)
    - Masseter
    - Temporalis
    - Medial pterygoid
    - Lateral pterygoid
    - Trapezius
    - Sternocleidomastoid.

2. **a. List six indications for diagnostic casts in planning for any prosthesis in a dentate patient? (3 marks)**
    - To study occlusion
    - Length and curvature of edentulous spaces
    - Occlusogingival dimensions
    - Orientation of abutment teeth
    - Wear facets
    - Positioning and super-eruption of opposing teeth
    - Prepare diagnostic wax-up.

   b. List four indications for taking radiographs in planning for any prosthesis in a dentate patient? (2 marks)
    - Caries: Interproximal and under the existing restorations
    - Periapical lesions
    - Quality of root canal treatments
    - Supporting bone level
    - Crown/root ratio
    - Length, configuration and direction of roots
    - PDL width (traumatic occlusion)
    - Retained root and any other pathology.

FUNDAMENTALS OF OCCLUSION

MULTIPLE CHOICE QUESTIONS

1. **The position of the condyle in centric relation is:**
   A. Anteriorly, superiorly braced position along the articular eminence of the glenoid fossa.
   B. Anteriorly, inferiorly braced position along the articular eminence of the glenoid fossa.
   C. Posteriorly, superiorly braced position along the articular eminence of the glenoid fossa.
   D. Posteriorly, inferiorly braced position along the articular eminence of the glenoid fossa.
   E. Posteriorly, medially braced position along the articular eminence of the glenoid fossa.
2. **The mandible makes a purely rotational opening and closing movement around the:**
   A. Vertical axis.
   B. Sagittal axis.
   C. Horizontal axis.
   D. Frontal axis.
   E. Orientation axis.
3. **A purely hinge movement of condyles within the range of 10 – 13 degree produces a separation of ....**
   A. 20 – 25 mm.
   B. 10 – 15 mm.
   C. 20 – 25 cm.
   D. 10 – 15 cm.
4. **A shield-shaped pattern has all distinct movement components except the:**
   A. Left lateral superior border
   B. Left lateral opening border
   C. Right lateral Inferior border
   D. Right lateral opening border.
5. **When the mandible moves laterally the nonworking side condyle will arc....**
   A. Forward and medially.
   B. Laterally and posteriorly.
   C. Forward and laterally.
   D. Medially and posteriorly.
   E. Laterally and anteriorly.
6. **When the mandible moves laterally the working side condyle will arc:**
   A. Forward and medially.
   B. Laterally and posteriorly.

C. Forward and laterally.
D. Medially and posteriorly.
E. Laterally and anteriorly.

7. The dentist has control over which one of the following determinants of mandibular movement?

A. Anterior determinants.
B. Posterior determinants and temporomandibular joints.
C. Anterior determinants and temporomandibular joints.
D. Posterior determinants.
E. Temporomandibular joints.

8. The working occlusal interference is more likely to occur on:

A. Mesial-facing cusp inclines of maxilla.
B. Lingual-facing cusp inclines of maxilla.
C. Buccal-facing cusp inclines of maxilla.
D. Distal-facing cusp inclines of mandible.
E. Mesial-facing cusp inclines of mandible.

9. The centric occlusal interferences are more likely to occur on:

A. Buccal-facing inclines of mandibular molars.
B. Mesial-facing inclines of maxillary molars.
C. Mesial-facing inclines of mandibular molars.
D. Distal-facing inclines of maxillary molars.
E. Lingual-facing inclines of mandibular molars.

10. Protrusive occlusal interferences are more likely to occur on:

A. Buccal-facing inclines of mandibular molars.
B. Mesial-facing inclines of maxillary molars.
C. Distal-facing inclines of mandibular molars.
D. Distal-facing inclines of maxillary molars.
E. Lingual-facing inclines of mandibular molars.

11. The nonworking occlusal interference is more likely to occur on:

A. Mesial-facing cusp inclines of maxilla.
B. Lingual-facing cusp inclines of maxilla.
C. Buccal -facing cusp inclines of maxilla.
D. Distal-facing cusp inclines of mandible.
E. Mesial-facing cusp inclines of mandible.

12. Mutually protected occlusion is otherwise called as:

A. Group function.
B. Incisor occlusion.
C. Molar occlusion.
D. Organic occlusion.

13. The concept of occlusion which is used in complete denture construction is:

A. Unilateral balanced occlusion.
B. Mutually protected occlusion.
C. Canine protected occlusion.
D. Bilateral balanced occlusion.

14. Mutually protected occlusion cannot be observed in patients with:

A. Class I occlusion.
B. Reverse occlusion.
C. Class I malocclusion.
D. Overjet occlusion.

15. During protrusive movement if the protrusive inclination is steep then the corresponding cuspal height is:

A. Shallow.
B. Flat.
C. Steep.
D. Undermined.

16. During immediate lateral translation movement if the translation is minimal then the corresponding cuspal height is:

A. Shallow.
B. Flat.
C. Steep.
D. Undermined.

17. If the vertical overlap is greater, then the posterior cuspal height is:

A. Shorter.
B. Flat.
C. Longer.
D. Undermined.

ANS : 1A 2C 3A 4C 5A 6B 7A 8B 9B 10D 11C 12D 13D 14B 15C 16C 17C

SHORT ANSWER QUESTIONS

1. **Name the determinants of mandibular movements. [2 marks]**
   - Posteriorly the right and left temporomandibular joints
   - Anteriorly the teeth
   - Overall the neuromuscular system.
2. **Describe the different types of occlusal interferences. [5 marks]**
   - Centric: Maxillary mesial-facing cusp inclines and mandibular distal-facing cusp inclines
   - Working: Maxillary lingual-facing cusp inclines and mandibular buccal-facing cusp inclines
   - Nonworking: Maxillary buccal -facing cusp inclines and mandibular lingual-facing cusp inclines
   - Protrusive: Maxillary distal-facing cusp inclines and mandibular mesial-facing cusp inclines.
3. **Describe the Okeson criteria for normal occlusion. [5 marks]**
   - In closure, the condyles are in the most superoanterior position against the discs on the posterior slopes of the eminences of the glenoid fossae. The posterior teeth are in solid and even contact, and the anterior teeth are in slightly lighter contact
   - Occlusal forces are in the long axis of the teeth
   - In lateral excursions of the mandible, working-side contacts (preferably on the canines) disocclude or separate the nonworking teeth instantly
   - In protrusive excursions, anterior tooth contacts will disocclude the posterior teeth
   - In an upright posture, posterior teeth contact more heavily than do anterior teeth.
4. **Discuss in detail the three recognized concepts of occlusion. [5 marks]**

   Bilateral Balanced Occlusion
   - Based on the work of von Spee and Monson
   - Dictates that a maximum number of teeth should contact in all excursive positions of the mandible
   - Useful in complete denture construction, in which contact on the nonworking side is important to prevent tipping of the denture.

   Unilateral Balanced Occlusion
   - Based on the work of Schuyler
   - Known as group function, distributes the occlusal load
   - Eliminate all tooth contact on the nonworking side, prevents those teeth from being subjected to the destructive, obliquely directed forces found in nonworking interferences
   - Saves the centric holding cusps and maintain the occlusion.

Mutually-protected Occlusion

- Based on the work of D'Amico, Stuart, Stallard, Stuart, Lucia
- Known as canine-protected occlusion or "organic" occlusion
- The anterior teeth bear the entire load and the posterior teeth are disoccluded in any excursive position of the mandible
- As a result of the anterior teeth protecting the posterior teeth in all mandibular excursions and the posterior teeth protecting the anterior teeth at the intercuspal position, this type of occlusion came to be known as a mutually-protected occlusion.

ARTICULATION AND ARTICULATORS

MULTIPLE CHOICE QUESTIONS

1. **Choose the correct ones**
   - a. **In an arcon articulator the condylar elements are placed on the lower member of the articulator.**
   - b. **In an arcon articulator, the condylar inclination becomes less steep when the teeth are separated or closed.**
   - c. **The most accurate method of locating the hinge axis is by trial and error method by McCollum and Stuart in 1921.**
   - d. **Arcon articulators are the most commonly used articulators for dentures.**
   - e. **Thickness of the interocclusal records is—3.0–5.0 mm.**
   - f. **The precise recording of the condylar paths is done by interocclusal recordings.**

   A. a, b and e.
   B. a, c and e.
   C. c, d and f.
   D. b, d and f.

ANS : 1B

EXTENDED MATCHING QUESTIONS

1. Theme: Articulation

A. Simple hinge articulator.
B. Semi-adjustable articulator.
C. Fully-adjustable articulator.
D. Face bow.
E. Fox plane.
F. Willis gauge.
G. Metal gauge.

Using a letter from A to G, choose the most appropriate articulator from the list above that best matches each of the following descriptions numbered 1 to 5 below. You may use each response A to G, once only or not at all.

1. The most suitable jaw simulator used in making short span bridges and complete dentures.
2. Device used to assess lower face vertical dimension.
3. Device used to assess parallelism of occlusal wax rims.
4. Device used to assess the thickness of crowns.
5. Device used to transfer the relationship between jaws and posterior hinge axis to the articulators.

Description	Response
1	B
2	F
3	E
4	G
5	D

SHORT ANSWER QUESTIONS

1. Name the type of mandibular movement in the tracings.

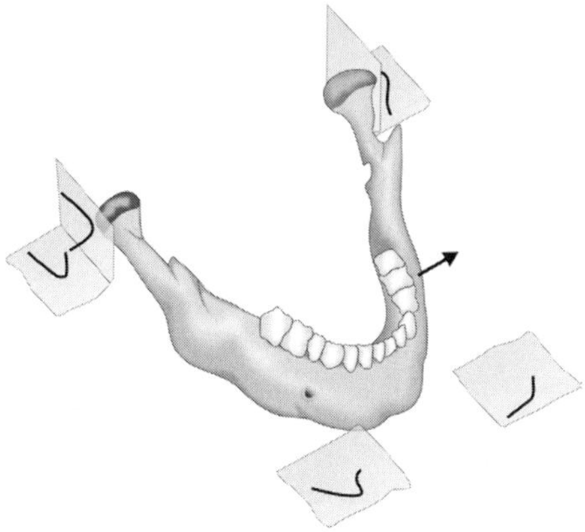

A. Left lateral excursion

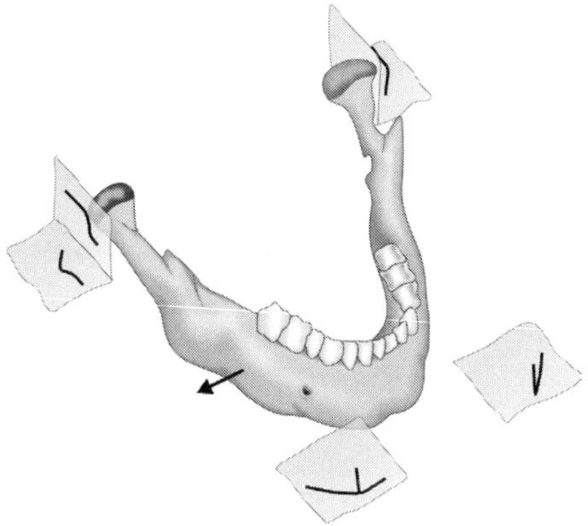

B. Right lateral excursion

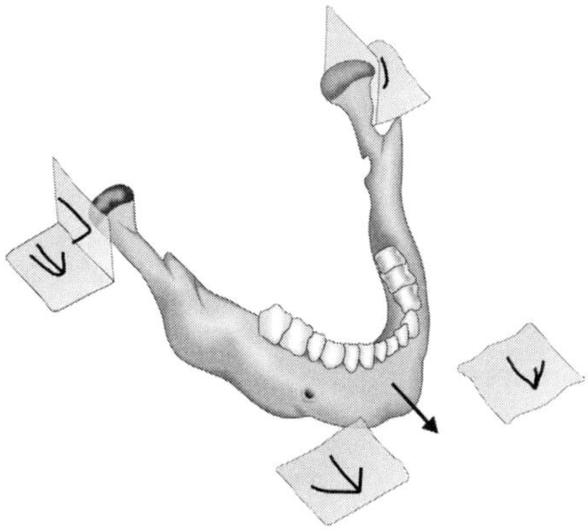

C. Protrusive excursion

INTEROCCLUSAL RECORDS

MULTIPLE CHOICE QUESTIONS

1. **The interocclusal record used to adjust the horizontal condylar guidance of a semi-adjustable articulator is the:**
   A. Centric relation.
   B. Lateral interocclusal.
   C. Protrusive.
   D. Maximum intercuspation.
   E. Retrusive.
2. **In what relation are study casts mounted for diagnosis and complex treatment, such as occlusal rehabilitation?**
   A. Eccentric relation.
   B. Maximum intercuspation.
   C. Centric relation.
   D. Canine relation.
   E. Protrusive relation.
3. **In what relation are study casts mounted for simpler treatment, such as single crown restorations?**
   A. Eccentric relation.
   B. Maximum intercuspation.
   C. Centric relation.
   D. Canine relation.
   E. Protrusive relation.
4. **The most consistent and repeatable method of obtaining centric relation is:**
   A. Chin point guidance.
   B. Unguided method.
   C. Bilateral manipulation.
   D. Physiologic method.
5. **The position of the condyle during the initial tooth contact with the mandible in the optimum position is called:**
   A. Eccentric relation contact position.
   B. Maximum contact position.
   C. Centric relation contact position.
   D. Protrusive contact position.

6. The bite registration material used for recording centric relation should be:

A. Elastic and brittle.
B. Rigid and flexible.
C. Rigid and brittle.
D. Elastic and flexible.
E. Rigid and elastic.

7. Occlusal clearance in a prepared tooth is best assessed by:

A. Visual examination.
B. Metal gauge.
C. Articulating paper.
D. Wax bite.
E. Bite registration paste.

ANS: 1C 2C 3B 4C 5C 6C 7D

SHORT ANSWER QUESTIONS

1. Name the three techniques for locating centric relation position. [2 marks]

- Chin point guidance—most posterior and superior position
- Unguided method—physiologic—not repeatable
- Bilateral manipulation—consistent, repeatable by Dawson.

TREATMENT PLANNING SINGLE TOOTH

MULTIPLE CHOICE QUESTIONS

1. **Which one of the following intra-coronal restoration is plastic in nature?**
   A. Metal inlay.
   B. Ceramic inlay.
   C. Complex amalgam.
   D. MOD onlay.
   E. Ceramic onlay.

2. **Which one of the following is a cemented intracoronal restoration?**
   A. Glass ionomer.
   B. Simple amalgam.
   C. Complex amalgam.
   D. Metal inlay.
   E. Ceramic veneer.

3. **Which one of the following materials should be protected (e.g. by resin) for 24 hours after restoring the tooth?**
   A. Glass ionomer cement.
   B. Zinc polycarboxylate.
   C. Resin-modified glass ionomer.
   D. Zinc oxide eugenol.
   E. Compomer.

4. **Which temporary restorative material is least favorable to use when it is to be replaced by a resin composite restoration?**
   A. Zinc polycarboxylate.
   B. Compomer.
   C. Zinc oxide eugenol.
   D. Conventional glass ionomer.
   E. Zinc phosphate.

5. **The choice of intracoronal restoration in an incipient lesion is:**
   A. Glass ionomer.
   B. Simple amalgam.
   C. Complex amalgam.
   D. Metal inlay.
   E. Ceramic onlay.

6. The intracoronal restoration of choice in class 4 lesions is:

A. Glass ionomer.
B. Simple amalgam.
C. Complex amalgam.
D. Composite resin.
E. Ceramic onlay.

7. The restorative material which releases fluoride is:

A. Glass ionomer.
B. Simple amalgam.
C. Complex amalgam.
D. Composite resin.
E. Metal inlay.

8. The restorative material which fails due to polymerization shrinkage is:

A. Glass ionomer.
B. Simple amalgam.
C. Complex amalgam.
D. Composite resin.
E. Metal inlay.

9. The choice of intracoronal restoration when the cusps are to be replaced:

A. Glass ionomer.
B. Simple amalgam.
C. Complex amalgam.
D. Composite resin.
E. Metal inlay.

10. The choice of intracoronal restoration when the teeth are endodontically treated:

A. Glass ionomer.
B. Simple amalgam.
C. Complex amalgam.
D. Composite resin.
E. Metal inlay.

11. The choice of intracoronal restoration when the isthmus is wider:

A. Metal inlay.
B. Ceramic inlay.
C. Complex amalgam.
D. Glass ionomer.
E. MOD Onlay.

12. Which one of the following intracoronal restoration is most appropriate in an esthetic zone where the isthmus preparation is narrower?

A. Metal inlay.
B. Ceramic inlay.
C. Complex amalgam.
D. MOD onlay.
E. Ceramic onlay.

13. An extracoronal restoration that requires minimal tooth preparation is the:

A. Metal-ceramic crown.
B. Ceramic veneer.
C. All ceramic crown.
D. All metal crown.
E. All acrylic crown.

14. The extracoronal restoration of choice when longevity is the main consideration is a:

A. Metal–ceramic crown.
B. Ceramic veneer.
C. All ceramic crown.
D. All metal crown.
E. All acrylic crown.

15. The choice of extracoronal restoration when it needs retention and esthetics:

A. Metal–ceramic crown.
B. Ceramic Veneer.
C. All ceramic crown.
D. Full metal crown.
E. Acrylic crown.

16. A large resin composite restoration was placed to replace a fractured buccal cusp; during the review appointment brown bands were noted on the buccal surface of the restoration. This is caused by:

A. The placement of a single increment of resin composite on the buccal surface.
B. The use of a metal matrix band constituents reacting with the uncured resin composite.
C. Polymerization contraction causing microspaces between increments that become stained.
D. Staining of resin composite due to a smoking habit.
E. White spot lesions becoming stained due to dietary constituents.

ANS: 1C 2D 3A 4C 5A 6D 7A 8D 9C 10C 11E 12B 13B 14D 15A 16C

TREATMENT PLANNING FOR MISSING TOOTH

MULTIPLE CHOICE QUESTIONS

1. **Which one of the following is an ideal crown–root ratio for an abutment tooth?**
   A. 3:2.
   B. 1:1.
   C. 2:3.
   D. 2:1.
   E. 3:1.
   Note: Minimum acceptable crown: root ratio is 1:1.
2. **Which one of the following root configuration is preferred for an abutment tooth?**
   A. Broader labiolingual roots.
   B. Conical and converged roots.
   C. Fused roots.
   D. Perfectly tapered roots.
   E. Round in cross section.
3. **Regarding the maximum occlusal force created by the natural dentition and different types of prosthesis, which one of following is correct?**
   A. Natural dentition > partial removable > fixed > complete removable.
   B. Natural dentition ≥ fixed > partial removable = complete removable.
   C. Natural dentition > fixed > partial removable > complete removable.
   D. Natural dentition = fixed > partial removable = complete removable.
   E. Natural dentition = fixed = partial removable = complete removable.

ANS: 1C 2A 3C

SHORT ANSWER QUESTIONS

1. **A 45-year-old patient presents with the following dentition. The patient would like to restore his missing upper left second premolar tooth [FDI 25]. The patient is healthy and medically fit.**

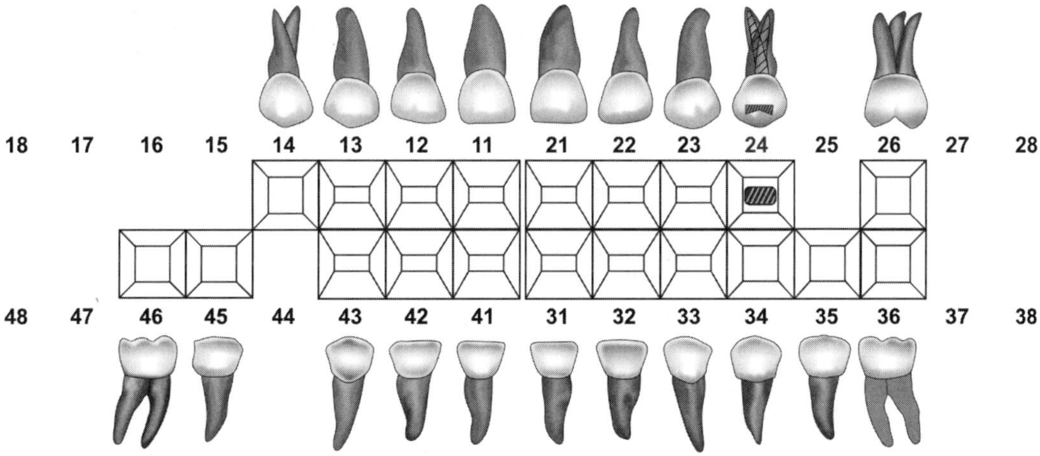

a. List six investigations you would carry out prior to restoring the missing FDI 25. (3 marks)

- OHI
- Mobility test
- Pocket depth
- Sensibility test on FDI 26
- Radiographic examination of the abutments
- Diagnostic casts.

b. What are two treatment options to consider in replacing the missing FDI 25. (2 marks)

- Crown for 24 and upper cast removable partial denture
- Crown for 24 and single unit implant to replace 25
- Three unit conventional bridge.

Cantilever bridge for 24 and 25

2. **20-years-old fit and healthy lady attends your practice complaining of gaps between her upper front teeth. History and examination reveals that there is space between her central incisors and canine on both sides because of her missing upper lateral incisors.**

   Fill in the given table with five treatment options that you may consider for this patient. Give one advantage and one disadvantage for each treatment option. (5 marks)

Table 1: Treatment options with their advantages and disadvantages

Treatment [2.5 marks]	Advantages [1.25 marks]	Disadvantages [1.25 marks]
1. Orthodontic treatment to close the spaces	1. No need for artificial teeth 2. Patient doesn't need any restorative treatment	1. Time period to complete the treatment 2. Reshaping the canine into laterals and color matching
2. Removable partial denture	1. Less treatment time 2. Less expensive 3. Less invasive to tooth structure	1. Not recommended for young patients 2. Compromise the gingival tissues
3. Resin bonded bridges	1. Fixed replacements 2. Minimum tooth preparation 3. Better esthetics	1. May debond 2. Replacement is necessary in long term
4. Conventional bridge	1. Fixed replacements 2. Better esthetics	1. More invasive procedure
5. Implants	1 Good esthetics as it looks like a real tooth 2. Fixed replacements	1. Expensive 2. Requires surgery

PRINCIPLES OF TOOTH PREPARATION

MULTIPLE CHOICE QUESTIONS

1. **Periodontal considerations are important when planning any fixed prosthodontic treatment. For optimum periodontal health, restoration finish lines should be placed:**
   A. Subgingival to not violate the biological width.
   B. Equigingival.
   C. Supragingival.
   D. Subgingival violating the biological width.
   E. Subgingival to gain maximum axial retention.
2. **Over contoured crown is primarily the result of:**
   A. Trying to strengthen the restoration.
   B. Gingival recession.
   C. Faulty impressions.
   D. Insufficient tooth reduction.
   E. Faulty casts.
3. **Retention of a complete crown preparation is increased by:**
   A. Decreasing the area of cement under shear strain.
   B. Decreasing the total preparation surface area.
   C. Decreasing the taper.
   D. Improving surface smoothness.
   E. Decreasing the length of preparation.
4. **What is the significance of bevelling a working cusp for a full veneer crown?**
   A. Enhances resistance to dislodgement by buccolingual forces.
   B. Aids in seating the casting during cementation.
   C. Relieves the stresses when the restoration is loaded by axial forces.
   D. Provides space for addition of metal in the area of heavy occlusal contact.
   E. Enhances resistance to dislodgement by horizontal forces.
5. **Which one of the following statements are correct in relation to extracoronal restoration?**
   A. Retention prevents dislodgment of restoration by force directed in an apical or oblique direction.
   B. The essential element of retention is luting cement.
   C. Crowns are retained in place by wedge retention.

D. Inlay and onlay restorations are retained in place by sleeve retention.
E. The essential element of retention is taper.
Note: Resistance prevents dislodgment by forces directed in an oblique direction
The recommended degree of taper for a molar is more than for a premolar.

6. **Which one of the following statements is correct about principle of tooth preparation?**
   A. A small tooth with short walls provides better retention than a large tooth with short walls.
   B. The recommended degree of taper for premolars is more than the anterior teeth.
   C. The optimum degree of taper for anterior teeth is around 17–24 degrees.
   D. The recommended degree of taper for a molar is less than an anterior tooth.
   E. The optimum degree of taper for a premolar is around 5–10 degrees.

7. **Which one of the following statements is correct with respect to a crown preparation?**
   A. The finish line of the preparation should be always located supragingivally.
   B. The finish line should be always 1mm away from alveolar crest.
   C. The path of insertion should be always parallel to the long axis of the prepared tooth.
   D. Knife edge is the choice of finish line on the lingual surface of lingually tilted lower molars
   E. Knife edge finish line produces maximal destruction on tooth preparation.
   Note: The finish line should be at least 2mm away from the alveolar bone crest.

8. **In which type of restoration preparation should all the angles and sharp edges be rounded and stress bearing areas flattened at right angles to the direction of load?**
   A. All ceramic.
   B. Metal-ceramic.
   C. All metal.
   D. Metal-acrylic.
   E. All acrylic.

ANS: 1C 2D 3C 4D 5E 6B 7D 8A

EXTENDED MATCHING QUESTIONS

1. Theme: Tooth Preparation

A. Functional cusp bevel.
B. Seating groove.
C. Axial reduction.
D. Wing.
E. Gingival bevel.
F. Chamfer.
G. Shoulder.

Using a letter from A to G, choose the most appropriate procedure from the list above that best matches each of the following descriptions numbered 1–5 below. You may use each option once only or not at all.

1. Maintains marginal integrity and periodontal preservation.
2. Provides structural durability.
3. Provides retention, resistance and structural durability.
4. Enhances retention and resistance.
5. Maintains marginal integrity.

Description	Response
1	F
2	A
3	C
4	B
5	E

2. Theme: Finish Lines

A. Chamfer finish line.
B. Flare.
C. Radial shoulder finish line.
D. Knife edge.
E. Deep knife edge.
F. Occlusal shoulder.
G. Chamfer with bevel.

Using a letter from A to G, choose the most appropriate code from the list above that best matches each of the following descriptions numbered 1–5 below. You may use each option once only or not at all.

1. Indicated for lingually tipped lower molars.
2. Indicated for metal restorations without inclinations.
3. Indicated for porcelain restorations.
4. Indicated on the functional cusp of onlay.
5. Indicated on the walls of a proximal box of onlay.

Description	Response
1	D
2	A
3	C
4	F
5	B

SHORT ANSWER QUESTIONS

1. **You are preparing a mandibular molar FDI 36 to receive a full gold crown restoration. What are the possible consequences of the following errors:**

   a. **Occlusal morphology during occlusal reduction is not maintained. (1 mark)**

   Adequate thickness of the material will not be there—heavy contact—leading to perforation

   b. **Excessive axial reduction. (2 marks)**

   - Destructive tooth preparation
   - Lead to pulpal exposure.

   c. **No definitive finish line. (2 marks)**

   The thin casting margin is more susceptible to distortion, leads to microleakage and secondary caries.

Overcontoured restorations—this affects periodontal health.

2. **You are preparing a mandibular molar FDI 36 to receive a full gold crown restoration. What are the possible consequences of the following errors:**

   a. **If the functional cusps are not beveled. [1 marks]**

   - Extremely thin casting leading to deformation of the restoration
   - Overcontoured casting with deflective occlusal contacts
   - If the preparation is tapered to compensate, it will lead to unnecessary destruction of tooth structure and loss of retention.

   b. **Inadequate axial reduction. [2 marks]**

   - Thin restoration leading to deformation of the restoration
   - Overcontoured restoration leading to disastrous effect on periodontium.

3. **You are preparing a mandibular molar FDI 36 to receive a full gold crown restoration.**

   a. **Explain the retention and resistance form in the crown preparation. (2 marks)**

   - Retention prevents removal of the restoration along the path of insertion or long axis of the tooth preparation
   - Resistance prevents dislodgement of the restoration by forces directed in an apical or oblique direction and prevents any movement of the restoration under occlusal forces.

   b. **List any three features that affects the retention and resistance form. (3 marks)**

   - Taper
   - Freedom of displacement
   - Length
   - Substitution of internal features
   - Path of insertion.

4. Which one on the following preparations on lower molar is correct? Discuss why the others are not correct. [3 marks]

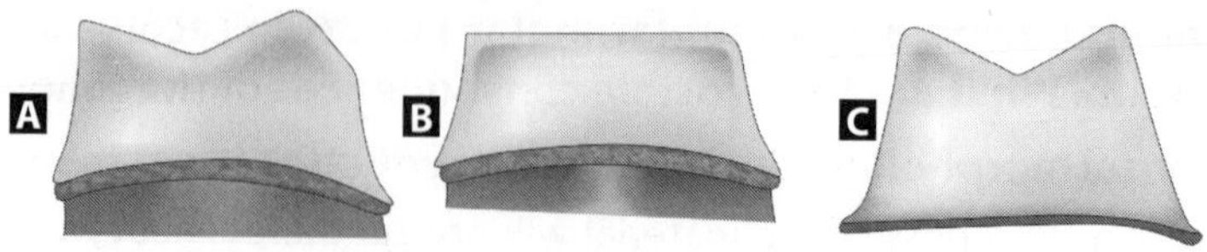

A. Correct—functional cusp bevel—adequate thickness of material.
B. Incorrect—basic inclined plane pattern to be maintained.
C. Incorrect—Functional cusp bevel is not present.

5. Explain how to survey the preparation visually. [3 marks]

Extra oral: One eye—distance of approximately 30 cm [12 inches].

Intra oral: Single crowns—mouth mirror held at an angle approximately ½ inch above the preparation—viewed with one eye.

Bridges: Firm finger rest—centered over one preparation and check for the other abutment preparation by pivoting on the same finger rest.

6. List the five principles that govern the design and execution of a crown/cast restoration. [2.5 marks]

1. Preservation of tooth structure.
2. Retention and resistance.
3. Structural durability.
4. Marginal integrity.
5. Preservation of the peridontium.

7. How retention of a preparation can be increased (at least two methods)? [2 marks]

- Taper —more parallel walls
- Freedom of displacement—reduced
- Preserving the length of the preparation
- Limiting the path of insertion
- Adding internal features.

8. How do you prepare a radial shoulder finish line? [2 marks]

Flat end tapered diamond; rounded internal line angle is done by end-cutting parallel-sided carbide finishing bur, specially modified bin-angle chisel, or radial fissure bur.

FILL IN THE BLANKS

Instructions: Fill up the blanks with appropriate answers.

1. **Fill the blanks.**
   A. Risk of marginal distortion is higher in ______________ finish line.
   B. Risk of overcontouring is higher in ______________ finish line.
   C. The preferred finish line for full ceramic crown preparation is ______________.

2. **Fill the following blanks with the name of the finish line shown on each picture.**

   A. ______________

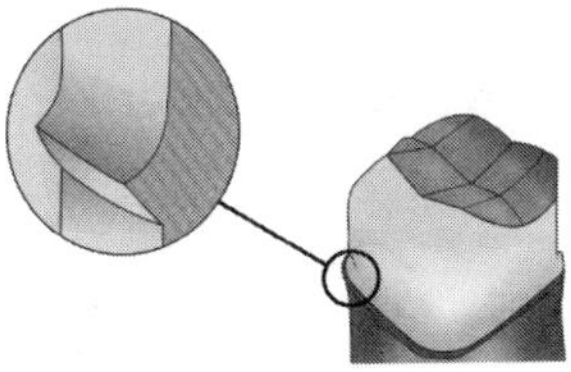

   B. ______________

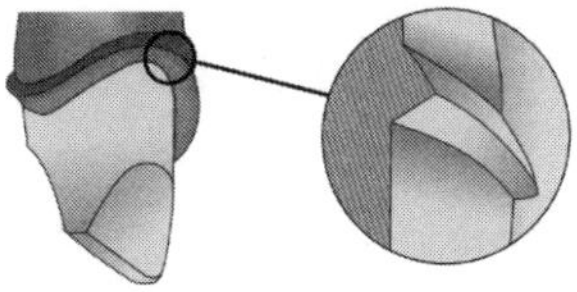

   C. ______________

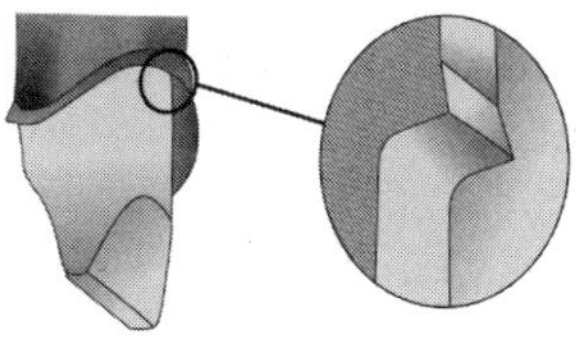

   D. ______________

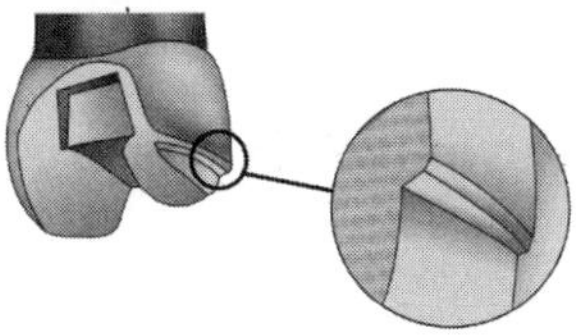

ANS: **1A**. knife edge **1B**. knife edge **1C**. radial shoulder **2A**. Chamfer **2B**. Shoulder **2C**. Radial shoulder **2D**. Shoulder with bevel

FULL COVERAGE RESTORATIONS

MULTIPLE CHOICE QUESTIONS

1. Occlusal clearance in a prepared tooth is best assessed by:

A. Visual examination.
B. Metal gauge.
C. Articulating paper.
D. Wax bite.
E. Bite registration paste.

2. The role of seating groove in a crown preparation is to provide:

A. Resistance and retention form.
B. Structural durability to the crown.
C. Marginal integrity and periodontal preservation.
D. Structural durability to the tooth.
E. Preservation of tooth structure.

3. The preferred finish line for a full-metal gold crown is knife edge:

A. Shoulder.
B. Radial shoulder.
C. Chamfer.
D. Deep chamfer.

4. A full coverage crown restoration has the advantage over a partial veneer restoration because the full crown restoration:

A. Preserves tooth structure.
B. Has more cleansable margins.
C. Allows for better retention.
D. Is associated with less periodontal irritation.
E. Results in fewer pulpal problems.

5. What is the possible consequence of preparation of labial surface of anterior teeth in one plane?

A. Compromising oral hygiene.
B. Compromising occlusion.
C. Compromising esthetics.
D. Compromising speech.
E. Compromising marginal integrity.

Note: Overcontouring of the restoration.
Over reduction of the labial surface.

6. Which one of the following statements about properties of full crown restorations is correct?

A. Most accurate fit: Full metal = metal–ceramic > full ceramic.
B. Most esthetic: Full ceramic = metal–ceramic > full metal.
C. Maximum tooth conservation: Full ceramic > metal–ceramic = full metal.
D. Most brittle: Metal–ceramic > full ceramic > full metal.
E. Better marginal integrity: Full ceramic > metal–ceramic = full metal.

ANS: 1D 2A 3C 4C 5C 6A

EXTENDED MATCHING QUESTIONS

1. **Theme: Crown preparation**

A. Chamfer finish line.
B. Cingulum reduction of anterior tooth.
C. Shoulder finish line.
D. Relieving the proximal contact.
E. Occlusal surface reduction.
F. Shoulder bevel.
G. Occlusal flare.

Using a letter from A to G, choose the most appropriate response from the list above that best matches each of the following descriptions numbered 1–5 below. You may use each response A–G, once only or not at all.

1. Established using a torpedo diamond bur.
2. Established using a flat end tapered diamond bur.
3. Established using a round end tapered diamond bur.
4. Established using a short needle diamond bur.
5. Established using a wheel diamond.

Description	Response
1	A
2	C
3	E
4	D
5	B

2. **Theme : Crown preparation**

A. Marginal integrity.
B. Periodontal preservation and structural durability.
C. Retention, resistance and preservation of tooth structure.
D. Structural durability.
E. Structural durability.
F. Retention, resistance and structural durability.
G. Marginal integrity and periodontal preservation.

The diagram illustrates preparation for posterior porcelain fused to metal crown. Match the name of the features with their function and location on the diagram.

1. Chamfer.
2. Functional cusp bevel.
3. Wing.

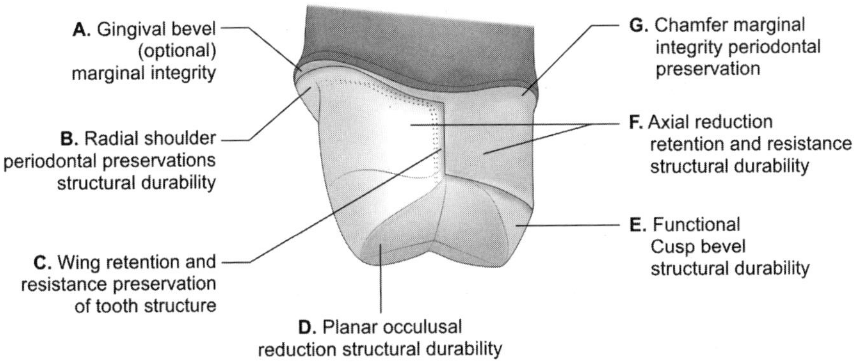

4. Radial shoulder.
5. Axial reduction.

Description	Response
1	G
2	E
3	C
4	B
5	F

3. Theme : Crown preparation

A. Periodontal preservation and structural durability.
B. Retention, resistance and preservation of tooth structure.
C. Structural durability.
D. Structural durability.
E. Structural durability.
F. Retention, resistance and structural durability.
G. Marginal integrity and periodontal preservation.

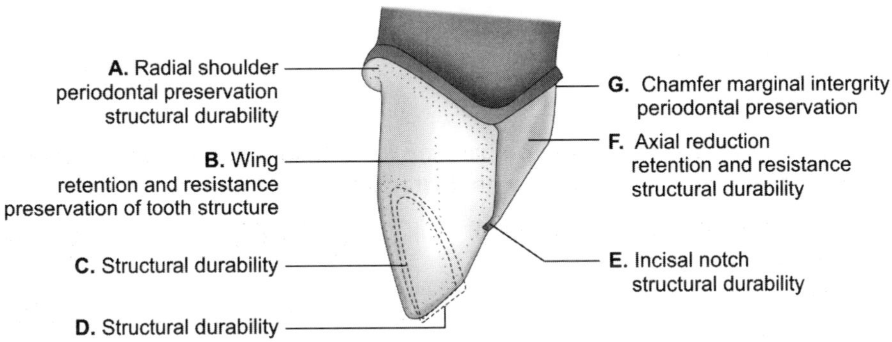

The above diagram illustrates preparation for anterior porcelain fused to metal crown. Match the name of the features with their function and location on the diagram.

1. Chamfer.
2. Incisal notch.
3. Wing.
4. Radial shoulder.
5. Axial reduction.

Description	Response
1	G
2	E
3	B
4	A
5	F

4. Theme : Crown preparation

A. Marginal integrity, structural durability, periodontal preservation and resistance
B. Retention, resistance and structural durability.
C. Structural durability.
D. Structural durability.
E. Structural durability.
F. Retention and resistance.

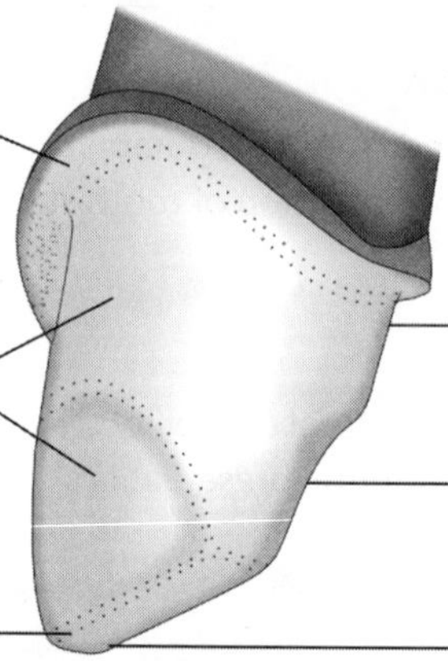

The above diagram illustrates preparation for anterior full porcelain (all ceramic) crown. Match the name of the features with their function and location on the diagram

1. Radial shoulder (round shoulder).
2. Axial reduction.
3. Incisal reduction.
4. Cingulum reduction.
5. Vertical lingual reduction.

Description	Response
1	A
2	B
3	D
4	E
5	F

SHORT ANSWER QUESTIONS

1. **Explain type of occlusal, buccal and lingual preparation for porcelain-fused-to-metal (with metal backing) crown preparation on posterior teeth mentioning depth of the preparation, type of finishing line and type of bur required for each part:**

   A. Occlusal: 2 mm reduction on functional cusp (1.5 mm + 0.5 occlusal bevel) and 1.5 non-functional cusps using round end tapered bur.

   B. Buccal reduction: 1.2–1.4 mm axial reduction with radial shoulder finishing line using flat and tapered bur followed by modified chisel.

   C. Lingual reduction: 0.7 mm axial reduction with chamfer using torpedo bur.

2. **What type of finish line is most suitable for full-ceramic crown and why?**

   Radial shoulder (round shoulder).

3. **Where the finishing line ideally should be prepared on a posterior tooth in relation to the gingival margin?**

   1 mm above the gingival margin. Because it is more hygienic (it is in self-cleaning area and will not retain plaque close to gingival margin).

4. **What are the possible consequences of preparing labial surface of central incisor in one plane (at least two points)? [2 marks]**

   - Extension of gingival plane: Bad shade match, over contoured
   - Extension of incisal plane: Over tapered and may encroach the pulp.

FILL IN THE BLANKS

Instructions: Fill up the blanks with appropriate answers.

1. **On the following schematic picture fill the blanks using the given options. [4 marks]**

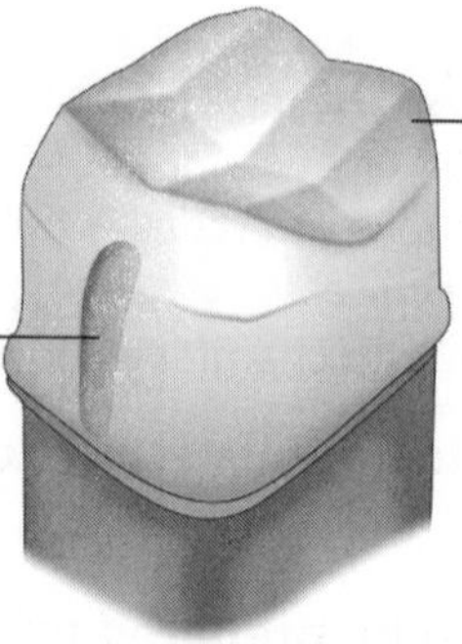

1.1. Which type of crown is this tooth prepared for: (refer to the picture)

A. Full ceramic.
B. Full metal–ceramic.
C. Full metal.
D. Partial metal.
E. Partial metal ceramic.

1.2. The type of finish line is __________ which is prepared by __________ bur.

A. Chamfer, round end tapered.
B. Shoulder, torpedo.
C. Radial shoulder, flat end tapered.
D. Chamfer, torpedo.
E. Radial shoulder, radial fissure.

1.3. The role of seating groove in crown preparation is to provide __________

A. Resistance and retention.
B. Structural durability.
C. Marginal integrity and periodontal preservation.
D. Strength.
E. Preservation of tooth structure.

2. **On the following schematic picture fill the blanks using the given options: [3 marks]**

2.1. Identify the type of labial finish line on the diagram below:

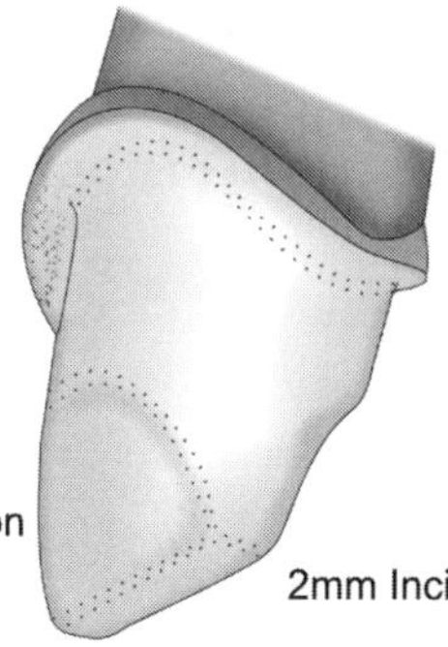

A. Chamfer.
B. Round edge.
C. Shoulder.
D. Deep chamfer.
E. Knife edge.

2.2. The above preparation is made for ____________ crown.

A. Full ceramic.
B. Full metal-ceramic.
C. Full metal.
D. Partial metal.
E. Partial metal ceramic.

2.3. The type of finish line is __________ which is prepared by __________ bur.

A. Chamfer, round end tapered.
B. Shoulder, torpedo and radial fissure.
C. Radial shoulder, flat end tapered and radial fissure.
D. Chamfer, torpedo.
E. Knife edge, long needle.

ANS: 1.1C 1.2D 1.3A 2.1C 2.2A 2.3C

PARTIAL COVERAGE RESTORATIONS

MULTIPLE CHOICE QUESTIONS

1. What are the advantages of using full crown restorations over partial veneer restorations?

A. Preserving tooth structure.
B. Easy cleaning of margins by patient.
C. Providing better retention.
D. Less periodontal irritation.
E. Less pulpal problems.

Note: Providing better resistance form also.

2. The proximal half crown.

A. Is indicated in a 60 degree rotated tooth.
B. Has the facial surface of the tooth left intact.
C. Is indicated in patients with good oral hygiene.
D. Is indicated in severely lingually inclined teeth.
E. Is indicated in a defective distal surface.

3. The mandibular reverse three-quarter crown.

A. Is indicated in severe labially inclined teeth.
B. Is indicated in 90 degree rotated teeth.
C. Tooth preparation includes an occlusal shoulder.
D. Has grooves that are placed at linguoproximal line angles.
E. Tooth preparation is extended to the non-functional cusps.

4. The seven-eighths crown.

A. Is indicated in a severely labially inclined tooth.
B. Is indicated in a 90 degree rotated tooth.
C. Is indicated in a tooth which needs the distofacial cusp to be covered.
D. Tooth preparation includes an occlusal shoulder.
E. Tooth preparation has poor resistance and retention form.

5. The most common cause of failure in resin bonded bridge is:

A. Inadequate taper.
B. Loss of retention.
C. Failure of connector.
D. Perforation.
E. Occlusal wear.

6. Which one of the following indirect restoration is less invasive?

A. Full metal crown.
B. Porcelain-fused-to-metal crown.
C. Resin-bonded bridge.
D. Full porcelain crown.
E. Three quarter metal crown.

7. A resin-bonded bridge is best suited to replace a:

A. Missing mandibular incisor.
B. Missing mandibular canine.
C. Missing mandibular 1st and 2nd premolar.
D. Missing maxillary canine.
E. Missing maxillary 1st and 2nd premolar.

8. The type of finish line for a resin-bonded bridge is:

A. Knife edge.
B. Shoulder.
C. Radial shoulder.
D. Chamfer.
E. Deep chamfer.

9. The placement of proximal groove will be on the ______ for a resin-bonded bridge:

A. Facioproximal line angle.
B. Lingual proximal line angle.
C. Mesioproximal line angle.
D. Distoproximal line angle.
E. Faciolingual line angle.

ANS: 1C 2C 3D 4C 5B 6C 7A 8D 9A

SHORT ANSWER QUESTIONS

1. **In the following picture, four different forms of proximal groove on 3/4 crown preparation are shown. Identify which groove preparation is correct and why? [3 marks]**

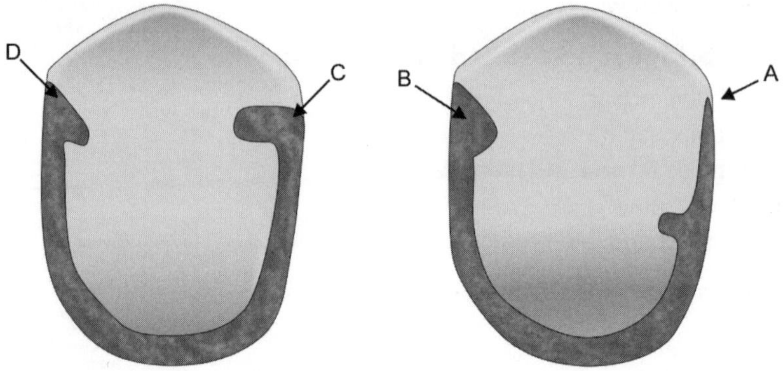

D is correct

Because of definite lingual wall which resist displacement.

2. **From the following picture answer the questions. [6 marks]**

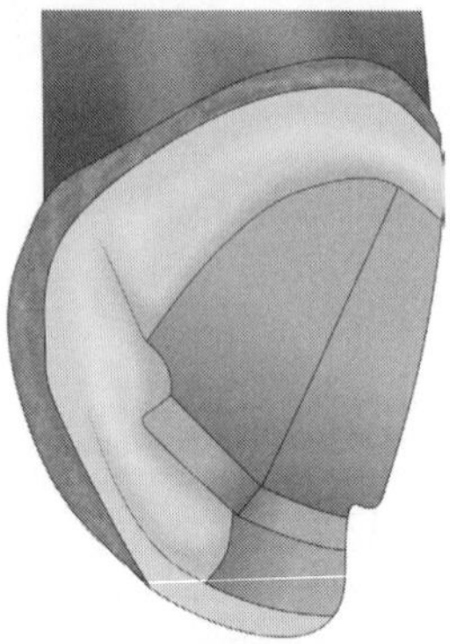

What is this type of preparation on upper canine called?

Three quarter restoration.

How should the axial surface and proximal grooves be related to the facial surface to improve retention and resistance form?

To improve on retention the axial surface and proximal grooves should be parallel to Incisal one-half to two thirds of the facial surface of the tooth.

What will happen if proximal grooves incline labially?

Retention and resistance is compromised.

What is the depth of lingual reduction? And what is the suitable bur to prepare this?

0.7 mm, small wheel diamond.

FILL IN THE BLANKS

1. On the following schematic picture of maxillary three-quarter crown preparation on premolar teeth state the function or name of each feature where indicated. [8 marks]

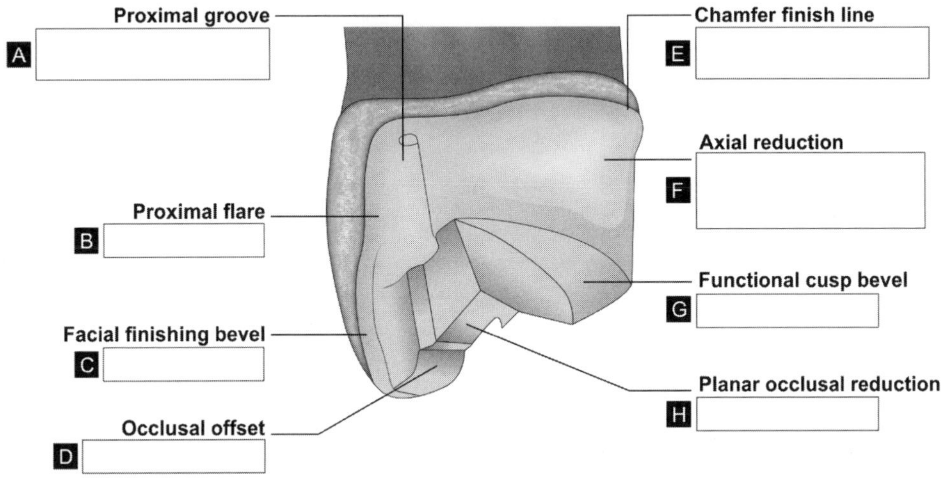

2. On the following schematic picture of maxillary three-quarter crown preparation on canine teeth state the function or name of each feature where indicated. [7 marks]

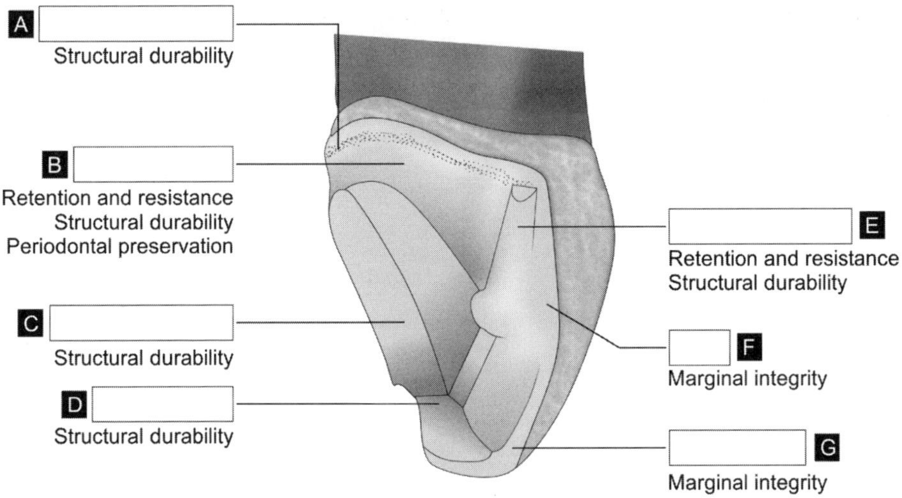

3. On the following schematic picture of mandibular three-quarter crown preparation on molar teeth state the function or name of each feature were indicated. [8 marks]

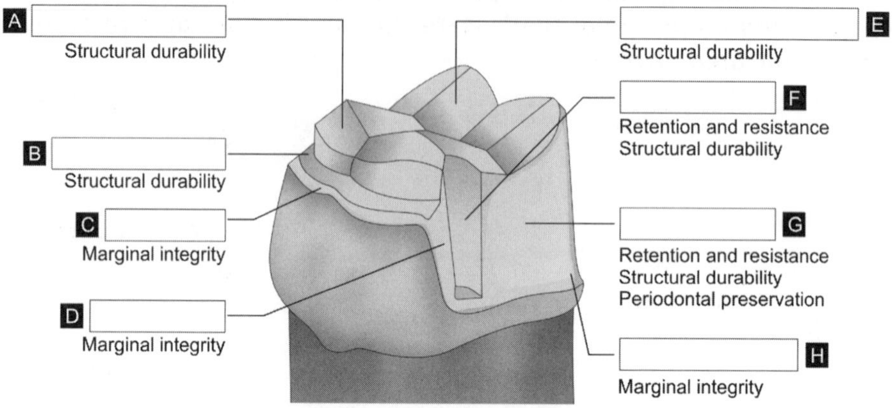

ANS:
1A. Retention and resistance, structural durability
1B. Marginal integrity
1C. Marginal integrity
1D. Structural durability
1E. Marginal integrity. Periodontal preservation
1F. Retention and resistance, structural durability, periodontal preservation
1G. Structural durability
1H. Structural durability
2A. Chamfer finish line
2B. Axial reduction
2C. Lingual reduction
2D. Incisal offset
2E. Proximal groove
2F. Flare
2G. Incisal bevel
3A. Function cusp bevel
3B. Occlusal shoulder
3C. Facial bevel
3D. Proximal flare
3E. Planar occlusal reduction
3F. Proximal groove
3G. Axial reduction
3H. Chamfer finish line

INTRACORONAL RESTORATIONS

MULTIPLE CHOICE QUESTIONS

1. **Which one of the following statements about the porcelain inlay restoration is correct:**
   A. It has poor esthetics.
   B. It is highly wear-resistant.
   C. It creates postoperative sensitivity.
   D. It undergoes polymerization shrinkage.
   E. It does not require cementation.

2. **Which one of the following statements is correct about an indirect onlay restorations:**
   A. It is indicated in root canal treated teeth with intact buccal and lingual cusps.
   B. The onlay preparation is more conservative than an inlay preparation.
   C. It is used as a retainer for long-span bridges.
   D. The retention mechanism is a "sleeve".
   E. Internal buccal and lingual walls should be convergent.
   Note: It is also indicated in a mesio-occluso-distal cavity with wide isthmus.

3. **Which following statements are correct about inlay preparation:**
   A. The width of Isthmus should be buccolingually about 1/2 of B-L width.
   B. Occlusal contact should be included in the outline.
   C. Bevel on gingival margins should be narrower and more acute than occlusal margins.
   D. Onlay restoration is recommended over MOD inlay on premolar.

ANS: 1B 2A 3D

EXTENDED MATCHING QUESTIONS

1. Theme : Tooth preparation

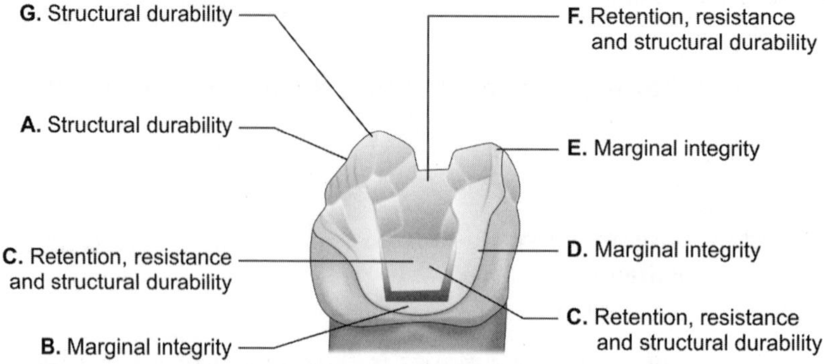

The above diagram illustrates preparation for a posterior metal only. Match the name of the features with their function and location on the diagram.

1. Gingival bevel.
2. Lingual flare.
3. Isthmus.
4. Occlusal shoulder.
5. Proximal box.

Description	Response
1	B
2	D
3	F
4	A
5	C

SHORT ANSWER QUESTIONS

4. **Name the type of retention provided by indirect metal inlay restorations.**

   Wedge retention.

5. **What is the role of dove tail in class II metal inlay preparation? And how much is its depth?**

   Horizontal retention and resistance to avoid horizontal dislodgment of the restoration, 1.5 mm.

6. **How much is the maximum width of isthmus?**

   About ¼ of buccolingual width of the tooth.

7. **In class II metal inlay what preparations should be carried out on the buccal, lingual and gingival margins?**

   Flare on buccal and lingual walls.
   Bevel on gingival wall (30–45°).

FILL IN THE BLANKS

Instructions: Fill up the blanks with appropriate answers.

1. **Fill the blanks: [3 marks]**
   A. In onlay preparation the function of occlusal shoulder is to provide________________.
   B. In onlay preparation the function of proximal box is to provide______________________.
   C. In onlay preparation the function of isthmus is to provide________________________.

ANS: **1A.** structural durability **1B.** retention and resistance, structural durability
1C. retention and resistance, structural durability

PROVISIONAL RESTORATION

MULTIPLE CHOICE QUESTIONS

1. **The percentage of shrinkage undergone by poly (methyl methacrylate) when it polymerizes is:**
   A. 8%.
   B. 12%.
   C. 15%.
   D. 20%.
   E. 2%.

2. **What type of provisional restoration is given for the patient after a small intracoronal inlay preparation?**
   A. Zinc oxide eugenol cement.
   B. Zinc phosphate cement.
   C. Calcium hydroxide cement.
   D. Glass ionomer cement.
   E. Composite restoration.

3. **One of the advantages of the direct technique of making a provisional restoration is:**
   A. Protection of the pulp.
   B. Reduction in polymerization shrinkage.
   C. Reduction in laboratory time.
   D. Providing a better marginal fit.
   E. Providing better esthetics.

4. **The external surface form in a provisional restoration:**
   A. Can be customized.
   B. Only preformed.
   C. Replicates the prepared tooth surface.
   D. Replicates the edentulous ridge.

ANS: 1A 2A 3C 4A

EXTENDED MATCHING QUESTIONS

1. Theme: Provisional restoration

A. Aluminium shell crown.
B. Cellulose acetate crown.
C. Preformed base-metal crown.
D. Cast metal restoration.
E. Polymethyl methacrylate crown.
F. Polycarbonate crown.
G. Polyvinyl ethyl methacrylate crown.

Using a letter from A to G, choose the most appropriate material from the list above that best matches each of the following descriptions numbered 1–5 below. You may use each option once only or not at all.

1. Customized provisional crown with poor color stability.
2. Customized provisional crown used as treatment restorations.
3. Preformed clear shell used to make direct provisional crowns.
4. Provisional preformed crowns used for posteriors in case of trauma.
5. Provisional crown which has significant presence of free monomer.

Description	Response
1	G
2	D
3	B
4	C
5	E

2. Theme: Provisional restoration

A. Alginate.
B. Zinc oxide eugenol.
C. Impression compound.
D. Polymethyl methacrylate.
E. Polycarbonate.
F. Type I plaster.
G. Type II plaster.

Using a letter from A to G, choose the most appropriate material from the list above that best matches each of the following descriptions numbered 1–5 below. You may use each option once only or not at all.

1. An impression material used to make dentate working models.
2. Material used to make indirect provisional crown.
3. Preformed shell used to make direct provisional crowns.

4. Material used to cement the provisional crown.
5. Material used to make the diagnostic models.

Description	Response
1	A
2	D
3	E
4	B
5	G

SHORT ANSWER QUESTIONS

1. **a. List two reasons as to why an indirect technique of fabricating a provisional restoration is preferred over a direct technique. (2 Marks)**
   - Accuracy
   - Avoid locking in undercuts
   - Protection to pulp
   - Improved fit or reduction in shrinkage
   - Improved marginal fit
   - Less clinical time [or more lab work].

   b. List any four requirements for a provisional restoration. (2 Marks)
   - Pulpal protection
   - Protects the remaining tooth structure
   - Positional stability
   - Occlusal function
   - Easily cleaned
   - Nonimpinging margins
   - Strength and retention
   - Esthetics.

   c. Name two different types of resin materials that can be used for fabricating custom provisional restorations. (1 Mark)
   - Poly (methyl methacrylate)
   - Poly (ethyl methacrylate)
   - Poly (vinyl ethyl methacrylate)
   - Bis-acryl composite resin
   - Visible light-cured (VLC) urethane dimethacrylate
   - Epimine resin.

2. **List the three techniques for fabricating an interim restoration.**
   - Indirect technique
   - Direct technique
   - Indirect–direct technique.

3. **Name the techniques for making a mold to form the outer surface of a custom provisional restoration that provides the appearance of a tooth where needed. [2 Marks]**
   - Overimpression
   - Template
   - Shell crown.

4. **When you think an overimpression is not possible to make intraorally? What is the procedure of making an overimpression in that case? [2 Marks]**

   Tooth with any defects— diagnostic cast—filled with utility wax— overimpression.

FILL IN THE BLANKS

Instructions: Fill up the blanks with appropriate answers.

1. Placing the poly (methyl methacryylate) provisional restoration in a pressure pot under 20 Psi for polymerization decreases ___________ and increases the ___________ .
2. The indirect technique of making a provisional restoration is preferred over the direct technique for its ___________.
3. ___________ is used to remove the excess cement from the interproximal region after crown cementation.

ANS: 1: porosity, transverse strength 2. accuracy 3. dental floss

FLUID CONTROL

MULTIPLE CHOICE QUESTIONS

1. **Which is the best fluid control technique when the lone dentist does a filling in the 14?**
   A. Saliva ejector.
   B. Svedopter.
   C. Rubber dam.
   D. High-volume vaccum.
2. **Which is the best fluid control technique when the lone dentist does a filling in the 41?**
   A. Saliva ejector.
   B. Svedopter.
   C. Rubber dam.
   D. High-volume vaccum.
3. **Which is the best fluid control technique when the dentist does an elastomeric impression of the maxillary arch?**
   A. Saliva ejector.
   B. Svedopter.
   C. Rubber dam.
   D. High-volume vaccum.
4. **Which is the best fluid control technique when the dentist does an elastomeric impression of the mandibular arch?**
   A. Saliva ejector.
   B. Svedopter.
   C. Rubber dam.
   D. High-volume vaccum.
5. **The most appropriate fluid control aid when taking an elastomeric impression of the maxillary arch is:**
   A. A saliva ejector.
   B. Cotton rolls.
   C. A tongue deflector.
   D. High-volume evacuator.
   E. Anti-sialagogues.

6. Name the antisialagogue which is an antihypertensive agent.

A. Banthine.
B. Propantheline bromide.
C. Clonidine hydrochloride.

7. To prevent lateral penetration of heat into the tissues with subsequent injury, the electrode should move at a speed of no less than __________ and if it is necessary to retrace the path of a previous cut, __________ should be allowed to elapse before repeating the stroke.

A. 7 mm per second/8–10 seconds.
B. 17 mm per second/18–20 seconds.
C. 20 mm per second/28–30 seconds.
D. 30 mm per second/38–40 seconds.

8. The most appropriate method for removing a limited amount of epithelial tissue to expose and record the finish line after crown preparation is:

A. Electrosurgery.
B. Rubber dam.
C. Antisialagogues.
D. Cotton rolls.
E. Rotary curettage.

9. The most appropriate method for removing inflamed tissue that has proliferated over the crown margin line is:

A. Electrosurgery.
B. Rubber dam.
C. Antisialagogues.
D. Copper band.
E. Rotary curettage.

10. Most effective isolation aid in fluid control [displaces gingiva by compression only].

A. Electrosurgery.
B. Rubber dam.
C. Antisialagogues.
D. Cotton rolls.
E. Rotary curettage.

11. Effectively carries the impression material and displaces the gingiva.

A. Electrosurgery.
B. Rubber dam.
C. Antisialagogues.

D. Copper bands.
E. Rotary curettage.

12. Which one of the following achieves gingival displacement by combining chemical and mechanical methods?

A. Electrosurgery.
B. Rubber dam.
C. Retraction cords.
D. Copper bands.
E. Rotary curettage.

13. The purpose of retracting the gingiva before making an impression is:

A. Improving the esthetics of final restoration.
B. Exposing the finish line only.
C. Recording the unprepared tooth surface below the finish line.
D. Recording the gingival margin below the finish line.
E. Protecting the soft tissue only.

ANS: 1A 2B 3A 4B 5A 6C 7A 8E 9A 10B 11D 12C 13C

EXTENDED MATCHING QUESTIONS

1. Theme: Fluid control and soft tissue management

A. Electrosurgery.
B. Copper bands.
C. Retraction cord.
D. Rubber dam.
E. Antisialagogues.
F. Cotton rolls.
G. Rotary curettage.

Using a letter from A to G, choose the most appropriate fluid control and soft tissue management aid from the list above that best matches each of the following descriptions numbered 1–5 below. You may use each option once only or not at all.

1. Limited removal of epithelial tissue in the sulcus to expose the finish line.
2. Removal of irritated proliferated tissue over the finish line.
3. Displaces gingiva only by compression.
4. Effectively carries the impression material and displaces the gingiva.
5. Displaces gingiva by combining chemical and pressure packing.

Description	Response
1	G
2	A
3	D
4	B
5	C

SHORT ANSWER QUESTIONS

1. **With regards to the gingival tissue management following tooth preparation:**

a. List three mechanical means of finish line exposure before taking the final impression. (1.5 marks)

- Copper band
- Rubber dam
- Plain cotton cord.

b. List three antisialagogues used in fluid control. (1.5 marks)

- Methantheline bromide (Banthine)
- Propantheline bromide (Pro-Banthine)
- Clonidine hydrochloride.

Note: Action—Gastrointestinal anticholinergics that act on the smooth muscle of the gastrointestinal, urinary and biliary tracts producing dry mouth as side effect.

c. What are the four signs of "epinephrine syndrome"? (2 marks)

- Tachycardia
- Rapid respiration
- Elevated blood pressure
- Anxiety, and postoperative depression.

2. **In relation to the gingival tissue management after tooth preparation**

a. What are the three factors which determine the suitability of gingiva for the use of rotary curettage?

- Absence of bleeding upon probing
- Sulcus depth less than 3.0 mm
- Presence of adequate keratinized gingival.

b. Name the four forms of currents used in electrosurgery and its tissue response.

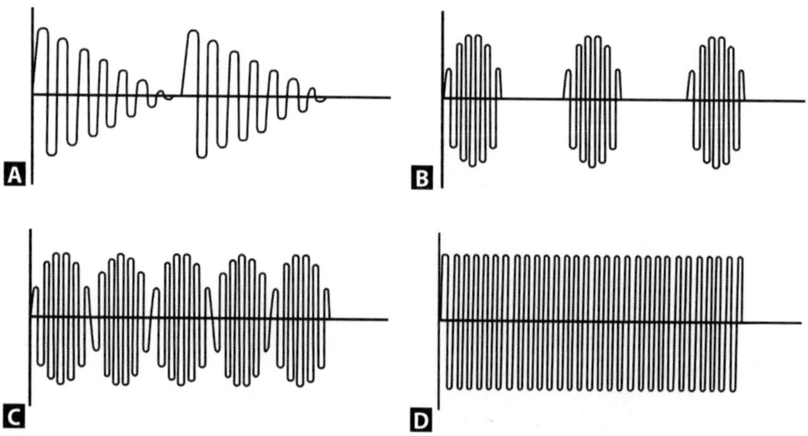

Four forms of electrosurgery current:

A. Unrectified, damped.
B. Partially rectified, damped (half-wave modulated).
C. Fully rectified (full-wave modulated).
D. Fully rectified, filtered (filtered).

3. Name the various methods used in fluid control. [2 marks]

- Rubber dam
- High-volume vaccum
- Saliva ejector
- Svedopter
- Antisialagogues.

4. What are the three factors which determine the suitability of gingiva for the use of rotary curettage? [2 marks]

- Absence of bleeding upon probing
- Sulcus depth less than 3.0 mm
- Presence of adequate keratinized gingival.

5. What are the disadvantages of Svedopter? [2 marks]

- Difficult access to lingual surface
- Bruising the floor of mouth
- Interference—presence of mandibular tori
- Provoke gag reflex.

6. What are the different methods of finish line exposure? [2 marks]

- Mechanical
- Chemicomechanical and surgical
- Rotary curettage and electrosurgery.

7. State the three criterias for a gingival retraction material. [2 marks]

- Effectiveness in gingival displacement and hemostasis
- Absence of irreversible damage to the gingiva
- Paucity of untoward systemic effects.

8. Name the electrodes. [5 marks]

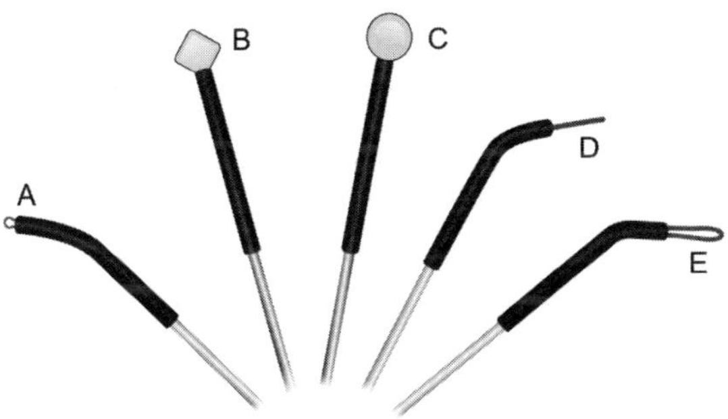

A. Coagulating.
B. Diamond loop.
C. Round loop.
D. Small straight.
E. Small loop.

FILL IN THE BLANKS

Instructions: Fill up the blanks with appropriate answers.

1. ______________ the most effective of all isolation devices utilized in dentistry.
2. Rubber dam should not be used with ______________ impression material.
3. Cord impregnated with ______________ is the most commonly used means of producing gingival retraction in chemicomechanical method.
4. Electrosurgery is contraindicated in patients with ______________.

ANS: **1.** Rubber dam **2.** polyvinyl siloxane **3.** 8% racemic epinephrine **4.** cardiac pacemakers

IMPRESSIONS

MULTIPLE CHOICE QUESTIONS

1. **Dimensional stability of an impression material depends on all the following factors except ______________.**
   A. By-product of setting reaction.
   B. Mixing technique.
   C. Storage condition.
   D. Continuity of setting reaction.
   E. Time length of storage.

2. **If you leave a condensation-cured silicone impression material at room temperature for 2 days without any coverage, what kind of error will occur?**
   A. Only the stone model becomes bigger.
   B. Only the restoration becomes bigger.
   C. The stone model and the restoration may become bigger and distorted.
   D. No changes will happen.
   E. The stone model becomes smaller, but the restoration becomes bigger.

3. **Which one of the following impression materials can record only the muco-compressive form of the tissue?**
   A. Zinc oxide eugenol.
   B. Impression plaster.
   C. Light body silicone impression materials.
   D. Impression compound.
   E. Alginate.

4. **Which one of the following impression materials should not be used with latex gloves and rubber dam?**
   A. Addition-cured silicone.
   B. Polysulphide.
   C. Polyether.
   D. Condensation-cured silicone.
   E. Zinc oxide eugenol.

5. **Which one of the following physical properties can be expected in an impression material without any setting by-products?**
   A. A higher degree of detail is recorded.
   B. Better handling characteristics.
   C. Hydrophobic behavior.

D. Better dimensional stability.
E. Better taste and odor.

6. Which one of the following impression materials is not suitable as a final impression material for tooth preparations?

A. Polyether.
B. Addition-cure silicone.
C. Condensation-cure silicone.
D. Polysulphide.
E. Alginate.

7. Which is the preferred order (from left to right) for disinfecting an impression?

A. Rinse, spray with disinfectant, pack and send it to the lab.
B. Rinse, immerse in disinfectant, pack and send it to the lab.
C. Rinse, immerse in disinfectant, rinse, pack and send it to the lab.
D. Spray with disinfectant, rinse, pack and send it to the lab.
E. Immerse in disinfectant, rinse, pack and send it to the lab.

8. What is the setting time of polysulfide rubber base?

A. 12–14 min.
B. 5 min.
C. 7–8 min.
D. 10 min.
E. 20 min.

9. Choose the material which has poor finish line readability.

A. Polysulfide rubber base.
B. Polyether rubber base.
C. Polyvinyl siloxane.
D. Reversible hydrocolloid.
E. Polymethyl siloxane.

10. Which is the radiopaque material?

A. Polysulfide rubber base.
B. Polyether rubber base.
C. Polyvinyl siloxane.
D. Reversible hydrocolloid.
E. Polymethyl siloxane.

11. Which one of the following materials has the poorest moisture tolerance?

A. Polysulfide rubber base.
B. Polyether rubber base.
C. Polyvinyl siloxane.
D. Reversible hydrocolloid.
E. Impression compound.

12. Choose the material which has poor odor/taste.

A. Polyether rubber base.
B. Polyvinyl siloxane.
C. Reversible hydrocolloid.
D. Polymethyl siloxane.
E. Polysulfide rubber base.

13. To achieve maximum adhesion of the impression material to the tray, allow the tray adhesive to dry for a minimum of ________________.

A. 15 minutes.
B. 15 seconds.
C. 15 hours.
D. 10 minutes.
E. 10 seconds.

14. Arrange these impression materials in their hydrophobic ascending order.

A. Polysulfide, polyvinyl siloxanes and condensation reaction silicones.
B. Polyvinyl siloxanes, polysulfide and condensation reaction silicones.
C. Polysulfide, condensation reaction silicones and polyvinyl siloxanes.

ANS: 1B 2C 3D 4A 5D 6E 7C 8A 9D 10A 11C 12A 13A 14A

EXTENDED MATCHING QUESTIONS

1. Theme: Impression Materials

A. Polysulfide.
B. Condensation-cured silicon.
C. Addition-cured silicon.
D. Polyether.
E. Compound.
F. Alginate.
G. Agar.

Using a letter from A to G, choose the most appropriate impression material from the list above that best matches each of the following descriptions numbered 1–5 below. You may use each response A–G, once only or not at all.

1. A radiopaque elastomeric impression material with the highest viscoelastic behavior.
2. The impression material of choice when there is poor moisture control.
3. The impression material with the highest dimensional stability.
4. A thermoplastic impression material.
5. An impression using a material that can be kept only for 2 hours in a humid environment before preparing the model.

Description	Response
1	A
2	D
3	C
4	E
5	F

SHORT ANSWER QUESTIONS

1. **a. List four varieties of addition-cure silicone impression materials based on their consistency. (2 marks)**

   Light body, medium body, heavy body and putty.

   b. Which one of the above mentioned types has the highest filler content? What are its advantages and disadvantages compared to others? (One point each) (3 marks)

   - Putty.
   - Low polymerization shrinkage, low coefficient of thermal expansion.
   - Less detailed record, less accuracy.

2. **What is the function of these modifiers in agar composition? [4 marks]**

   - Sodium tetraborate increases the strength of the gel and viscosity of the gel
   - Borax retarder
   - Potassium sulfate counteracts borax; increases rupture strength, and improve plastic deformation
   - Thymol—Bactericidal.

3. **a. You are about to make final impression and send it to a dental lab to produce a cast partial denture. The impression is expected to reach the lab after three days. There are relatively deep hard and soft tissue undercuts. Which impression material will you use? Why? (2 marks)**

   A. Addition-silicon impression material.

   B. Good dimensional stability.

   b. What kind of error may occur when impression is debonded from the tray? How this can be prevented? (2 marks)

   The impression will be distorted.

   It can be prevented by using perforated tray or using tray adhesive.

   c. Explain one technique to minimise the distortion of impression when removing from patient mouth. (1 mark)

   Fast removing (sharp tug) of the impression from mouth.

FILL IN THE BLANKS [16 MARKS]

Instructions: Fill up the blanks with appropriate answers.

1. Impression materials can be classified as readily wettable by gypsum ___________ and resistant to wetting ___________.
2. The use of a ___________ is effective in reducing both the contact angle and the number of voids trapped in the resulting cast.
3. A material that exhibits this property of becoming more fluid when the shear rate is increased by deforming or "disturbing" it (shaking, spatulating, or injecting through a syringe) is described as ___________.
4. The mechanisms by which the hydrocolloids can lose water by ___________ or by ___________.
5. The mechanism by which the hydrocolloids can absorb water ___________.
6. The dimensions for the tissue stops in a customized tray is ___________.

ANS: **1.** hydrophilic, hydrophobic **2.** surfactant on impression surface **3.** thixotropic **4.** syneresis [water seeping from the surface], evaporation **5.** imbibition **6.** 3 × 3 mm

WORKING CAST AND DIES

MULTIPLE CHOICE QUESTIONS

1. **The disadvantage of using a working cast with a separated die is:**
   A. Poor finishing line.
   B. Distortion of the wax pattern.
   C. Over extension of the finishing line.
   D. Poor esthetics.
   E. Weak restoration.

2. **Pindex machine in pindex system of preparing working cast and die is used for:**
   A. Locating and paralleling the pin holes.
   B. Inserting the pins in the pin holes.
   C. Gluing the pins in the pin holes.
   D. Ditching (trimming) below the finishing line.
   E. Splitting the die.

3. **The thickness of the relief agent for coating over a die is:**
   A. 20–40 mm.
   B. 60–80 mm.
   C. 0–10 cm.
   D. 20–40 µm.
   E. 60–80 µm.

4. **When a working cast with a removable die is used to prepare a wax pattern, the risk of which one of following errors is highest:**
   A. Distortion of the wax pattern.
   B. Discrepancy between the die and working cast.
   C. Discrepancy in thickness of the die spacer and working cast.
   D. Improper reseating of the die on the working cast.
   E. Over extension of the finishing line.

5. **During the die preparation the finish line should not be highlighted with a sharp colorbrite ________________ pencil.**
   A. Red.
   B. Black.
   C. Blue.
   D. Green.

6. When a cut was made on the mesial and distal side of each die, the cuts should taper towards each other slightly from:

A. Occlusal to gingival.
B. Mesial to distal.
C. Gingival to occlusal.
D. Distal to mesial.

7. What is the recommended thickness of the working cast to have a adequate handle on the die?

A. 1 inch.
B. 1 feet.
C. 1 centimeter.

ANS: 1B 2A 3D 4D 5B 6A 7A

SHORT ANSWER QUESTIONS

1. **Explain the basic difference between working cast with separated die and with a removable die.**

   Working cast with separated die: Preparing a segmental cast (die) and a full arch cast separately in a two pour technique.

   Working cast with removable die: Preparing a full arch cast in a single pour and separating each individual abutment tooth (die) on that cast.

2. **Why working die should be trimmed under finishing line?**

   To gain access for carving the wax on the finishing line.

3. **List different techniques of working cast with a removable die (two techniques).**

   - Straight dowel pin
   - Curved dowel pin
   - Pindex system
   - Di-lok tray.

CEMENTATION

MULTIPLE CHOICE QUESTIONS

1. **The internal configuration in an extracoronal restoration allows:**
   A. The restoration to seat completely without binding.
   B. Intimate contact of the restoration with the distal wall of the tooth.
   C. Intimate contact of the restoration with the occlusal surface of the tooth.
   D. An internal surface that is conducive to a weaker cement bond.
   E. Intimate contact of the restoration with the mesial wall of the tooth.
2. **The microcrystalline surface layer formed by the abraded surface material, filling into the surface irregularities is known as:**
   A. Beilby layer.
   B. Abraded layer.
   C. Filled layer.
   D. Surface layer.
   E. Lailby layer.
3. **In terms of bond strength, which one of the following luting cements should be the material of choice to cement an all-ceramic crown?**
   A. Zinc polycarboxylate cement.
   B. Glass ionomer cement.
   C. Zinc phosphate cement.
   D. Zinc oxide eugenol cement.
   E. Resin cement.
4. **Which step you will not evaluate before you cement a fixed restoration in the patient's mouth.**
   A. Proximal contacts.
   B. Internal fit.
   C. Margins.
   D. Stability.
   E. Taper.
5. **Which one is not called a defective margin in a fixed restoration?**
   A. Overextended margins.
   B. Underextended margins.
   C. Thick margins.
   D. Open margins.
   E. Closed margins.

6. What is the obtainable or acceptable marginal gap in the fixed restorations?

A. 30–50 μm.
B. 50–60 μm.
C. 60–70 μm.
D. 70–80 μm.
E. 80–90 μm.

7. The best instrument used to detect the marginal gap of a metal crown clinically is:

A. William periodontal probe.
B. Sharp straight explorer.
C. CPITN probe.
D. Gingival marginal trimmer.
E. Wax carver.

8. The long-term success of any cemented fixed restoration is not influenced by:

A. Dispensing of appropriate cleaning aids.
B. Length and width ratio of the preparation.
C. Type of the restorative material.
D. Type of the luting cement.

ANS: 1A 2A 3E 4E 5E 6A 7B 8A

SHORT ANSWER QUESTIONS

1. **List any five factors that are essential for the long-term success of the cemented fixed restoration.**
    - Dispensing of appropriate cleaning aids
    - Home care instructions
    - Quality of patient's oral hygiene
    - Removal of the excess cement
    - Pulpal and periodontal status of the tooth
    - Taper of the preparation
    - Length and width ratio of the preparation
    - Type of the restorative material
    - Type of the luting cement.
2. **You have prepared a mandibular molar FDI 36 to receive a full gold crown restoration.**

    a. List down six things that you want to evaluate before you cement it on the patient's mouth. [3 marks]
    - Proximal contacts
    - Internal fit
    - Margins
    - Stability
    - Occlusion
    - Contours
    - Esthetics.

    b. On examination you have found there is a defective margin List the four different types of defective margins in a fixed restoration?
    - Overextended margins
    - Underextended margins
    - Thick margins
    - Open margins.
3. **You are evaluating a full gold crown received from the laboratory prior to permanently cementing this on a mandibular molar tooth FDI 46.**

    a. Which instrument will you use to detect the marginal gap clinically [1 mark]

    Sharp explorer.

    List four different types of defective margins in a fixed restoration [2 marks]
    - Overextended margins
    - Underextended margins
    - Thick margins
    - Open margins.

List two causes for a poorly adapted crown margin. [2 marks]

- Too tight proximal contact preventing the complete seating of the restoration
- Distortion of the restoration
- Internal discrepancies or nodules on the inner side of the restoration.

4. **A patient who had his vital tooth FDI 21 prepared for a metal ceramic crown a week ago attends for cementation of the final crown. The patient reports symptoms in the prepared tooth.**

a. What symptoms may force you to delay the permanent cementation? (1 mark)

Patient complaining of hypersensitivity/pain following the provisional restoration.

b. What are the possible causes for the patient to become symptomatic? (2 marks)

- Hyperocclusion of provisional restoration
- Deficiency in the provisional restoration
- Pulpal exposure/trauma during preparation.

c. What clinical investigations would you carry out in sequence for the patient during this appointment? (1 mark)

- Sensibility test, percussion test and TTP (tooth tender to percussion), if positive
- Periapical radiograph.

d. How will you manage the tooth further if your attempts of non-invasive managements were going to fail? (1 mark)

If the non-invasive management fails then the tooth is indicated for root canal treatment

5. **List the five preparatory procedures that need to be performed on any type of cemented restoration after it is fabricated from the laboratory. [5 marks]**

- Preliminary finishing
- Try-in and adjustment
- Precementation and polishing
- Cementation
- Postcementation finishing.

6. **List the four advantages of having a correct internal configuration in a fixed restoration. [2 marks]**

- To seat completely without binding
- Provides space for the luting cement
- Allows the margins to lie in intimate contact with the finish line
- Provides an internal surface that is conducive to a strong cement bond.

7. **What are the consequences of not having proper proximal contacts before you cement a fixed restoration in the patient's mouth? [4 marks]**

1. If it is too tight—interfere with correct seating of the restoration

- Produce discomfort to the patient
- Difficulty to floss
- Fracture of ceramic in an all ceramic or metal ceramic restoration.

2. If it is too light
   - Impaction of strands of food which is deleterious to gingiva.

8. Can you explain the steps in doing the occlusal adjustments in a fixed restoration before you cement the crown? [5 marks]

1. Compare the occlusal contact in the adjacent tooth before and after placement of the crown with the help of shim stock, if there is a variation correct the crown occlusal surface with the help of articulating papers till the patient can hold the shim stock on the adjacent tooth same way before and after crown placement.
2. Then check if the patient can hold the shim stock also with the crown same way as the adjacent tooth to make sure there is no any overreduction in the occlusal surface of the crown.
3. Once the centric relation is corrected use two different colors to correct the deflective contacts in the eccentric relation.

PONTICS

MULTIPLE CHOICE QUESTIONS

1. **The preferred material of choice on the tissue surface of a pontic is:**
   A. Polished metal.
   B. Polished porcelain.
   C. Resin bonded to metal.
   D. Polished self-cure resin.
   E. Polished heat-cure resin.

2. **The saddle pontic is also called as:**
   A. Ridge lap.
   B. Hygienic.
   C. Conical.
   D. Ovate.
   E. Prefabricated pontic.

3. **The Perel pontic is also called as:**
   A. Ridge lap.
   B. Hygienic.
   C. Conical.
   D. Ovate.
   E. Prefabricated pontic.

4. **The occlusogingival thickness of the hygienic pontic should not be less than:**
   A. 3.0 mm.
   B. 3.0 cm.
   C. 3.0 inch.
   D. 3.0 m.
   E. 3.0 µm.

5. **The preferred pontic design over thin ridges in the non-esthetic zone is:**
   A. Ridge lap.
   B. Hygienic.
   C. Conical.
   E. Ovate.
   F. Prefabricated pontic.

6. **The preferred pontic design in the mandibular posterior region is:**
   A. Ridge lap pontic.
   B. Hygienic pontic.

C. Conical pontic.
D. Ovate pontic.
E. Prefabricated pontic.

7. What type of pontic design would you use in a patient with a high esthetic demand for a fixed partial denture?

A. The ridge lap pontic.
B. The sanitary pontic.
C. The modified ridge lap pontic.
D. An ovate pontic.
E. Bullet-shaped pontic.

8. Which one of the following pontic designs is indicated when replacing a missing upper central incisor for a patient with a high smile line?

A. Ridge lap.
B. Sanitary.
C. Saddle.
D. Ovate.
E. Bullet shaped.

9. The treatment of choice to correct a reduced pontic space due to tilting of abutment teeth is:

A. Repositioning the teeth orthodontically.
B. Modifying abutment teeth with full coverage retainers.
C. Modifying abutment retainers to eliminate the need for a pontic.
D. Accommodating the pontic in the available space.
E. Increasing the thickness of connectors.

ANS: 1B 2A 3B 4A 5C 6B 7C 8D 9A

EXTENDED MATCHING QUESTIONS

1. Theme: Pontics

A. Saddle pontic.
B. Modified ridge lap pontic.
C. Hygienic pontic.
D. Conical pontic.
E. Ovate pontic.
F. Metal ceramic pontic.
G. Prefabricated pontic facing.

Using a letter from A to G, choose the most appropriate pontic design from the list above that best matches each of the following descriptions numbered 1–5 below. You may use each option once only or not at all.

1. Preferred over thin ridges of the nonesthetic zone.
2. Forms a large concave contact with the ridge.
3. Used only in the nonesthetics zone.
4. Used where esthetics is a primary concern.
5. Has tissue contact which does not extend lingually.

Description	Response
1	D
2	A
3	C
4	E
5	B

SHORT NOTE QUESTIONS

Instructions: Write briefly to the point answers.

1. **Draw and explain the different types of ridge deformities given by Siebert [5 marks]**

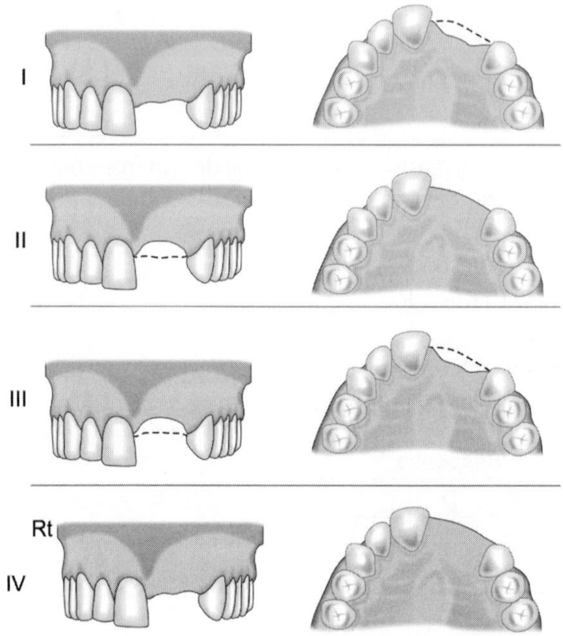

Ans:

- I–Faciolingual loss of tissue width with normal ridge height
- II–Loss of ridge height with normal ridge width
- III–Combinations of loss in both dimensions
- IV–Minimal deformity.

2. Regarding pontic contact with the tissues, which picture is wrong and why? [3 marks]

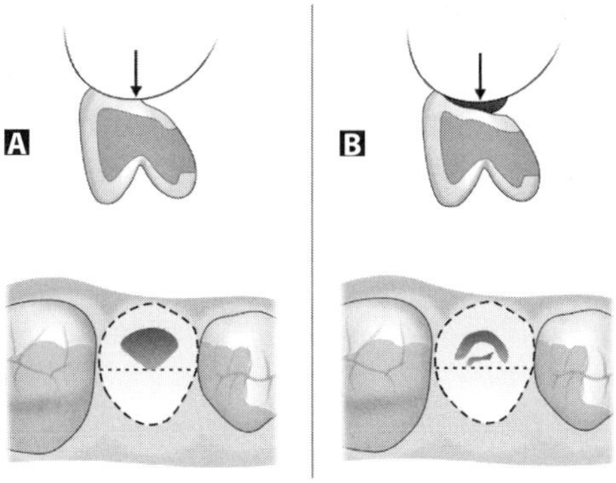

B—Wrong
Reason—Food entrapment

FILL IN THE BLANKS [3 MARKS]

Instructions: Fill up the blanks with appropriate answers.

1. **The occlusal forces exerted against the prosthetic appliances has been shown to be ______ lb for removable partial dentures: ______ lb for fixed partial denture : ______ lb for natural teeth.**

ANS: 26, 54.5, 150

FAILURES

MULTIPLE CHOICE QUESTIONS

1. The commonest cause of failure in the minimum preparation bridges is:

A. Inadequate taper.
B. Loss of retention.
C. Failure of connector.
D. Perforation.
E. Occlusal wear.

2. Which one of this is a mechanical failure in relation to crown and bridges?

A. Distortion.
B. Porcelain fracture.
C. Fracture of connectors.
D. Fracture of acrylic facings.
E. All of the above.

3. Which one of the following is a design failure in relation to crown and bridges?

A. Over-prescribed bridges.
B. Inadequate abutment preparation.
C. Under-prescribed bridges.
D. All of the above.

4. Which one of this is a clinical or laboratory failure in relation to crown and bridges?

A. Overhang on the margins.
B. Poor shape or color.
C. Marginal defect.
D. All of the above.

5. In metal–ceramic restorations, failures usually occur:

A. In the porcelain.
B. At the porcelain–metal interface.
C. In the metal.
D. At the metal–tooth interface.
E. In the tooth.

ANS: 1B 2E 3D 4D 5A

EXTENDED MATCHING QUESTIONS

1. Theme: Crown and bridge failures

A. Periodontal disease.
B. Distortion of the bridge/crown.
C. Inadequate type of retainer.
D. Poor shape or color.
E. Occlusal problems.
F. Pericoronitis.

For each of the following failure, choose the most appropriate type from the list above. You may use each option once or not at all.

1. Mechanical failure.
2. Design failure.
3. Inadequate clinical technique.
4. Abutment failure.
5. Inadequate laboratory technique.

Description	Response
1	B
2	C
3	E
4	A
5	D

SHORT ANSWER QUESTIONS

1. **A 40-year-old patient presents complaining of movement of his three unit fixed-fixed bridge in which teeth FDI 15 and 17 are abutments and tooth FDI 16 is replaced by a pontic.**

   a. How can you clinically identify the failed retainer? (1 mark)
   - Pressing the bridge and look for small bubbles in the saliva at the margins of the retainers.

   b. List any two causes for this failure. (1 mark)
   - Cementation failure
   - Nonretentive preparations
   - Secondary caries
   - Poor design.

   c. List any three solutions to manage this failure. (3 marks)
   - Recementation with chemically adhesive cement
   - Cut off one retainer and convert to cantilever
   - Preparations are redone and the retainer(s) are remade
   - If needed, add additional abutments
   - Change the design.

2. **A 40-years-old patient reports to your dental office with a complaint that his anterior metal ceramic crown is fractured. On examination it is found that the fracture surface is ceramic.**

   a. Explain whether the fracture is cohesive or adhesive failure. (1 mark)
   - Cohesive failure.

   b. How do you manage the fractured ceramic if the other features of the crown are satisfactory? (2 marks)
   - Repair with composite and follow-up—temporary management
   - Redo—permanent management.

   c. How to prevent this type of fracture? (2 marks)
   - Proper crown/bridge design
   - Adequate preparation to have enough thickness for metal-ceramic or all ceramic to avoid distortion
   - Extension of porcelain to the lingual side of pontic.

3. **A 40-years-old patient reports to your dental office with a complaint that his anterior metal–ceramic crown is fractured. On examination it is found that the fracture surface is between metal and ceramic.**

   a. Explain whether the fracture is cohesive or adhesive failure. (1 mark)
   - Adhesive failure.

b. Explain how ceramic is bonded to the underlying metal. (2 marks)

- Through metal oxide layer.

c. How can you prevent this type of failure? (2 marks)

- Proper crown/bridge design
- Adequate preparation to have enough thickness for metal–ceramic or all ceramic to avoid distortion
- Extension of porcelain to the lingual side of pontic.

LAMINATE VENEERS

Definitions

Veneer

Veneer is a protective or ornamental facing—(GPT 7).

Laminate Veneer

It is a thin veneer facing which is laminated (adhesive bonded) to etched tooth structure by using resin cements.[1]

Introduction

In 1928 Dr Charles Pincus used veneers for movie stars. He used porcelain onto platinum foils and fixed them for actors with denture adhesives.

Indications for Veneers

- Cosmetic —for stained tooth that cannot be bleached and for shaping anterior teeth
- Restorative—fractured, worn or traumatized anterior teeth and for avoiding composite fillings
- Functional—to correct diastema, malaligned and malformed teeth. To reconstruct anterior canine-guided occlusion.

Contraindications of Laminate Veneers

- Large diastemas
- Bruxism
- Poor oral hygiene
- Severe malocclusions
- Severe fracture of tooth
- Severe tooth rotations.

Types of Laminate Veneers

- Hollow ground denture teeth
- Preformed stock acrylic laminates
- Custom made veneers—composite or porcelain.

Hollow ground denture teeth

Advantages—Easy to prepare, less expensive.
Disadvantages—They are opaque and only minimal color corrections are possible.

Preformed stock acrylic laminates (E.g. Componeer by Coltene)

Advantages—Readymade veneers.
Disadvantages—May not be available in all shapes and shades, expensive.

Custom-made Veneers (Types)

a. Composite resin

Advantage—Direct clinical technique—simple and less time consumption.
Disadvantage—May acquire stains and difficult to polish.

b. Porcelain laminate veneers

Advantage—Highly esthetic, least plaque retention and characterization is possible.
Disadvantages—Indirect technique, requires lab support, expensive and technique sensitive.

PORCELAIN LAMINATE VENEERS

Indications

Same as general indications, such as discolored tooth, fractured tooth, diastema closure, malformed teeth, defective restorations, adolescent teeth (have large pulps), worn teeth (erosion/abrasion/attrition), root exposures, stained restorations, to lengthen short crowns and smile designing (Fig. 1).

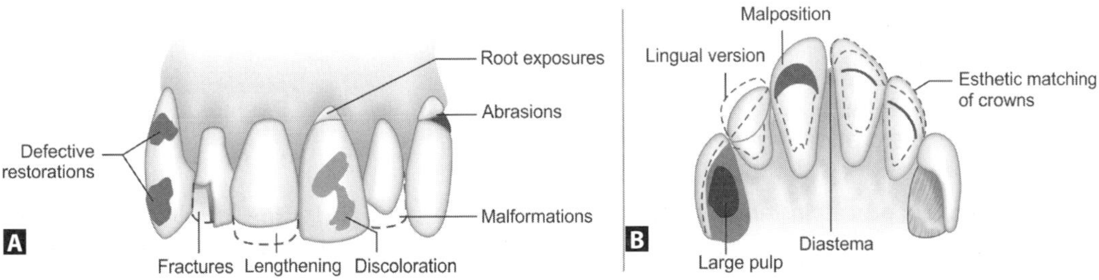

Figs 1A and B: Indications for laminate veneers

Porcelain materials used

Pressable ceramic, lithium disilicate [E.g. Emax (Ivoclar Vivadent)] is the most favored core material —340MPa.

Alumina (690Mpa) or zirconia (1200–1400Mpa) may also be used as core for laminate veneer. But they are opaque, cannot be etched and hence, are not frequently used as the core.

Procedure

- Ceramic blocks (ingots) of lithium disilicate are heated at 1150 °C
- The softened ceramic is slowly injected under pressure into the mold at high temperature under vacuum
- The core is retrieved and layered with feldspathic porcelain and is stained and characterized
- This core is etchable with hydrofluoric acid and may be used in crowns, veneers, inlays and onlays.

Selection of veneer cases

- At least 50% enamel should be present on the tooth surface to be bonded (for effective bonding of the veneer)[2]
- 1mm circumferential principle'—Atleast one millimeter of the peripheral margins of the prepared tooth should have enamel, this ensures a proper marginal seal[3]
- Shade selection is done before the preparation
- Selecting a lighter than the desired shade is desirable.

Mouth preparation before laminate preparation[4]

If there are other carious surfaces, defective restorations, isolated discolored tooth areas, or any, class 3 cavities present restore them with composite before the veneer preparation.

Steps in preparation of a veneer

- Facial preparation/Finish line
- Proximal preparation
- Incisal preparation
- Finishing of preparation
- Gingival retraction
- Impression making
- Provisional restoration—generally not required
- Try-In
- Preparation of porcelain veneer for bonding—(HF acid etching and silane coupling application)
- Preparation of tooth for bonding—37% phosphoric acid etch followed by bonding agent application
- Application of resin on veneer
- Seating and setting of veneer
- Check occlusion.

Facial preparation (Fig. 2)

- Gingival half of labial surface = 0.3mm reduction
- Labioincisal half = 0.5mm reduction
- Finish line = Chamfer
- Finish line termination : At crest of gingiva (equigingival)/slightly subgingival
- No sharp internal line angles—helps to avoid stress concentration on the porcelain
- Respect the facial convexity during tooth preparation.

Why chamfer finish line?

- Chamfer provides a definitive seat for accurate laminate positioning
- Chamfer is easily distinguishable in impressions and by the lab
- Provides adequately thick porcelain at margins
- Exposes enamel prisms near the cervical region at correct angle thereby increasing the surface area of enamel for better etching
- Chamfer make no internal line angles—less stress on porcelain
- Less destructive of tooth structure than shoulder preparation
- Chamfer provides gradual transition from tooth to veneer.

Proximal preparation (Fig. 2)

- Is the extension of facial reduction
- Should just end facial to contact area
- Should not break contact area
- Change to a smaller diameter bur (to prevent damage to adjacent tooth, if required).

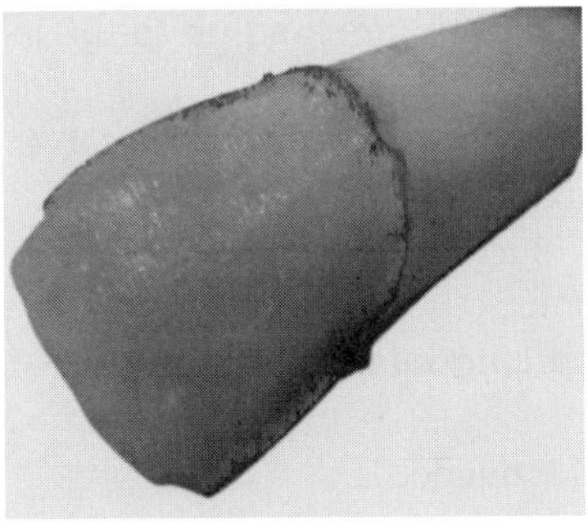

Fig. 2: Proximal and facial preparation

Proximal reduction—when to break contact?

Contact is broken when existing proximal restoration are at the contact region in malpositioned teeth and diastemas.

Incisal preparation

The design varies in regard to the incisal preparation. The different types of incisal preparation are

- Window design preparation
- Feather edge preparation
- Incisal bevel preparation
- Incisal overlap/Incisal wrap/Lingual wrap design.

Incisal preparation—Different designs (Fig. 3)

- Window design
- Feather edge
- Incisal bevel
- Incisal wrap/lingual wrap.

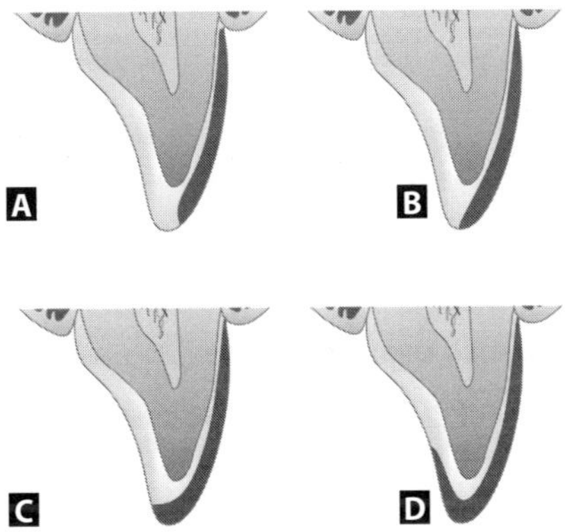

Figs 3A to D: Different incisal preparations

a. **Window design preparation**—Preparation is close but not up to the incisal edge
Limitations—Difficult to hide joint between the veneer and the tooth and hence, not a preferred design.

b. **Feather edge preparation**—Tooth prepared up to the incisal edge without incisal edge reduction.
   Indications—When the existing crown length is acceptable.
   Advantages—Maintains guidance on natural tooth.
c. **Incisal bevel preparation**—Buccopalatal bevel given and hence, more control over incisal esthetics. Not commonly done.
d. **Incisal over lap/Incisal wrap/Lingual wrap design (Fig. 4)**
   Indications
   - When crown lengthening is needed
   - When the faciolingual thickness of tooth is too thin
   - Fractured incisal edges.

   Advantages
   - Provides vertical stop
   - Less stress concentration at incisal edge
   - Increases the surface area for bonding
   - Lingual reduction for incisal overlap—keeps porcelain under compression (in mandibular tooth)
   - Chamfer 0.5 mm deep
   - Bur is held parallel to lingual surface and the two proximal finish lines is connected to produce a mesial and distal notch
   - Lingual finish line should be 1 mm away from centric contacts.

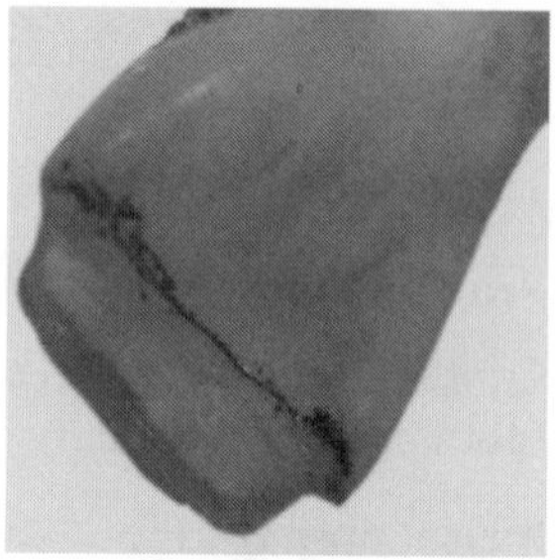

Fig. 4: Incisal/Lingual wrap

Finishing the preparation

- Remove all sharp line angles
- No sharp corners/angles.

Stump shade selection done (Fig. 5)— communicated to the lab (supported by a good photograph).

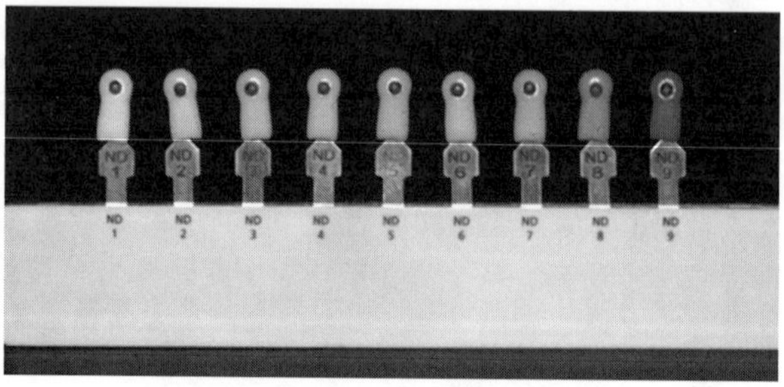

Fig. 5: Stump shade guide

Gingival displacement—Gingival retraction done to expose finish line so that impression flows into sulcus—To record the tooth profile beyond finish line.

Impression material—Addition silicone (polyvinyl siloxane)—good dimensional stability.

Provisional restoration—Not usually required since the preparation is mostly in enamel there is less chances of postoperative sensitivity. In case temporary restoration is given eugenol-based preparations should not be used as eugenol remnant can hamper the polymerization of the resin cement.

Try- in—Try in pastes have the same optical properties as luting composite. So it is helpful to determine how the shade of the porcelain laminate veneer will be beforehand.

Adhesive Bonding of Veneer[5]

The monoblock effect—Tooth + resin cement + ceramic restoration— is the key to the success towards the longevity of the restoration.

Preparation of the porcelain laminate veneer for bonding (Fig. 6)

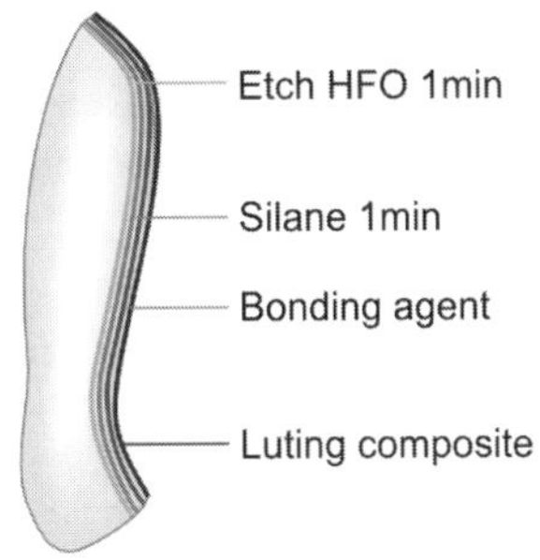

Fig. 6: Preparation of porcelain laminates veneer prior to bonding

- Hydrofluoric acid etching (2.5–10% for 1minute)—Hydrofluoric acid (HF) is a porcelain etchant. It selectively dissolves the glassy matrix from the applied surface which when washed away exposes the rough crystals thereby increasing the surface area for bonding
- Silane coupling agent application—is a major factor for resin cement bonding on to silica-based ceramics. Silanes are bifunctional molecules that bonds silicon dioxide with the OH groups on the ceramic surface. They also have a degradable functional group that copolymerizes with the organic matrix of the resin

Preparation of the tooth for bonding porcelain laminate veneer (Fig. 7)

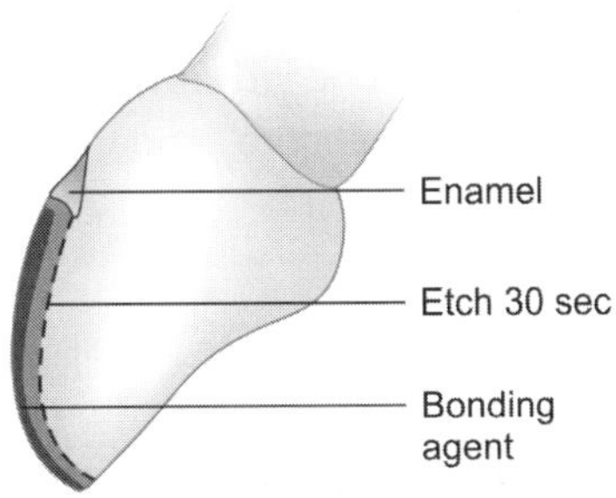

Fig. 7: Preparation of the tooth for bonding porcelain laminate veneer

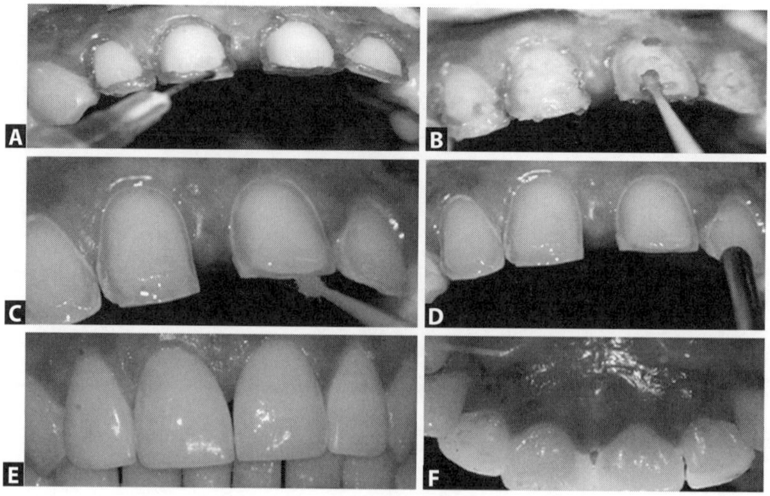

Figs 8A to F: A completed case of porcelain veneer

- Etching the tooth with total etch (37% phosphoric acid) and or self etch philosophies
- Then the bonding agent is applied on the tooth and not cured (it is cured through the laminate veneers which are thin restorations).

Other steps for bonding laminate veneers

- The veneer is uniformly loaded with low viscosity resin
- Ensure complete seating of the veneer
- Laminate veneers are very thin restorations and need gentle handling as they are brittle before bonding
- They are carried to the tooth for bonding using special sticks with glue (e.g. Optrastick by Ivoclar) which could be removed after the veneer is cured
- Remove gross excess resin
- The margins where resin cement is exposed to air is applied with glycerin/vaseline to prevent oxygen from coming into contact with resin as contact of resin cement with oxygen in the air could inhibit the polymerization of the resin cement. This may lead to marginal leakage, discoloration and disintegration)
- Adjust occlusion—Check all excursion movements
- Eliminate interferences especially in lengthened crowns
- Ensure that there is no centric contact at enamel—porcelain margins (Fig. 8).

Other Types of Veneers: Lumineers

- Lumineers are 'no prep veneers'. They are marketed by Dent-Mat corporation, California as Cerinate Lumineers
- No local anesthetic administration nor tooth preparation is recommended here.

Advantages

- Patients are more comfortable with the idea of no preparation
- Temporaries are often unnecessary, lowering the cost of treatment
- Restorations bond strongly to enamel, so these stay
- Procedures are reversible if the results are not satisfactory
- There is minimal damage to the dental pulp.

Disadvantages

- Esthetic changes are limited
- Limited potential for color change
- Difficulties manufacturing, inserting and bonding the restorations
- Patient complaints about excessive bulk
- Flat esthetics due lack of room to create deep embrasures.

References

1. Tylman's theory and practice of fixed prosthodontics.
2. Albers H. Tooth colored restoratives, ed 7. Coatai, California: Alto books 1985;pp 7-1 to 7-31.
3. Jordan R. Ethetic Composite Bonding. St. louis: The CV Mosby Co; 1986. p 28.
4. Galip Gurel. The science and art of porcelain laminate veneers. Quintessence Publishing Co. Ltd; 2003.
5. Markus B, et al. Resin –Ceramic bonding: A review of literature. JPD;2003.

FIXED PARTIAL DENTURES—AN INSIGHT

Introduction

Scientific advancements in the treatment of fixed partial denture prosthesis has taken place at all levels starting with diagnosis and treatment planning to options in types of restoration, to recent advances in equipments, soft tissue management, impression making, articulators, shade selection and newer materials for provisional prosthesis, luting and the definitive prosthesis.

Literature search was carried out using PubMed and Google scholar from 1993 to 2013 on review articles and evidence-based studies related to all the above mentioned aspects of the fixed prosthesis denture and has been projected as a summary in this article.

Advancements in Diagnosis

Latest advancements have been in form of caries detection systems, such as[1]

1. **DIAGNODent Laser Device** (KaVo, Lake Zurich,Ill.) uses laser fluorescence to detect incipient caries. The device measures the fluorescence of bacterial products within carious lesions. (Fig. 9).

   Advantages: A valuable device when combined with a visual examination to detect demineralization. It is capable to ascertain demineralization under sealants also.

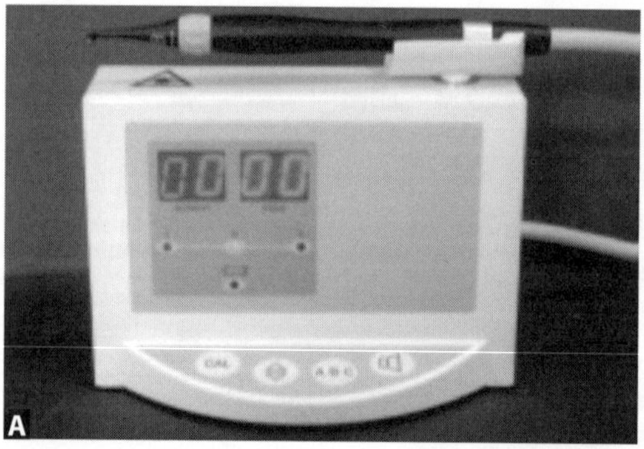

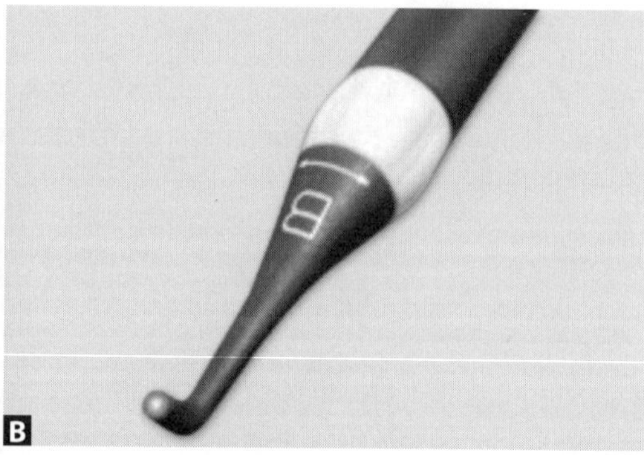

Figs 9A and B: DiagnoDent Laser Device

   Limitations: The readings can be recorded in the patient's chart but cannot be used for comparison or large scale studies.

2. **Digital Imaging Fiber-Optic Transillumination Device (DIFOTI) (Fig. 10)**
   - It allows images from all tooth surfaces to be digitally captured and stored
   - The principle behind transilluminating teeth is that demineralized areas of enamel or dentine scatter light more than sound areas
   - Incipient caries appear as darker areas in the resultant images.

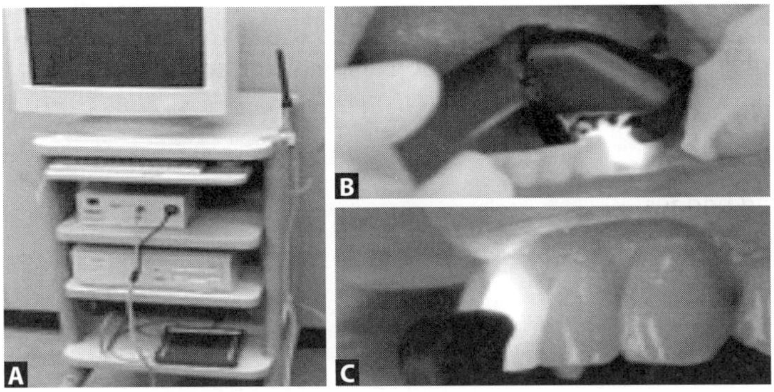

Figs 10A to C: DIFOTI device and clinical use

Advantages—Simple to use and the instantly available images are easily interpreted. It can also be used as a patient education tool.

Limitations—Image interpretation is difficult, because the results are not directly quantified.

3. **Quantitative Light-induced Fluorescence (1995)**
   - QLF is a more versatile system than either DIAGNODent or DIFOTI and can measure absolute mineral loss along with a number of other applications
   - Good reproducibility of QLF methods clinically with reliability greater than 0.95 was reported after training
   - Bacterial products appear as red fluorescence, determine the activity of lesions
   - QLF can be used as a diagnostic system, rather than a detection device.

Advantages: Ability to detect root caries and early orthodontic demineralization.

Other caries detection methods include electronic caries monitor, fiberoptic transillumination, bite wing radiographs.

Advancements in Restorative Options

Shortened Dental Arch Concept

The shortened dental arch (SDA) may be defined as having an intact anterior region but a reduced number of occluding pairs of posterior teeth.[2]

In 1992, the World Health Organization stated that the retention, throughout life, of a functional, esthetic, natural dentition of not less than 20 teeth and not requiring recourse to prostheses should be the treatment goal for oral health.[3]

The above concept adopts the fact that if the patient is having an intact anterior region but a reduced number of occluding pairs of posterior teeth with good occlusal stability and correct vertical dimension there is no need to restore the posterior edentulous spaces.

SDA protocol terminates the occlusal platform at the second premolar region. But the remaining teeth should be closely monitored and oral hygiene is to be well maintained with periodic recalls.

Minimally Invasive Prosthodontics/Microdentistry

This concept highlights maximum preservation of remaining sound teeth.[4]

Types

- Partial veneer crowns
- Resin-bonded bridges
- Laminate veneers
- Inlay/Onlay
- Anchor systems.

Advantages

- Less destructive
- Good esthetics
- Fixed restoration
- More comfort for the patient
- Less time
- Easy marginal finishing and cleaning.

Disadvantages

- Only can restore short span
- Commonly used materials are IPS E max, Zirpress (Zirconium oxide).

Anchor systems (CBW—Crown less bridge work)

In anchor system titanium anchors are adhesively bonded to the proximal sides of the abutment tooth and pontic is attached to this anchor.

Systems are—UDA and Delta bridge systems

Advantages
Minimal preparation, esthetic, less interference with existing occlusion and it is a reversible and repairable process.

Disadvantages

Difficult to clean, only in short span, cannot be used in free end saddles and in parafunctional habit cases, requires good skill and experience.

Resin-bonded Fixed Partial Dentures (RBFPD)

First introduced in the 1970s by Rochette presently more advanced bonding and bridge materials such as fiber-reinforced composites and Zirconium has increased the longevity of resin-bonded restoration.

Good bonding with minimal abutment preparation increase the bond strength of the RBFPD.

Advantages

- Minimal tooth preparation
- Decreased pulpal trauma

- Minimal periodontal irritation
- Anesthesia is often not needed
- Easy margin placement and cleaning due to supragingival margin
- Improved esthetics
- Reduced cost with less chair time
- Provisional restoration not required
- Re bonding is possible.

Limitations

- Debonding is the commonest cause of failure
- Design is outside the dimensions of the natural tooth hence, bulky contours
- "Graying out" of teeth that are thin labiolingually at the incisal surfaces
- Good alignment of abutments is required
- No space correction
- Good lab precision required
- Restricted to single teeth replacements.

Advancement in materials includes coating of zirconia with a glass infiltration agent by heating above the glass transition temperature. This is called selective infiltration etching emerged in 2006.[5] This technique creates sliding and splitting of the surface grains creating nano porosities where the adhesive resin can infiltrate and interlock. This technique increases the bond strength.

Advancements in Tooth Preparation/Equipments

Equipments: Recent advances in hand pieces.

Laser treatment for hard tissues

Goldman et al., in 1964 introduced laser into dentistry.[6]

Amongst the type of lasers the Er: YAG laser was tested in 1988 on hard tissues

Advantages—Decreased vibrations and noise causing more comfort to the patient, low pulpal temperatures, reduces amount of bacteria in surgical field, good control of bleeding, improved visualization of the surgical field, and can be performed with less injectable anesthesia. Burkes etal reported that even without water-cooling the prepared cavities showed no cracks and low or no charring.[7]

Gimbel observed that the Er: YAG laser is capable of removing cement, composite resin and glass ionomer which can be used in removal of crowns and bridges.[8]

Limitations—Although they are useful for caries removal and tooth preparation, the erbium lasers are unable to remove gold and porcelain, accessibility to the treatment area is limited, and apart from the line supply an additional air supply is required. It is presently used only as an adjunct to conventional technique.

DJP Evans et al. observed that though patients were comfortable with lasers, dentist preferred the conventional method because after using laser they had to use conventional handpieces to complete the cavity due to difficulty in access and slow speed of cutting.[9]

Dental Air Abrasion Handpiece (KaVo PROPHYflex 3)

Indications

- Cleaning of enamel before etching for subsequent fissure sealing
- Cleaning before using DiagnoDent caries detector
- Cleaning of implant surfaces
- Fast and pain-free removal of plaque and stains
- Preparation of cavities for improved bonding.

Advancements in Soft Tissue Management

Gingiva Pastes and Gels

Recent advances in soft tissue management include cordless gingival retraction methods using injectable materials such as Expasyl (Kerr Corporation) (Fig. 11) and magic foam (ColteneWhaledent) (Fig. 12). These materials ensure hemostasis and open the sulcus.

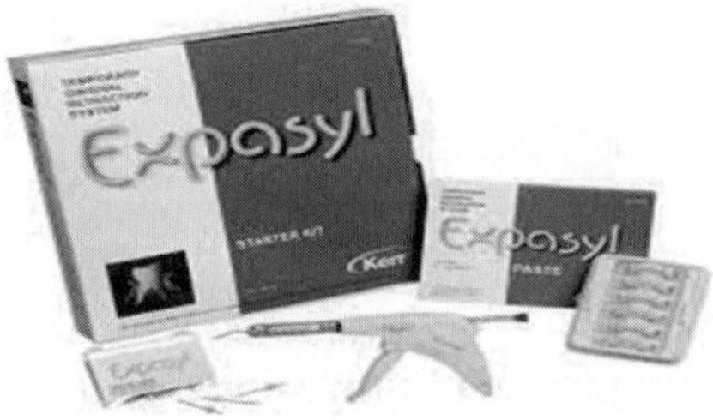

Fig. 11: Gingival retraction Expasyl injectable

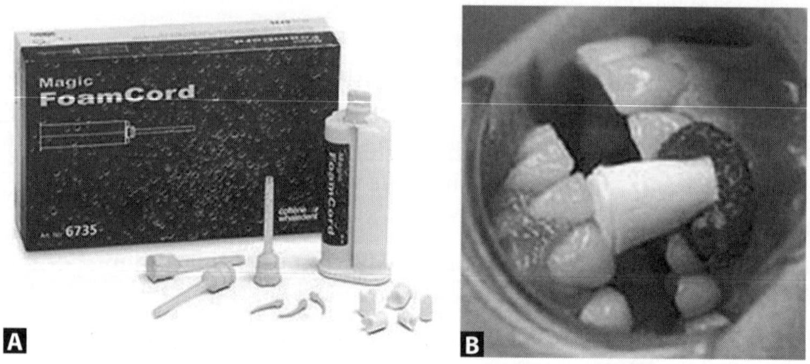

Figs 12A and B: Magic foam injectable types

Other cordless techniques are Traxodent Hemodent Paste Retraction System (Premier Products Company) and Gingitrac (Centrix).

Modified impression techniques, such as matrix system and modified shell system are also presently employed.[10]

Advancements Impression Materials

More recently the three-dimensional (3D) digital scanners are being used to capture 3D virtual images of tooth preparations, from which restorations are fabricated directly (CAD/CAM systems) or indirectly (dedicated impression scanning systems for the creation of accurate master models).

The computer-aided design/computer-aided manufacture (CAD/CAM)

- They feed data obtained from accurate digital scans of teeth directly into milling systems
- The milling systems carve restorations out of ceramic or composite resin blocks without the need for a maxillary and mandibular model
- Another modified way is to scan the master models poured from elastic impressions digitally and to create stereolithic models on which the restorations are made.

Principles Behind 3d Surface Imaging

These devices contain a digital map of the surface of an object and collect data on its three dimensional size and shape which form a point cloud representing the 3D coordinates of the digitized surface (Fig. 13).

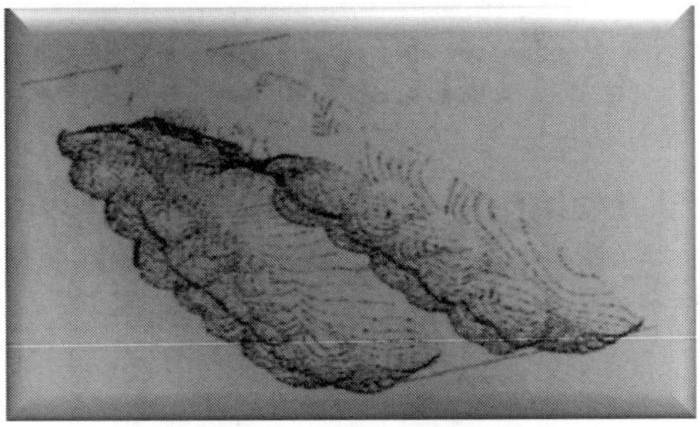

Fig. 13: Digital image

Two types of 3D surface scanners are available:

Coordinated Measuring Machines (CMM)—in which a measuring probe moves over the surface to determine the coordinates of the points comprising the surface.

Non-contact scanners—A laser beam is incident on the surface to be scanned and a camera-like device, such as a charged coupled device or a position sensitive detector, records the location of the point at which the laser beam strikes the device.

Systems available

- CADENT iTero
- 3M ESPE Lava COS
- CEREC by Sirona
- E4D by D4D Technologies
- The Cadent and 3M ESPE machines produce models that are sent to the lab to produce the restoration of choice
- Sirona and D4D include milling units for immediate chair side fabrication of the final restoration.

CEREC AC can be used for fabrication of a model-only system by purchasing it without the milling center. It uses blue LED optical scanner and requires the use of powder.

E4D's system includes the interoffice milling center to produce same-day single crowns using Culp's database of dental anatomy. It uses a LASER scanner and does not require powder. Here scanning can be done intraorally, on the conventional impression or the poured model..

LAVA COS (chair side oral scanner) is a video format that uses the blue LED scanning system that requires powder. The downloaded scan information produces a model that allows for fabrication of any type of restoration (Fig. 14).

iTero is an optically assisted laser scanner that does not require powder. This optics allows real-time imaging, which produces a milled model allowing for fabrication of restorative needs.

Glidewell developed a scanning system that was introduced at the 2011 Chicago Midwinter Meeting. The system uses an optical scanning platform.

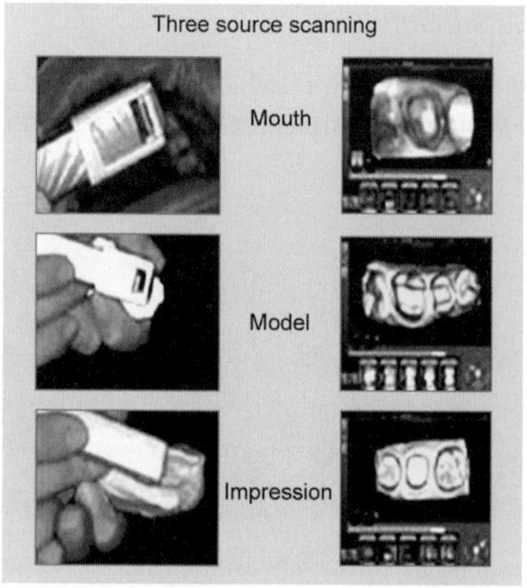

Fig. 14: Final computer image of 3D model after scanning

Comparison of digital impression and conventional impression

1. Digital impression is more efficient than conventional impression.
2. Overall treatment time is longer for conventional impression technique.
3. Treatment comfort of the digital impression technique was higher.

Advancements in Articulators

- Virtual articulators by simulation of real patient data allows analyses with regard to static and dynamic occlusion as well as to jaw relation
- The virtual articulator requires digital 3D representations of the jaws and the specific data on jaw movements
- It then simulates jaw movements and provides a dynamic visualization of the occlusal contacts. They are of two types, completely adjustable and mathematically simulated.

Completely Adjustable Virtual Articulator

- Records/reproduces paths of the mandible using an electronic jaw registration system called jaw motion analyser
- The entire mandibular movements and their recorded paths can be viewed in the computer screen from different planes
- The software calculates and visualizes both static and kinematic occlusal collisions and is used in designing and correction of occlusal surfaces in computer-aided designing systems.

Eg. Kordass and Gartner virtual articulators.

Mathematically-simulated Virtual Articulator

- Records/reproduces movements of the articulator based on mathematical simulation of articulator movements
- These virtual articulators allow for additional settings, such as curved Bennett movement or other movements for adjustment in ideal settings.
- The main disadvantage is that it behaves as a mean value articulator and it is not possible to obtain individualized movement paths of each patient.

Eg. Stratos 200, Szentpetery's virtual articulator.

Advantages of Digital Articulators over Mechanical Dental Articulator

- The main goal of the digital articulator is to improve the design of dental prosthesis, adding kinematic analysis to the design process
- Commonly used semiadjustable articulators, cannot represent the effects of resilience of the soft tissue or the time-dependent muscle-guided movement pattern of mastication
- Also they cannot represent the real dynamic condition of the occlusion in mouth.

Advancements in Shade Matching

The first shade guide was introduced in 1956 by Vita Zahnfabrik for the measurement of ceramic color systems.

The development from visual analysis to spectrophotometers was a milestone in shade matching.

Types of Spectrophotometeric Shade Guides

Easy shade standard
Easy shade compact

- The Vita easy shade is one of the latest spectrophotometers available for clinical use
- The instrument's software gives absolute CIE lab* color values for natural teeth
- When assessing the color of a ceramic, the spectrophotometer provides the differences from color value presets in the instrument database (Figs 15 and 16)
- The easy shade compact introduced in 2009 was smaller, wireless and easier to handle

- The difference between the compact and standard was that the compact has a single spectrophotometer whereas standard has two
- The tip of the instrument is placed on the buccal surface of the tooth and the LCD screen at the base of the instrument displays the absolute CIElab* values of the tooth.

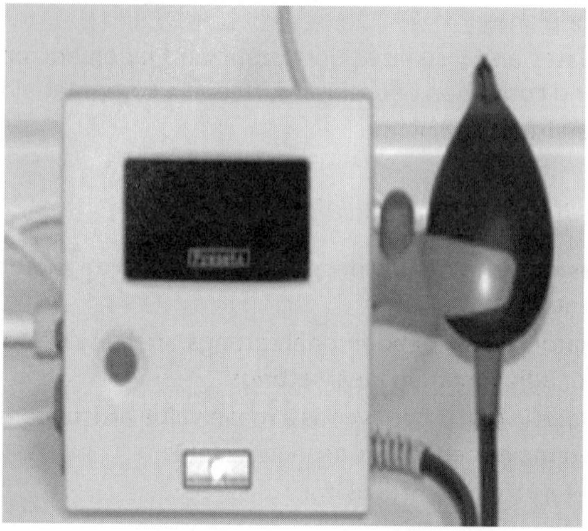

Fig. 15: Vita-easy shade

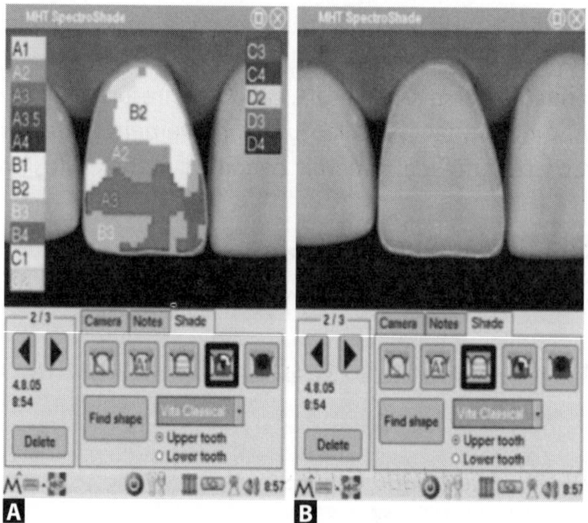

Figs 16A and B: Vita easy shade display

Advancements in Provisional Restoration Materials

A provisional prosthesis is prosthesis designed to enhance esthetics, provide stabilization and/or function for a limited period of time, and should be replaced by a definitive prosthesis after a period of time (G.P.T-8).

The materials commonly used are polymethylmethacrylate, polyethylmethacrylate, bisacryl composites, polyvinylmethyl methacrylate and visible light cured urethane dimethacrylate (Table 2).

Table 2: Materials used for provisional restoration

Material	Advantage	Disadvantage
Polymethyl methacrylate	• Durable • Good transverse strength • Good marginal fit • Good polishability	• High exothermic heat • Low abrasion resistance • Free monomer content • High volumetric shrinkage
Polyethyl methacrylate	• Good polishability • Minimal exothermic heat • Good stain resistance • Low shrinkage	• Low surface hardness • Low transverse strength • Durable
Bis-acryl composite	• Good marginal fit • Low exothermic heat • Good abrasion resistance • Good transverse strength	• Low surface hardness • Less stain resistance • Limited shade selection • Limited polishability
Polyvinyl methyl methacrylate	• Flexibility • Good stain resistance • Good polishability • Minimal exothermic heat	• Low fracture toughness • Compromised esthetics • Low transverse strength • Low surface hardness
Visible light cured urethrane Dimethacrylate	• High surface hardness • Good transverse strength • Good abrasion resistance and color stability • Controllable working time	• Expensive • Less stain resistance • Limited shade selection • Poor marginal fit and brittle

Advancements in Luting Agents

Temporary Cement

Luting the temporary/provisional/treatment restoration is done with a class of eugenol and eugenol-free cements.

Eugenol-free luting agents are Ora TempNE, Kavitan®CEM, Centrix access, TempSpan® Transparent, TempSpan® CMT, Embonte, GC Fuji TEMP LT™—GC America
Integrity® TempGrip™ —Dentsply Caulk, RelyX™ Temp—3M ESPE.

OraTempNE (Fig. 17)

- Radioopaque eugenol free, self curing cement based on zinc oxide
- Working time 1–2 mins
- Setting time 3–4 mins.

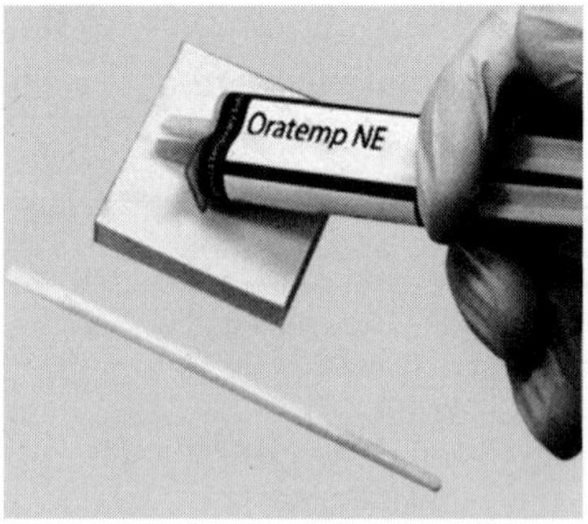

Fig. 17: OraTempNE

Kavitan®CEM

Gel-based consistency and extraordinary adhesion to tooth structure. Its the ideal material for cementing crowns and bridges, inlays and onlays onto a metal base.

- Optimal film thickness
- Excellent fixation consistency
- High compressive strength
- Low solubility and disintegration
- Anti-caries effect due to long-time fluoride release
- Optimal biocompatibility.

Centrix access

- A softer, semi-elastic set allows for easier removal and minimal clean up
- Eugenol-free temporary cement with calcium hydroxide
- Does not influence the setting of resin-based filling and luting materials
- Working time ≥2 minutes
- Setting Time (37°C) = 4 – 10 minutes.

TempSpan® Transparent

- Transparent—ideal for the highly esthetic anterior zone
- Ideal retention—securely retains provisional restorations and facilitates easy removal
- Non-eugenol—ensures compatibility with resin-based permanent cements
- Auto-mix delivery—provides accurate placement into the provisional with minimal waste
- Dual-Cure—offers ideal working time with on command cure.

TempSpan® CMT

Apart from the above properties it contains three desensitizers (potassium nitrate, sodium fluoride and calcium phosphate).

Embonte

ZOE-based used for temporary crowns, splints and for trial cementation of permanent restorations. Has a 30-second mix time and working time of 4 minutes at 72°F.

GC Fuji TEMP LT™—GC America (Fig. 18)

- The first glass ionomer provisional and implant cement
- Provides versatility, reliability, durability and ease of use
- Greater fluoride release
- Excellent seal and low patient sensitivity
- Two minutes working time and one minute set time in the mouth
- Paste–paste automix syringe delivery system
- Smooth consistency and low film thickness.

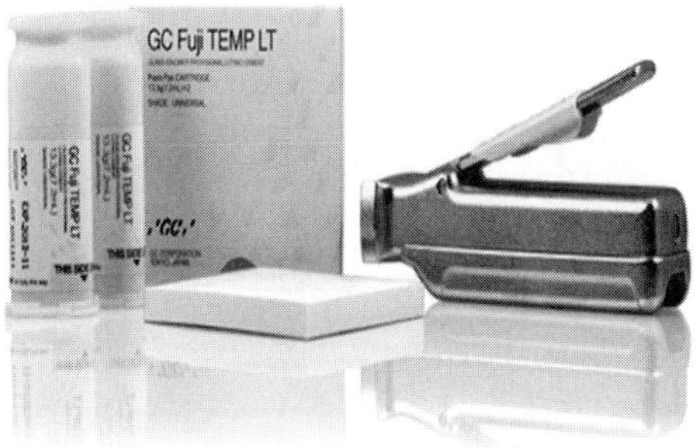

Fig. 18: GC Fuji Temp LT

Integrity® TempGrip™ —Dentsply Caulk

- Smooth seating from optimal flow
- Fast procedure with short set time
- Easy removal with cement that stays in crown—not on the tooth
- Reliable mixing with automix syringe delivery
- Reliable strength from high compressive and flexural strength and low film thickness.

Contains 2–9 g syringes and 20 mixing tips.

RelyX™ Temp—3M ESPE

Advantages

- Extremely low film thickness for use with precision fitting restorations
- High retention to tooth yet easy removal.

Advancements in Definitive Restorative Materials[11]

Duceram LFC ('hydrothermal low fusing ceramic) (Fig. 19)

- Composed of an amorphous glass containing hydroxyl ions
- Greater density, higher flexural strength, greater fracture resistance and lower hardness than feldspathic porcelain
- Due to the absence of leucite crystals, the hardness of the material and its ability to abrade the opposing natural tooth structure is claimed to be reduced

- Duceram LFC has two layers. A base layer leucite containing porcelain which is placed on a refractory die and then baked at 930°C
- The second layer, is applied over the base layer using powder slurry technique and baked at 660°C. This material is available in a variety of shades and can be characterized with surface stains and modifiers.

Uses

Ceramic inlays, veneers and full contour crowns.

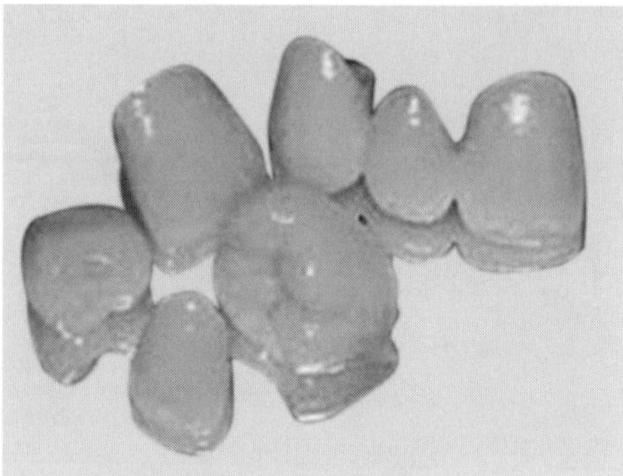

Fig. 19: Duceram LFC

Injection moulded glass ceramic/Leucite-reinforced hot pressed glass ceramic (Optec OPC)

- This system was first described by Wohlwend et al. and became available commercially as IPS Empress (Fig. 20) and Optec OPC
- It is a preceremmed glass reinforced with leucite that prevents crack propagation without diminishing its translucency
- The available ingots are heated and injected under pressure and temperature into a mold created by the lost wax technique to produce a restoration
- Less susceptible to fatigue failure than conventional feldspathic porcelain but shows a lower compressive strength than metal ceramics or In-ceram restorations.

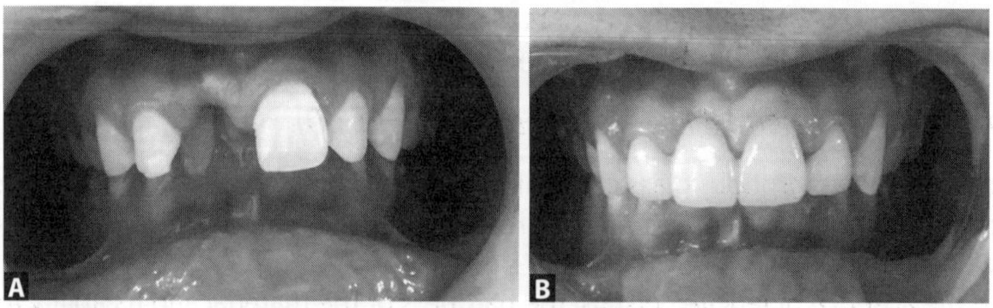

Figs 20A and B: IPS Empress restoration

Advantages

- Lack of metal or opaque ceramic core
- Moderate flexural strength
- Excellent fit
- Excellent esthetics.

Disadvantages

- Potential to fracture in posterior areas
- Need for special equipment (pressing oven and die material).

Uses

Indicated for single anterior crowns, inlays, onlays and veneers.

Infilterable ceramic/High alumina ceramic (in Ceram) (Fig. 21)

- The fine grained alumina powder particles are mixed with water to form a suspension or slurry referred to as a 'slip' and painted onto an absorbent refractory die
- The die draws excess water from the slurry and forms a layer of solid alumina on the surface which is sintered at 1120°C for 10 hours to produce an opaque porous core
- In the second phase, glass infiltration material of appropriate shade is applied onto the core and fired at 1100°C for 3–5 hours
- This molten glass infiltrates into the residual pores by capillary action, and results in a dense composite structure which has 20 times the strength of the core material
- Its flexural strength is 450 MPa when compared to any other dental ceramic
- The core is then veneered with conventional dentin and enamel feldspathic porcelains
- A compositional analysis has revealed alumina to be 99.56 wt% and the infiltration glass to be lanthanum aluminosilicate with small amounts of sodium and calcium
- Lanthanum decreases the viscosity of the glass to assist infiltration and increases its index of refraction to improve the translucency of ceramic
- Disadvantage with high alumina ceramics is their high opacity, which limits their use to the construction of high strength substructures

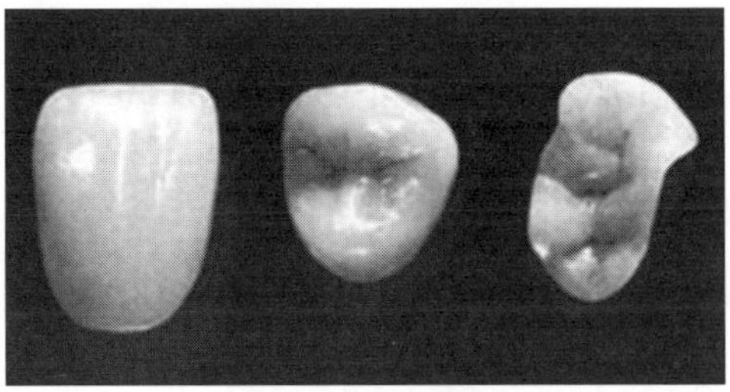

Fig. 21: Inceram

Inceram spinel (Fig. 22)

Spinel is used instead of alumina which contains aluminum and magnesium oxide ($MgAlP_4$) Because of the lower refractive index of spinel compared to alumina, the translucency of ceramic is improved but has low flexural strength. The fabrication process is similar to In-ceram.

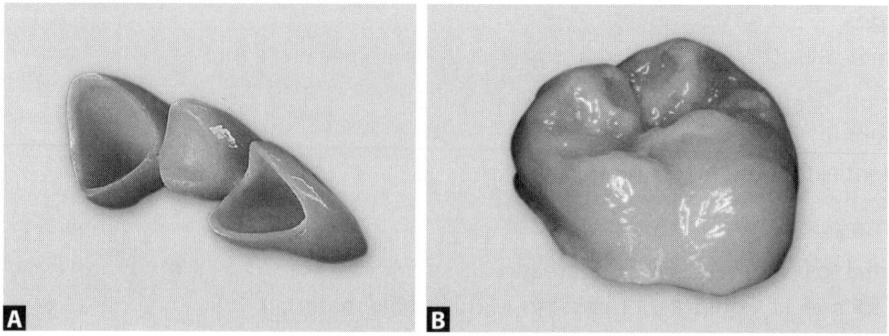

Figs 22A and B: Inceram spinel

Advancements in Permanent Luting Cement

The most recent development in the field of dental cements was the introduction of resin cements, they are Bis-GMA based resins which bond with micromechanical type of adhesion. Later systems bonded chemically to tooth structure, e.g. META.

Resin Cements

- Resin cements in combination with a dentin bonding agent, give superior bonding but due to concerns for postoperative sensitivity a total etch is still a concern as many bonding agents need a total etch
- A combination bonding agent that bonds to tooth structure and resin cement that adheres to the bonding agent and to silane-treated porcelain is also observed to give superior bonding properties.

Resin-modified Glass Ionomer (RMGI) cements

Uses—Luting of crowns and bridges, inlay and onlay restorations. They are hybrid formulations of resin and glass ionomer components.

Disadvantages—Excess water sorption, ceramic fracture. E.g. RelyX Luting, RelyX Luting Plus (3 M/ESPE), Fuji Plus (GC) and UltraCem RRGI Luting Cement.

Adhesive Resin Cements

They are self-adhesive giving good bonding. E.g: MaxCem (Kerr), RelyX Unicem (3 M/ESPE).

Hybrid Acid-based CaAl/Glass Ionomer[12]

- Is based on calcium aluminate/glass ionomer. E.g: Ceramir C and B (Doxa Dental AB, Uppsala, Sweden)
- *Uses*—is a new dental luting agent intended for permanent cementation of crowns and bridges, gold inlays and onlays, prefabricated metal, cast post and cores, all-zirconia or all-alumina crowns

- The cement is a water-based hybrid composition comprising of calcium aluminate and glass ionomer and after setting (3–4 hours) it reaches a basic pH of ~8.5
- This basic PH makes it bioactive and it has unique properties, such as apatite formation and remineralization which develop quickly and continue to be active.

References

1. Bennett T. Amaechi" Emerging technologies for diagnosis of dental caries: The road so far." J Appl Phys. 2009;105.
2. Kayser AF. Shortened dental arches and oral function. J Oral Rehabil. 1981;8:457-62.
3. World Health Organization. Recent advances in oral health. WHO Technical Report Series No. 826. WHO, Geneva; 1992. p. 16-17.
4. Murdoch-Kinch CA, McLean ME. "Minimally invasive dentistry" JADA. 2003;134.
5. Aboushelib MN, Kleverloan CJ, Feilzer AJ. Selective infiltration etching for a strong and a durable bonding with Zirconia based restorations. J Prosthet Dent. 2007;98:379-88.
6. Goldman L, Hornby P, Meyer R, Goldman B. Impact of the laser on dental caries. Nature. 1964;203: 417.
7. Burkes EJ, Hoke J, Gomes E, Wolbarsht M. Wet versus dry enamel ablation by Er: YAG laser. J Prosthet Dent. 1992;67:847-51.
8. Gimbel CB. Hard tissue laser procedures. Dental Clinics of North America 2000;44(4):931-53.
9. DJP Evans "A clinical evaluation of an Erbium: Yag Laser for dental cavity preparation". Br Dent J. 2000; 188:677-9.
10. Livadits GJ. The matrix impression system for fixed prorthodontics. J Prosthet Dent. 1998;79:208-16.
11. Conrad HJ, Wook-Jin Seong, et al. Current ceramic materials and systems with clinical recommendations: A systemic review. J Prosthet Dent. 2007;98:389-404.
12. Lööf J, Svahn F, Jarmar T, Engqvist H, Pameijer CH. A comparative study of the bioactivity of three materials for dental applications, Dental Materials, vol. 24, no. 5. 2008; pp. 653-9.

References

Index

Page numbers followed by *f* refer to figure and *t* refer to table.

D